D0294983

WITHDRAWN

THE LIBRARY
SWINDON COLLEGE
NORTH STAR

LIBRARIES

REHABILITATION OF SPORTS INJURIES:
SCIENTIFIC BASIS

IOC MEDICAL COMMISSION

SUB-COMMISSION ON PUBLICATIONS IN THE SPORT SCIENCES

Howard G. Knuttgen PhD (Co-ordinator)
Boston, Massachusetts, USA

Harm Kuipers MD, PhD
Maastricht, The Netherlands

Per A.F.H. Renström MD, PhD
Stockholm, Sweden

REHABILITATION OF SPORTS INJURIES: SCIENTIFIC BASIS

THE LIBRARY
SWINDON COLLEGE
NORTH STAR

VOLUME X OF THE ENCYLOPAEDIA OF SPORTS MEDICINE

AN IOC MEDICAL COMMITTEE PUBLICATION

IN COLLABORATION WITH THE

INTERNATIONAL FEDERATION OF SPORTS MEDICINE

EDITED BY

WALTER R. FRONTERA

Blackwell
Science

© 2003 International Olympic Committee
Published by Blackwell Science Ltd
a Blackwell Publishing company
Blackwell Science, Inc., 350 Main Street, Malden, Massachusetts 02148-5018, USA
Blackwell Science Ltd, Osney Mead, Oxford OX2 0EL, UK
Blackwell Science Asia Pty Ltd, 550 Swanston Street, Carlton South, Victoria 3053, Australia
Blackwell Wissenschafts Verlag, Kurfürstendamm 57, 10707 Berlin, Germany

The right of the Author to be identified as the Author of this Work has been asserted
in accordance with the Copyright, Designs and Patents Act 1988.

All rights reserved. No part of this publication may be reproduced, stored in a retrieval system,
or transmitted, in any form or by any means, electronic, mechanical, photocopying, recording or otherwise,
except as permitted by the UK Copyright, Designs and Patents Act 1988, without the prior permission of the publisher.

First published 2003

Library of Congress Cataloging-in-Publication Data

Rehabilitation of sports injuries : scientific basis / edited by
Walter R. Frontera.
    p. cm. — (The Encyclopaedia of sports medicine ; v. 10)
"An IOC Medical Commission publication in collaboration
with the International Federation of Sports Medicine."
Includes bibliographical references and index.
    ISBN 0-632-05813-7
    1. Sports injuries.   2. Athletes—Rehabilitation.
I. Frontera, Walter R., 1955–   II. IOC Medical Commission.
III. International Federation of Sports Medicine.   IV. Series.
    RD97 .R439 2002
    617.1′027—dc21

                              2002007253

THE LIBRARY
SWINDON COLLEGE
NORTH STAR

ISBN 0-632-05813-7

A catalogue record for this title is available from the British Library

Set in 9/12 Palatino by Graphicraft Limited, Hong Kong
Printed and bound in Great Britain by MPG Books Ltd, Bodmin, Cornwall

Commissioning Editor: Andrew Robinson
Production Editor: Julie Elliott
Production Controller: Kate Charman

For further information on Blackwell Science, visit our website:
www.blackwellpublishing.com

54050000175026

Contents

List of Contributors

J. AUDETTE MD, *Instructor, Department of Physical Medicine and Rehabilitation, Spaulding Rehabilitation Hospital, Harvard Medical School, Boston MA, USA*

A.-X. BIGARD MD, *Department of Human Factors, Centre de Recherches du Service de Santé des Armées, BP 87 La Tronche, 38702, France*

B.W. BREWER PhD, *Associate Professor, Department of Psychology, Springfield College, Springfield, Massachusetts 01109, USA*

K.-M. CHAN MD, *Chair Professor and Chief of Service, Hong Kong Centre of Sports Medicine & Sports Science, Department of Orthopaedics & Traumatology, Chinese University of Hong Kong, Prince of Wales Hospital, Hong Kong*

T.J. CHANDLER EdD, *Associate Professor, Exercise Science, Sport, and Recreation, Marshall University, Huntington WV, USA*

A.E. CORNELIUS PhD, *Center for Performance Enhancement and Applied Research, Department of Psychology, Springfield College, 263 Alden Street, Springfield, MA 01109, USA*

A. ESQUENAZI MD, *Director, Gait and Motion Analysis Laboratory Moss Rehabilitation Hospital, Department of Physical Medicine and Rehabilitation, Jefferson College School of Medicine and Department of Bioengineering, Drexel University, Philadelphia PA, USA*

E. FINK PhD, *Department of Human Factors, Centre de Recherches du Service de Santé des Armées, BP87, La Tronche, 38702, France*

W.R. FRONTERA MD, PhD, *Chairman, Department of Physical Medicine and Rehabilitation, Spaulding Rehabilitation Hospital, Harvard Medical School, Boston MA, USA*

J.J. GONZÁLEZ ITURRI MD, *Department of Physical Medicine and Rehabilitation, University of Navarra, 31007 Pamploma, Spain*

G. GRIMBY MD, PhD, *Professor Emeritus, Department of Rehabilitation Medicine, Göteborg University, Göteborg, Sweden*

S.A. HERRING MD, *Clinical Professor, Departments of Orthopedics and Rehabilitation Medicine, University of Washington, Seattle, Washington, USA*

H.C.L. HO MBChB, *Department of Orthopaedics and Traumatology, The Chinese University of Hong Kong, Prince of Wales Hospital, Hong Kong*

W.B. KIBLER MD, *Medical Director, Lexington Sports Medicine Center, Lexington, KY 40504, USA*

W. MICHEO MD, *University of Puerto Rico, Medical Sciences Campus, School of Medicine, Department of Physical Medicine, Rehabilitation and Sports Medicine, San Juan PR 00936-5067*

I. MUJIKA PhD, *Department of Research and Development, Medical Services, Athletic Club of Bilbao, Basque Country, Spain*

B.W. OAKES MD, *Associate Professor, Department of Anatomy and Cell Biology, Faculty of Medicine, Monash University, Clayton 3168, Melbourne, Australia*

S. PADILLA MD, PhD, *Department of Research and Development, Medical Services, Athletic Club of Bilbao, Basque Country, Spain*

C.T. PLASTARAS MD, *Rehabilitation Institute of Chicago, Center for Spine, Sports and Occupational Rehabilitation, 1030 N. Clark Street, Chicago, IL 60610, USA*

J.M. PRESS MD, *Rehabilitation Institute of Chicago, Center for Spine, Sports and Occupational Rehabilitation, 1030 N. Clark Street, Chicago, IL 60610, USA*

M.R. SAFRAN MD, *Co-Director Sports Medicine, Department of Orthopaedic Surgery, University of California San Francisco, San Francisco, California 94143, USA*

M.L. SCHAMBLIN MD, *Department of Orthopaedic Surgery, University of California, Irvine, California, USA*

M. SCHWELLNUS MD, PhD, *Associate Professor, Sports Science Institute of South Africa, The University of Cape Town, Cape Town, South Africa*

J.K. SILVER MD, *Assistant Professor, Department of Physical Medicine and Rehabilitation, Spaulding Rehabilitation Hospital, Harvard Medical School, Boston, MA, USA*

C.J. STANDAERT MD, *Clinical Assistant Professor, Department of Rehabilitation Medicine, University of Washington, Seattle, Washington, USA*

R. THOMEÉ PhD, *Department of Rehabilitation Medicine, Göteborg University, Göteborg, Sweden*

C.W.C. TONG MBChB (Hons), *Department of Orthopaedics and Traumatology, The Chinese University of Hong Kong, Prince of Wales Hospital, Hong Kong*

S.L. WIESNER MD, *Chief, Occupational Health Department, The Permanente Medical Group, 280 West MacArthur Boulevard, Oakland, California 94611-5693, USA*

Forewords

The sports medical care of athletes is often wrongly assumed to comprise simply the immediate treatment of injuries and of systemic medical problems. The considerable time and the extensive effort devoted by medical and allied health personnel, both to the prevention of injuries and to the rehabilitation of athletes from injuries which curtail or prevent training and competition, are frequently overlooked.

This new volume in the Encyclopaedia of Sports Medicine series addresses all of the important issues related to the rehabilitation of the injured athlete. Dr Frontera and his team of expert contributing authors present the cutting edge of knowledge relative to the basic science and accompanying practical considerations regarding tissue injury and repair.

This volume provides an excellent complement to the volumes already published. The series now includes the preparation of an athlete for competition, the prevention of sports injuries, the immediate treatment of injuries, and the rehabilitation that must occur to bring an athlete back to training and competition.

My congratulations go to the editor and authors for their excellent work and to the IOC Medical Commission for providing this admirable contribution to sports medicine literature.

Dr Jacques ROGGE
IOC President

The general aim of the Encyclopaedia of Sports Medicine series is to present the latest and most authoritative information available relative to a broad range of topic areas included under the rubric of Sports Medicine. The earlier volumes of the Encyclopaedia series have addressed a wide variety of areas of interest relative to both sports medicine and the sport sciences. Following the general interest publication of Vol. I, *The Olympic Book of Sports Medicine*, succeeding volumes were devoted to the more definitive topics of endurance, strength and power, prevention and treatment of injuries, the child and adolescent athlete, sports nutrition, women in sport, and biomechanics.

The publication of this volume further reinforces the intense interest that the IOC Medical Commission has in the health and welfare of the athletes of the world. Not only does optimal rehabilitation assist in returning an injured athlete to training and competition, but a carefully administered programme of rehabilitation serves to prevent the recurrence of the same injury or the occurrence of additional injuries. A high-quality programme of rehabilitation is of importance to all athletes, their coaches, and the teams and nations that they represent.

This volume will stand for many years as the most comprehensive and authoritative reference on sports injury rehabilitation available both for clinicians and sports scientists. I extend both my appreciation and my congratulations to Dr Frontera and each of the contributing authors.

Princes Alexandre de MERODE
Chairman, IOC Medical Commission

Preface

Conceptual framework

Rehabilitation is, by definition, the restoration of optimal form (anatomy) and function (physiology). It is a process designed to minimize the loss associated with acute injury or chronic disease, to promote recovery, and to maximize functional capacity, fitness and performance. The process of rehabilitation should start as early as possible after an injury and form a continuum with other therapeutic interventions such as the use of pharmacological agents. It can also start before or immediately after surgery when an injury requires a surgical intervention. The rehabilitation of the injured athlete is managed by a multidisciplinary team with a physician functioning as the leader and coordinator of care. The team includes, but is not limited to, athletic trainers, physiotherapists, psychologists, and nutritionists. The rehabilitation team works closely with the athlete and the coach to establish the rehabilitation goals, to discuss the progress resulting from the various interventions, and to establish the time frame for the return of the athletes to training and competition.

Injuries during sports competitions may result from high forces during actions or movements inherent to the sport. The rehabilitation plan must take into account the fact that the objective of the patient (the athlete) is to return to the same activity and environment in which the injury occurred. Functional capacity after rehabilitation should be the same, if not better, than before injury since avoiding the conditions associated with the injury is not, in many cases, an alternative.

The sequence of events resulting from a sports-related injury that may lead to a reduction or inability to perform in sports can be framed using a disability model widely used in the field of rehabilitation medicine (Fig. 1). In this context, the ultimate goal of the rehabilitation process is to limit the extent of the injury, reduce or reverse the impairment and functional loss, and prevent, correct or eliminate altogether the disability.

From a clinical perspective it is possible to divide the rehabilitation process into three phases. The goals during the initial phase of the rehabilitation process include limitation of tissue damage, pain relief, control of the inflammatory response to injury, and protection of the affected anatomical area. The pathological events that take place immediately after the injury could lead to impairments such as muscle atrophy and weakness and limitation in the joint range of motion. These impairments result in functional

Pathology (injury)	Impairment	Functional loss	Disability
Strain	Contracture	Inability to	Inability to
Sprain	Muscle atrophy	run, jump	compete
Fracture	and weakness		in sports

Fig. 1

losses, for example, inability to jump or lift an object. The extent of the functional loss may be influenced by the nature and timing of the therapeutic and rehabilitative intervention during the initial phase of the injury. If functional losses are severe or become permanent, the athlete now with a disability may be unable to participate in his/her sport.

The goals during the second phase of rehabilitation include the limitation of the impairment and the recovery from the functional losses. A number of physical modalities are used to enhance tissue healing. Exercise to regain flexibility, strength, endurance, balance, and coordination become the central component of the intervention. To the extent that these impairments and functional losses were minimized by early intervention, progress in this phase can be accelerated.

The final phase of rehabilitation represents the start of the conditioning process needed to return to sports training and competition. Understanding the demands of the particular sport becomes essential as well as communication with the coach. This phase also represents an opportunity to identify and correct risk factors, thus reducing the possibility of re-injury. The use of orthotic devices to support musculoskeletal function and the correction of muscle imbalances and inflexibility in uninjured areas should receive the attention of the rehabilitation team.

Structure of this volume

This volume contains a total of 15 chapters divided into four sections. The first section covers relevant basic concepts of the epidemiology and pathology of sports injuries. The implications of the patterns of sports injury for rehabilitation are discussed and the physiological and cellular response to tissue injury reviewed in detail. The second section contains three chapters on the basic science of tissue healing and repair of the five most frequently injured tissues in sports: muscles, tendons, ligaments, bones,

and/or cartilage. Section three includes three chapters on practical issues of great significance to the outcome of the rehabilitation process. The treatment and rehabilitation of injuries in athletes requires, in many cases, the reduction or complete cessation of training. Injuries and detraining alter basic physiological mechanisms and the functional capacity of the athlete. These effects must be taken into consideration especially at the beginning of the second phase of the rehabilitation process. It is a common mistake to consider the physical rehabilitation of the athlete disconnected from the psychological recovery. The last chapter of this section addresses relevant emotional and psychological aspects of sports rehabilitation.

The last section of the book includes seven chapters that discuss the most commonly used interventions in clinical rehabilitation. The use of pharmacological agents, physical modalities, and the various types of therapeutic exercise are all discussed in detail. Particular attention is given to the use of orthotic devices and to functional rehabilitation and issues related to the return to training and competition.

All authors have made a serious attempt to summarize the relevant scientific literature. It is our interest to discuss the evidence, if any, that supports current rehabilitative strategies.

Acknowledgements

I would like to thank all authors for their time and excellent contributions to this volume. I also wish to express special thanks to Professor Howard Knuttgen, Chair of the Sub-commission on Publications of the IOC Medical Commission for his guidance. Final thanks to the IOC Medical Commission and the International Federation of Sports Medicine for having established this important Encyclopedia of Sports Medicine.

Walter R. Frontera
Boston, Massachusetts

PART 1

EPIDEMIOLOGY AND PATHOLOGY

Chapter 1

Epidemiology of Sports Injuries: Implications for Rehabilitation

WALTER R. FRONTERA

Introduction

The study of the relationships among the various factors determining the frequency and distribution of diseases and/or injuries in a human community is known as epidemiology. The basic elements of epidemiology have been applied to the study of a frequent, albeit unintended, consequence of the practice of sport; i.e. injuries to the musculoskeletal system.

Understanding the incidence and prevalence of injuries based on variables such as type and nature of the injury, age group, nature of the sport, gender and time since the onset of symptoms, among others, has contributed to the development of programmes aimed at the prevention and treatment of injured athletes (Walter & Hart 1990). Most importantly, these studies have resulted in the identification of risk factors for sports injuries (Macera *et al.* 1989) and modifications in the competitive rules in various sports. Although research in epidemiology has proved essential for the development of preventive and therapeutic interventions, the relationship between the epidemiology of sports injuries and the process of rehabilitation of the injured athlete has not received similar attention.

Some authors have proposed a model that uses epidemiological information to generate preventive strategies (Van Mechelen 1993). The sequence of prevention is illustrated in Fig. 1.1. In this model, the identification of the problem and description using epidemiological outcomes leads to the study of the mechanisms of injury and the naming and grouping of risk factors. Based on that information, preventive measures

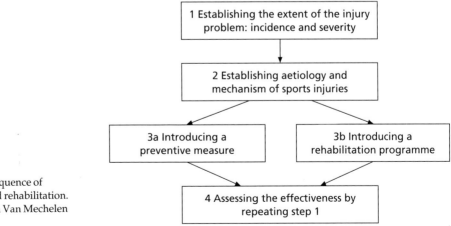

Fig. 1.1 The sequence of prevention and rehabilitation. (Adapted from Van Mechelen 1993.)

1 Establishing the extent of the injury problem: incidence and severity

2 Establishing aetiology and mechanism of sports injuries

3a Introducing a preventive measure

3b Introducing a rehabilitation programme

4 Assessing the effectiveness by repeating step 1

designed to reduce the risk and/or severity of the injuries are designed and implemented. Finally, the measures are evaluated by repeating the description of the problem (step 1) after the intervention. We suggest that this useful model could be expanded by including, as part of the intervention strategies, effective rehabilitation programmes that contribute to symptom resolution, limit functional losses, and restore physiological function and performance.

From a clinical point of view, an analysis of sports injuries by pattern, type, incidence and severity, together with an improved understanding of the physiological losses associated with these injuries, could help us design better rehabilitative interventions. Further, this knowledge could help us explain the extent to which the lack of effective rehabilitation itself becomes a risk factor predisposing injured athletes to the recurrence of an existing injury or to new injuries in a different, but related, anatomical area. For example, a high incidence of chronic injuries could indicate that proper rehabilitation did not follow the treatment of the symptoms in the acute inflammatory phase. It should be understood that, for the competitive athlete, resolution of the acute symptoms, such as pain, and clinical signs, such as swelling, is not the goal of the sports medicine practitioner. Restoration of form, and more importantly, function after resolution of the symptoms is necessary for optimal sports performance. Further, as our understanding of the physiological losses associated with the most common sports injuries improves, it will be possible to anticipate the functional deficits resulting from those injuries. Thus, the implementation of appropriate rehabilitation programmes will be feasible.

The purpose of this chapter is to illustrate how data on the pattern of injuries in various sports populations can help us restore form and function after injury. It is not the author's intention to present an exhaustive and critical review of the literature on the epidemiology of sports injuries but to interpret some existing data in the context of the goals of a standard rehabilitation programme. It will suffice to demonstrate

a reasonable association between the two. Further, most of the observations included in this chapter are descriptive of a sports injury clinic located in a sports training centre and not in a hospital or medical centre. The descriptive nature of these observations limits the extent to which we can draw conclusions and only allows us to make preliminary observations and speculations. Finally, it is not intended to present an analysis of the incidence of sports injuries with considerations of the population at risk or the difference in exposure (hours during which an athlete risks injury) (Wallace 1988). These factors appear to be less relevant in clinical rehabilitation.

Patterns of sports injuries

It is common to examine the distribution of injuries in relation to other variables of interest like age group, type of injury (traumatic vs. overuse), time since onset of symptoms, whether the injury occurred during training or competition, anatomical area, specific diagnosis and severity of injury. These variables are of significant interest when rehabilitation is our main focus. Let us examine briefly the influence of these factors on our rehabilitation strategies.

Type of injury (traumatic vs. overuse)

Roughly 45–60% of all injuries treated in a sports medicine clinic can be classified as overuse injuries. This is particularly true in sports like gymnastics (Fig. 1.2) where soft tissues and joints are subject to unusual positions and stresses. Risk factors for overuse injuries include muscle weakness, muscle strength imbalance and anatomical misalignment (Knapik et al. 1991). An examination of these risk factors suggests that properly designed rehabilitation programmes and the use of rehabilitation devices such as foot orthotics could contribute to a reduction in the incidence and prevalence of overuse sports injuries.

Clearly, the situation may be different when the analysis is restricted to clinical encounters

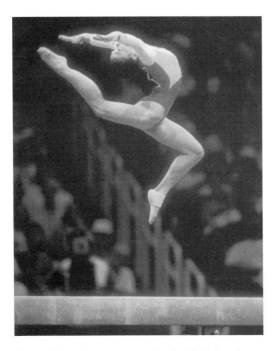

Fig. 1.2 Repetitive stress associated with high-volume training results in overuse injuries in many athletes in various sports including gymnastics. M.O. Huilan at Atlanta, 1996. (© Allsport, Doug Pensinger, 1996.)

in an emergency department. Many traumatic injuries (Fig. 1.3) are more acute and severe, resulting frequently in immobilization and prolonged rehabilitation.

Time from onset

Epidemiological studies show that, when the time from onset of symptoms is considered, most (70.2% of a total of 1650) injuries treated in an ambulatory sports medicine clinic are chronic in nature (Frontera *et al*. 1994). In other words, the time between the onset of symptoms and the evaluation in the clinic is longer than 2 weeks. There are several potential reasons or scenarios that could explain this observation. As mentioned above, an insidious onset in the absence of obvious trauma with a slow progression of the injury could result in a delay in making a clinic appointment to get the signs and symptoms evaluated. This is typical of the overuse injuries that have become so prevalent in sports like running, swimming and baseball.

Another possibility could be that the symptoms are not well defined, at least initially, making the diagnosis by a physician difficult. It is also conceivable that the incorrect therapeutic modality or rehabilitation intervention was chosen to initiate treatment or that the patient did not complete the treatment as prescribed by the physician for other reasons. These two situations could prolong the acute stage resulting in the persistence of symptoms. Moreover, many injuries occur during training sessions when health care professionals may not be available to immediately treat

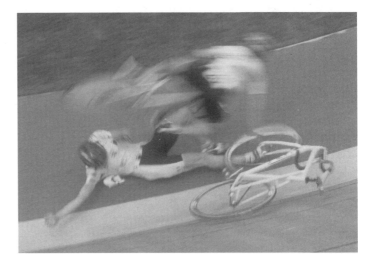

Fig. 1.3 Falls in cycling can result in significant traumatic injuries.

the injured athlete. The athlete may delay seeking help or may initiate treatment him/herself if the symptoms are not severe or disabling, and tissue damage may increase in the absence of acute therapeutic intervention. Finally, it is also possible that the correct treatment was applied resulting in resolution of the symptoms but that proper rehabilitation of impairments and functional losses did not follow the therapeutic interventions. In other words, the athlete is allowed back into training and competition based on the absence of pain and inflammation but not on the recovery of strength, flexibility or endurance needed for successful performance in sports.

In the absence of appropriate rehabilitation, acute, subacute or chronic injuries frequently result in significant physiological and functional losses that place the affected anatomical area (and adjacent tissues and joints) at risk for reinjury. Recovery from these losses becomes one of the most important goals of the rehabilitation programme. The extent of these losses is illustrated by a clinical epidemiology study published by Holder-Powell and Rutherford in 1999. These authors evaluated the strength of various muscle groups in asymptomatic subjects with history of a sports injury. The injuries occurred between 0.75 and 42 years before the evaluation (mean = 9.7 ± 11 years).

The most important observation in that study was a decrement of concentric, eccentric and static strength in the knee extensor muscles of the injured limb many years after the injury (Fig. 1.4). This was the case even when the muscle group was distant from the injured area. In other words, the authors of the study observed weakness of the knee extensors in patients with injuries such as fractures of the leg and sprains of the ankle ligaments. The degree of weakness present in the hamstrings, on the other hand, was minor in some cases and non-existent in others, suggesting that the rehabilitation approach must be muscle specific.

In another study, Croisier et al. (2002) demonstrated that athletes with strains of the hamstrings had significant strength deficits. More importantly, these investigators showed that if those that

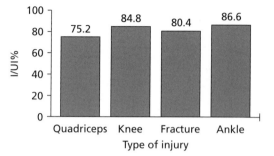

Fig. 1.4 Concentric peak torque of the knee extensors of the injured side measured at 30 degrees per second and expressed as a percentage of the uninjured side (I/UI) in subjects with different types of injuries. The injuries occurred an average of 9.7 years before the evaluation. (Adapted from Holder-Powell & Rutherford 1999.)

have significant deficits complete a rehabilitation programme, in this study consisting of isokinetic strengthening concentric and eccentric exercises, muscle weakness is reversed. Further, the incidence of postrehabilitation injuries in the 12 months following return to their sport was zero.

Anatomical distribution of injuries

When the incidence of sports injuries is analysed by anatomical region, the most frequently injured areas are the knee (Fig. 1.5), shoulder and ankle (Garrick 1985; DeHaven & Lintner 1986; Frontera et al. 1994). Of course the anatomical

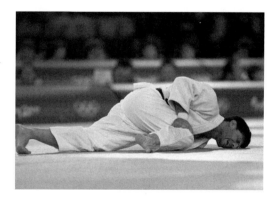

Fig. 1.5 An acute knee injury in a judo player, Girolamo Giovinazzo of Italy at Sydney, 2000. (© Allsport, Clive Brunskill, 2000.)

distribution of injuries in a particular sport can be very specific. In other words, basketball players may suffer more injuries to the knee than to the shoulder but the situation in swimmers is the reverse.

Knowledge of the anatomical distribution of injuries in a particular sport is essential to develop a training programme that maximizes sport-specific conditioning and minimizes the risk of injury. Further, because deconditioning associated with rest could potentially affect muscle groups proximal and distal to the injured area, knowledge of this anatomical distribution of injuries by sport could be vital for the rehabilitation of the injured athlete. A well-planned rehabilitation programme should include exercises for the injured area as well as for those areas at risk of injury in the specific sports activity.

Most frequent diagnoses

Most sports injuries are relatively mild and do not require surgical intervention. Independent of the level of competition, the most frequent diagnoses are in descending order: tendonitis (or tendinosis), first degree strains (muscle tendon unit), first degree sprains (ligament and capsular injuries), patellofemoral pain and second degree sprains. The best course of action in these cases is appropriate conservative intervention to control symptoms such as pain and swelling, followed by comprehensive rehabilitation. The indications for surgery in these cases are few and rehabilitation becomes the most effective intervention when fast return to practice or competition and prevention of future injuries are the most important goals (DeHaven & Lintner 1986; Matheson *et al.* 1989).

Severity of injury

The severity of the injury can be judged by the nature of the diagnosis, the duration and nature of the treatment, the time lost from sports training or competition, and/or the presence and degree of permanent damage (Van Mechelen 1993). There is usually a positive correlation between severity, functional loss and the need for extended rehabilitation. Clearly, when the severity is high, longer periods of immobilization or rest are needed for tissue healing. As a result, larger physiological losses are experienced by the athlete and deconditioning of uninjured areas is more extensive. Under these conditions, it should be anticipated that rehabilitation will last longer.

Rehabilitation and the preparticipation exam

Every competitive athlete must undergo a preparticipation medical examination on a regular basis. The preparticipation exam is an ideal situation in which to: (i) treat existing medical conditions early before the competition; (ii) anticipate the health care needs of the athlete; (iii) educate the athlete and his/her coach regarding health issues such as vaccinations and prevention of disease and injury; and (iv) discuss topics such as doping in sports.

Another important element of the preparticipation exam is the identification of risk factors for medical conditions in general and for sports injuries in particular. The process of identifying risk factors can make use of the epidemiological evidence published in the sports medicine literature. Findings such as joint contractures or reduced flexibility, muscle weakness and muscle strength asymmetry represent ideal opportunities to do 'preventive rehabilitation'. The restoration of normal form and function in these cases does not necessarily follow a sports injury but may be important in the prevention of future injuries. In addition, rehabilitation may prove to be beneficial for sports performance because an enhanced level of flexibility, cardiovascular endurance and muscle strength and endurance, alone or in combination, are required in almost any sport.

Health services in international competitions

The study of the pattern of disease and injuries in international sports competitions can help the team physician make plans regarding, among

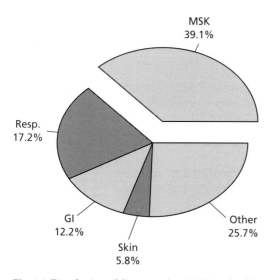

Fig. 1.6 Distribution of diagnoses (*n* = 2468) in a health clinic during international sports competitions by system. GI, gastrointestinal; MSK, musculoskeletal. (Adapted from Frontera *et al.* 1997.)

other things, the composition of the health care team travelling with sports delegations, the equipment and medical supplies necessary to deliver health care (including rehabilitation services) in an Olympic village, the most commonly used and permitted medications, and the therapy modalities needed for rehabilitation (Frontera *et al.* 1997).

As the number of athletes and competitions increase and new transportation methods facilitate travel, health professionals will be challenged to respond to the needs of the travelling athlete exposed to different environmental conditions, pathogens and demanding training regimes.

Although disorders of the respiratory and gastrointestinal tracts are very common among travelling athletes, the main cause of morbidity during an international competition is injuries to the musculoskeletal system (Fig. 1.6).

The five most common injuries or disorders affecting the musculoskeletal system (total number of diagnoses = 966) include: first degree strains (23.1%), tendinitis/tendinosis (18.7%), contusion (12.7%), myositis (10.9%) and first degree sprains (10%). All of these diagnoses could benefit from rehabilitative interventions to control the symptoms in the acute stage and to restore physio-

logical and functional capacity in later stages. In fact, in the above study, typical rehabilitation interventions such as physical therapy modalities (cold packs, hot packs, ultrasound, transcutaneous electrical stimulation, massage, therapeutic exercises) were needed in 23.1–36.9% of the total number of cases.

It is important to note that, just like in the case of the sports injury clinic discussed above, the onset of symptoms preceded the competition in many cases. Thus many injuries could be classified as chronic in nature. High-performance athletes often continue to train and compete even in the presence of symptoms and signs of injury, and may delay proper treatment and rehabilitation of an injury to participate in important competitions. Thus, it is reasonable to speculate that some of the injured athletes did not receive appropriate rehabilitation after the initial insult. These two observations make the inclusion of rehabilitation services in precompetition assessment and plans for a sports delegation an absolute necessity.

Conclusion

The study of the epidemiology of sports injuries can be as valuable to rehabilitation as it is to prevention. Many injuries may occur because the rehabilitation of a previous injury was not complete. Understanding risk factors associated with sports injuries can help in the design of rehabilitation strategies resulting in a lower incidence and severity of injuries. Rehabilitation principles can be applied in a sports injury clinic but also as part of the health care services for a travelling team. The following chapters will discuss the scientific basis of current rehabilitation practices. Every sports medicine practitioner should be familiar with these principles and apply them in their work with athletes.

References

Croisier, J.-L., Forthomme, B., Namurois, M.-H., Vanderhommen, M. & Crielaard, J.-M. (2002) Hamstring muscle strain recurrence and strength performance disorders. *American Journal of Sports Medicine* **30**, 199–203.

DeHaven, K.E. & Lintner, D.M. (1986) Athletic injuries: comparison by age, sport, and gender. *American Journal of Sports Medicine* **14**, 218–224.

Frontera, W.R., Micheo, W.F., Aguirre, G., Rivera-Brown, A. & Pabon, A. (1997) Patterns of disease and utilization of health services during international sports competitions. *Archivos de Medicina del Deporte* **14**, 479–484.

Frontera, W.R., Micheo, W.F., Amy, E. *et al.* (1994) Patterns of injuries in athletes evaluated in an interdisciplinary clinic. *Puerto Rico Health Sciences Journal* **13**, 165–170.

Garrick, J.G. (1985) Characterization of the patient population in a sports medicine facility. *Physician and Sportsmedicine* **13**, 73–76.

Holder-Powell, H.M. & Rutherford, O. (1999) Unilateral lower limb injury: its long-term effects on quadriceps, hamstring, and plantarflexor muscle strength. *Archives of Physical Medicine and Rehabilitation* **80**, 717–720.

Knapik, J.J., Bauman, C.L., Jones, B.H., Harris, J.M. & Vaughan, L. (1991) Preseason strength and flexibility imbalances associated with athletic injuries in female collegiate athletes. *American Journal of Sports Medicine* **19**, 76–81.

Macera, C.A., Pate, R.R., Powell, K.E., Jackson, K.L., Kendrick, J.S. & Craven, T.E. (1989) Predicting lower-extremity injuries among habitual runners. *Archives of Internal Medicine* **149**, 2565–2568.

Matheson, G.O., Macintyre, J.G., Taunton, J.E., Clement, D.B. & Lloyd-Smith, R. (1989) Musculoskeletal injuries associated with physical activity in older adults. *Medicine and Science in Sports and Exercise* **21**, 379–385.

Van Mechelen, W. (1993) Incidence and severity of sports injuries. In: *Sports Injuries: Basic Principles of Prevention and Care* (Renström, P.A.F.H., ed.). Blackwell Scientific Publications, Oxford: 3–15.

Wallace, R.B. (1988) Application of epidemiologic principles to sports injury research. *American Journal of Sports Medicine* **16** (Suppl. 1), 22–24.

Walter, S.D. & Hart, L.E. (1990) Application of epidemiological methodology to sports and exercise science research. In: *Exercise and Sports Sciences Reviews* (Pandolf, K.B. & Holloszy, J.O., eds). Williams & Wilkins, New York: 417–448.

Chapter 2

Pathophysiology of Injury

MARK L. SCHAMBLIN AND MARC R. SAFRAN

Introduction

No matter what the age of an athlete, the level of competition or the sport, inflammation is likely to affect an individual at some point in their endeavours. Whether an injury is one of chronicity, related to repetitive movements, or one of acute onset, related to trauma, the detrimental effects on athletic performance are well documented. Too frequently the complexity of the inflammatory process is not fully understood and inflammation is treated as an unwanted hindrance to athletic performance, however, it is truly a complex network of vascular and cellular responses designed to facilitate the repair of traumatized tissue (Bryant 1977; Gamble 1988; Martinez-Hernandez 1988).

The development of an inflammatory reaction to an injury is complex, utilizing many of the body's systems to mediate its purpose. The goal of any inflammatory reaction is to resolve the pathological insult and restore the anatomy to a level of physiological function identical or nearly identical to preinjury status. Ideally this can be accomplished by removing diseased or damaged tissue with the subsequent regeneration of normal anatomical tissue. However, this is often not the case. Too frequently the insult is far too great or perpetrated over too long a period, resulting in increased tissue destruction. This often leads to scar tissue formation that in turn may propagate a continued inflammatory reaction. A persistent inflammatory action, therefore, may be harmful to an individual's athletic performance, as well as to the individual.

Although in the recent past, understanding of the mediators of inflammation has vastly improved, many factors responsible for induction, regulation and resolution remain indefinable. This lack of understanding remains an elusive cornerstone in treatment for both the physician and the athlete. The purpose of this chapter is to provide an understanding of our current knowledge of the complex nature of the pathophysiological mechanisms, which function to mediate a host's response to tissue injury. This knowledge is then utilized in later chapters to understand specific tissue responses to injury as related to the athlete.

Cytokines

Inflammation may be seen in a variety of circumstances that affect the human body. It may occur as a defensive response to foreign material or as a response to mechanical trauma, toxins or in the face of abnormalities such as neoplasia. The accumulation and activation of leucocytes seems to play an essential role in nearly all forms of inflammation. Following the influx of leucocytes in the acute phase of inflammation, its propagation and amplification is mediated by both humoral and cellular components of the immune system.

Cytokines are cellular proteins that are the mediators of physiological activity, including the inflammatory process. There are proinflammatory and anti-inflammatory cytokines, which modulate their effect by binding to receptors on target cells. Through this interaction the up-regulation or down-regulation of cellular activity may be propagated. In the acute phase response of inflammation, cytokines appear to be responsible for a myriad of physiological modifications occurring both locally at the site of the pathology and also at regions distant from the insult (Rosenberg & Gallin 1993).

The functions of cytokines are varied. A given cytokine may initiate and regulate cellular activities in numerous cells simultaneously. At the same time, more than one cytokine may induce a particular biological activity (Table 2.1). Interleukin 1 (IL-1), a common cytokine seen in inflammation, acts on virtually all leucocytes, endothelial cells, monocytes and hepatocytes to up-regulate the expression of adhesion molecules, cytokines and arachidonic acid metabolites (Rosenberg & Gallin 1993). It results in neutrophil accumulation, fibroblast proliferation, angiogenesis, acute phase protein synthesis and metabolic alterations such as fever. Similar activity is seen in other proinflammatory cytokines, such as tumor necrosis factor alpha (TNF-α), IL-6, IL-4, IL-10 and transforming growth factor beta (TGF-β). An excellent example of this biological redundancy can be seen with IL-1 and TNF-α. Both of these cytokines result in the up-regulation of adhesion molecules, accumulation of leucocytes, protein synthesis and angiogenesis (Rosenberg & Gallin 1993; Bemelmans *et al.* 1996).

Local cytokines react with their receptors in an autocrine, paracrine and endocrine fashion (Fig. 2.1). The autocrine pathway allows for the amplification of the cytokine-induced inflammatory process. The paracrine pathway allows cytokines to influence cells in the local environment, leading to the accumulation of inflammatory cells. The induction of acute phase protein synthesis in the hepatocytes is an example of an endocrine mechanism of peripherally circulating cytokines (Akira *et al.* 1993; Dinarello 1996). By utilizing these three mechanisms of action, the cytokine is able to alter the local tissue as well as the acute phase response in the face of inflammation.

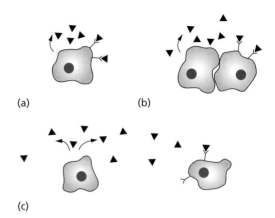

(a) (b) (c)

Fig. 2.1 Cytokines mediate their effects via three mechanisms of action. (a) Autocrine: the release of cytokines by a cell allows binding to receptors on the cell of origin. (b) Paracrine: most cytokines have a small radius of activity and mediate their effects on adjacent cells. (c) Some cytokines (IL-1 and TNF) mediate their activity via endocrine mechanisms.

The regulation of cytokine function is of critical importance. Secondary to a cytokine's powerful ability to modify biological behaviour, the body has evolved numerous cellular and molecular mechanisms to control their activity. The predominant mechanism of regulation occurs at the level of gene transcription. Cytokines are not stored, but rather created *de novo* following cellular activation. Antigen stimulation leads to increased transcription within 30 min. A steady-state level is seen in anywhere from 4 to 8 h (McDonald *et al.* 1993; Jain *et al.* 1995; Serhan 1997). With the cessation of the stimulus, return to the baseline will usually occur in 24 h. A second form of regulation is the conversion of an inactive form of the cytokine to the active form. This mechanism is seen in the conversion of a procytokine within the cytosol to the cytokine IL-1β, as well as the formation of TNF-α, which is formed in its active state but limited to the cell membrane. Cleavage of the membrane-bound TNF-α by converting enzymes facilitates secretion.

The ability to down-regulate the inflammatory process is as important as the ability to initiate it. Chronic inflammation or failure to control an

Table 2.1 The actions of selected cytokines including source, targets and activities.

Cytokine	Cell source	Cell target	Biological activity
IL-1α IL-1β	Monocytes Macrophages	All cells	Up-regulation of adhesion molecule expression Macrophage emigrations Acute phase protein synthesis
IL-2	T-cells	T-cells B-cells Monocytes Macrophages	T-cell activation and proliferation Enhanced monocyte and macrophage cytolytic activity
IL-3	T-cells Mast cells NK cells	Monocytes Macrophages Mast cells Eosinophils	Stimulation of haematopoietic progenitors
IL-4	T-cells Mast cells Basophils	T-cells B-cells Monocytes Macrophages Neutrophils Eosinophils	Stimulates T-cell and B-cell differentiation Anti-inflammatory action on T-cells, B-cells and monocytes
IL-5	T-cells Mast cells Eosinophil	Eosinophils Basophils	Regulates eosinophil migration and activation
IL-6	Monocytes Macrophages B-cells	T-cells B-cells Epithelial cells	Induction of acute phase proteins T-cell and B-cell differentiation
IL-8	Monocytes Macrophages T-cells Neutrophils	Neutrophils T-cells Monocytes Macrophages	Induces neutrophil, monocyte and T-cell migration Neutrophil adherence Angiogenesis Histamine release
IL-10	Monocytes Macrophages T-cells B-cells	Monocytes Macrophages B-cells T-cells Mast cells	Inhibits macrophage proinflammatory cytokine production Inhibits differentiation of T-cells Inhibits NK cells
TNF-α	Monocytes Macrophages Mast cells Basophils NK cells B-cells T-cells	All cells	Fever, anorexia and proinflammatory cytokine production Enhanced capillary permeability Acute phase protein synthesis
TNF-β	T-cells B-cells	All cells	Cell cytotoxicity
TGF-β	Most cell types	Most cell types	Down-regulates T-cell and macrophage responses Stimulates angiogenesis
IFN-α	All cells	All cells	Stimulates T-cell, macrophage and NK cell activity Direct antitumour effects Antiviral activity
IFN-γ	T-cells NK cells	All cells	Regulates macrophage and NK cell activation T-cell differentiation Immunoglobulin production by B-cells

IFN, interferon; IL, interleukin; NK, natural killer; TGF, transforming growth factor; TNF, tumour necrosis factor.

inflammatory process may lead to host tissue damage. There are several mechanisms utilized in the down-regulation of inflammation. These include production of activated complement inhibitors, apoptosis of inflammatory cells and production of anti-inflammatory cytokines such as IL-4, IL-10, IL-13 and TGF-β (Feng *et al.* 1996). IL-4 and IL-10, perhaps the best known of the anti-inflammatory cytokines, appear to mediate an anti-inflammatory effect on the T-cell predominantly, but also B-lymphocytes, mast cells, basophils and endothelial cells, as well as a variety of others (Feng *et al.* 1996).

Cytokines are potent proteins in the initiation, propagation and regulation of the inflammatory process. In this regard they are not alone, as the body synthesizes various types of proteins to mediate these same functions. Among these are prostaglandins and leukotrienes, which will be discussed in the subsequent sections.

Prostaglandins

Along with cytokines, prostaglandins are amongst the best-defined mediators of the inflammatory response. Since their discovery in 1931, advances in their structure, function and physiological mechanisms have afforded an increased understanding of these molecules (Kurzok & Lieb 1931). Independent work by two groups demonstrated arachidonic acid conversion to prostaglandin E2 via the enzyme cyclooxygenase (Goldblatt 1933; Von Euler 1935; van der Pouw *et al.* 1995). From this finding it was thought that essential fatty acids served merely as a precursor to prostaglandin synthesis. This has subsequently been shown to be only one of the many functions of fatty acids, albeit an important one.

There are many ways of inducing prostaglandin synthesis that appear to be cell specific. In macrophages, prostaglandin E_2 (PGE_2) and thromboxane A_2 (TxA_2) are stimulated by the presence of antigen–antibody complexes (Poranova *et al.* 1996). Cytokine receptors on mast cells stimulate the synthesis and secretion of PGD_2 (Murakami *et al.* 1994). IL-1 and TNF-α stimulation of endothelial cells and fibroblasts leads to PGE_2 as well as PGI_2 production. The production of prostaglandins is accomplished by the breakdown of membrane phospholipids by phospholipase A_2 with the subsequent formation of arachidonic acid. Arachidonic acid is then converted to PGG_2 via cyclooxygenase 1 and 2. PGG_2 then may be converted into various prostaglandins by prostaglandin synthase (Fig. 2.2).

Investigations of the role of prostaglandins within the inflammatory cascade are extensive. In general, their function has been delineated by their injection into both animal and human subjects with subsequent monitoring of their effects. Another area of focus is the role of nonsteroidal, anti-inflammatories in the regulation

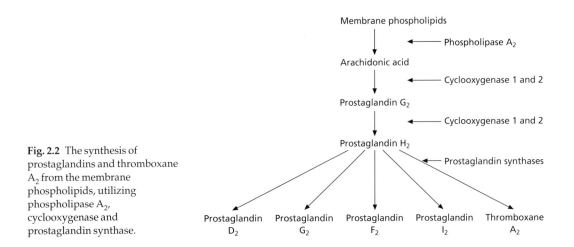

Fig. 2.2 The synthesis of prostaglandins and thromboxane A_2 from the membrane phospholipids, utilizing phospholipase A_2, cyclooxygenase and prostaglandin synthase.

of cyclooxygenase function. Throughout these studies, one thing has remained clear, the biological responses instigated by the presence of prostaglandins are wide ranging and varied in nature. In an attempt to simplify their function, their actions may be broken down into four general areas of the inflammatory process: fever, pain, oedema and leucocyte regulation.

Fever appears to be a complex neuroendocrine response to both infection and inflammation. A variety of proinflammatory mediators appear to serve as a stimulant to fever production. Various cytokines, which will be discussed in later sections, assist in the stimulation of the thermoregulatory centre by stimulating both the synthesis of the PGE family as well as mediating a direct effect on the thermoregulatory centre itself. Increased levels of PGE_2 have been demonstrated in the cerebral spinal fluid of febrile animals. This PGE_2 is most probably synthesized within the central nervous system as a result of bacterial-induced cytokine release. PGE_2 appears to modulate its effect on thermoregulatory centres within the hypothalamus; however, the specific receptor of action remains elusive (Feldberg & Saxena 1971; Milton & Wendlandt 1971). Cyclooxygenase inhibitors, specifically cyclooxygenase 2 inhibitors, given to human subjects modulate an antipyretic effect, lending further support to the role of prostaglandins in the induction of a febrile state.

In experimental models, the injection of prostaglandins in itself does not induce a painful response. However, in the presence of prostaglandins, particularly PGE_2 and PGI_2, the response to painful stimuli is greatly increased (Ferreira et al. 1978). It is unclear which of these two prostaglandins serves to accentuate the painful stimuli to the greatest extent or if different individuals respond to different stimuli in altered manners. In some experimental studies, PGE_2 appears to predominate while in others PGI_2 appears to be the prime mediator of an increase in the nociceptive response (Mnich et al. 1995; Plemons et al. 1996).

Similar to the response seen in pain, the injection of prostaglandins alone does not stimulate oedema. In states of inflammation, however, an increase in oedema is seen by the ability of prostaglandins to dilate the vasculature leading to increased blood supply to traumatized areas (Moncada et al. 1973; Wheeldon & Vardey 1993). In the presence of inflammation, increased vascular permeability is present secondary to the action of many proinflammatory mediators; this increased permeability coupled with increased blood flow stimulates excessive oedema. Experimental models also support this finding, as the injection of prostaglandins, specifically PGE_2 and PGI_2, coupled with bradykinin or platelet-aggregating factor (PAF) (powerful stimulants to increased permeability) stimulate oedematous states (Von Euler 1934).

In an apparent contradiction, the systemic administration of prostaglandins appears to mediate an anti-inflammatory effect (Kunkel et al. 1979; Fantone et al. 1980). Circulating prostaglandins (PGE_2 and PGD_2) inhibit neutrophils, monocytes and circulating T-lymphocytes. The inhibition of neutrophils is accomplished by inhibition of activation as measured by chemotaxis and superoxide production (Wedmore & Williams 1981). The inhibition of monocytes is mediated via the decreased production of various proinflammatory mediators such as TNF-α (Kunkel et al. 1986). T-lymphocyte inhibition is seen as a decrease in T-cell proliferation, a decrease in released cytokines and a decrease in the number of migrating T-cells (Goodwin et al. 1977; Shaw et al. 1988; Betz & Fox 1991; Trinchieri 1995). Through these three mechanisms, systemic prostaglandins appear to inhibit the inflammatory reaction, whereas, as discussed previously, the local accumulation of prostaglandins accentuates the inflammatory response.

As one can see, in recent years, the role of prostaglandins has been greatly elucidated and their involvement in the inflammatory reaction has been well documented. Secondary to their complex nature, however, it is highly probable that their involvement is even more significant than is currently known. Recent advances in understanding the nature of these molecules have led to improved pharmacological agents, such as specific cyclooxygenase inhibitors in anti-inflammatory medications. Despite the success of these agents, one thing is clear—prostaglandins are merely a fraction of the known types of pro-inflammatory mediators that affect the human body in the face of pathology.

In addition to mediators such as cytokines and prostaglandins, the body's immune system is composed of a highly complex series of cellular and plasma-derived components. The cellular component consists of a variety of cell types, each with a specific function. These cells interact in a well-orchestrated manner to improve the efficiency of the immune response. The cell types are variable and functions range from stimulating the aggregation of leucocytes to presenting foreign material to the actual destruction and removal of the offending pathogen. Some of the more important cellular components of the inflammatory process will be outlined in the following pages.

Mast cells and basophils

Several components of the immune system play a critical role in inflammatory reactions. Tissue mast cells and circulating basophils are haematopoietically derived cells, which express a variety of surface receptors that allow them to migrate to specific tissue locations, interact with cells and tissues, and respond to activation molecules. Both types of cells contain granules, which serve as storage for histamine, serotonin, cytokines and proteases. When IgE-sensitized mast cells or basophils are stimulated by either antigens or C3a and C5a (complement anaphylatoxins), the granules are released resulting in the secretion of these mediators. These in turn induce a reversible cell contraction in the endothelium, leading to the formation of gap junctions (Black *et al.* 1972; Arrang *et al.* 1983). This increases the permeability of the vasculature leading to increased tissue oedema. Both mast cells as well as basophils may be induced to release histamine and serotonin by other means, including physical stimuli such as trauma or proteins secreted by activated platelets and neutrophils.

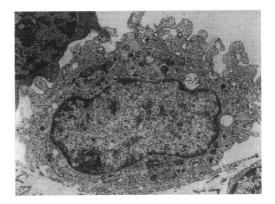

Fig. 2.3 Electron micrograph of a macrophage.

Macrophages

Macrophages are present throughout a variety of host tissues (Fig. 2.3). These cells are able to react to abnormalities such as ischaemia or metabolic disturbance by initiating an inflammatory reaction. When local processes are insufficient and unable to remove the host tissue of the initiating stimuli, macrophages along with other cells can mobilize other forms of leucocytes (polymorphonuclear neutophils in particular) by the activation of local endothelium and by the production of a variety of chemokines, cytokines and other lipid mediators of the inflammatory reaction (Table 2.2) (Bacon & Schall 1996). If the pathology continues and becomes one of chronicity, macrophages are able to up-regulate their microbicidal activity (Bell *et al.* 1994). When considering the role of macrophages in the initiation, propagation and resolution of inflammation, it is important to remember that each macrophage contains variable receptors on its membrane, allowing it to regulate the biosynthesis and secretion of substances in response to stimuli from the host tissue (Peterson *et al.* 1987).

As noted previously, macrophages interact with a variety of cells within the human body. These interactions are complex and reciprocal in nature. Non-haemopoietic cells, such as endothelium, are dramatically affected by the secretory products of the macrophage, and in turn have a profound effect on the ever-adapting macrophage itself.

Table 2.2 Macrophage-derived secretory products.

Cytokines	
IL-1	Multiple local and systemic host defence functions
TNF-α	Multiple local and systemic host defence functions
IFN-α/β	Antiviral, immune modulation
IL-6	Acute phase response
IL-10	Inhibits proinflammatory cytokines
TGF-β	Inhibits activation of macrophages and other cells
Complement proteins	
Most components	Local opsonization and complement activation
Coagulation factors	Initiation and regulation of clot formation
Adhesion and matrix molecules	Localization and migration
	Modulates cellular interactions and phagocytosis
Bioactive lipids	
Cyclooxygenase, lipoxygenase	Mediators of inflammation
Platelet-activating factor	
Antimicrobic activity	
Superoxide anion	Killing and stasis of microbial targets
Hydrogen peroxide	
Nitric oxide	

In this way, one can see how the macrophage is an important component in the regulation of the inflammatory process.

Neutrophils

These cells maintain the ability to mobilize from the blood to the tissue with subsequent degranulation in a matter of seconds. Their major function in the inflammatory cascade is one of endocytosis (eating) or exocytosis (secreting) (Bainton 1980). In the normal adult human, a polymorphonuclear neutrophil is found in one of three environments: bone marrow, blood or tissues. The bone marrow is the site where proliferation and maturation occurs. Following the phase of proliferation and maturation, the neutrophils are released into the blood where they circulate for approximately 10 days. They then migrate into the tissues where they survive for approximately another 1–2 days. Their ultimate fate after this is unknown (Bainton 1980).

Four distinct populations of granules have been identified within neutrophils by cytochemical and cell-fractionation procedures (Borregaard &

Cowland 1997). The azurophil granules contain myeloperoxidase (an antibacterial enzyme), lysozyme and lysosomal enzyme, as well as a variety of other agents (Table 2.3) (Klebanoff & Clark 1978). Specific granules by definition do not contain peroxidase (Cramer & Breton-Gorius 1987; Livesey et al. 1989; Mutasa 1989; Path et al. 1996). These granules contain numerous agents including lysozyme and lactoferrin (Bretz & Baggiolini 1974). Gelatinase granules are subsets of specific granules, and are therefore peroxidase negative (Borregaard & Cowland 1997). They are named for their high content of gelatinase found in their granules (Borregaard et al. 1993; Kjelsen et al. 1993; Borregaard & Cowland 1997). Secretory vesicles are a group of vesicles that are easily mobilized to the surface; they are remarkable for the presence of alkaline phosphatase within the membrane as well as the presence of albumin (Borregarrd et al. 1990; Borregaard 1996).

The degranulation of neutrophils is mediated by the presence of an injury. The azurophil and secretory granules can be released independently (Williams & Morley 1973; Wright et al. 1977; Presentey 1984). However, depending on

Table 2.3 Contents of neutrophil granules and vesicles.

Azurophil granule	Specific granule	Gelatinase granule	Secretory vesicle
Cd63	Cd66	Cd11b	Alkaline phosphatase
Cd68	Cd67	Cytochrome b558	Cytochrome b558
β-glycerophosphatase	Cytochrome b558	Diacylglycerol-deacylating enzyme	Cd11b
Acid mucopolysaccharide	Fibronectin-R	Plasminogen activator-R	Cd14
α_1-antitrypsin	G-protein subunit	Acetyltransferase	Cd16
α-mannosidase	Laminin-R	β_2-microglobulin	Plasminogen activator-R
Heparin-binding protein	Thrombospondin-R	Gelatinase	Albumin
Bactericidal permeability	Plasminogen	Lysozyme	Tetranectin
increasing protein	activator-R		
β-glycerophosphatase	Collagenase		
β-glucuronidase	Gelatinase		
Cathepsins	Histaminase		
Defensins	Heparanase		
Elastase	Lactoferrin		
Lysozyme	Lysozyme		
Myeloperoxidase	Sialidase		
Proteinase-3	β-microglobulin		
Sialidase	TNF-R		

TNF, tumour necrosis factor.

the stimuli, concomitant release is required to accentuate the bactericidal effects. There appears to be a hierarchy in ability to mobilize granules (Borregaard *et al.* 1993). The hierarchy for mobilization for excretory function appears to be secretory vesicles, gelatinase granules, specific granules and finally azurophilic granules being the least likely to be mobilized (Borregaard 1996). When activated, the specific granules, gelatinase granules and the secretory vesicles bind to the plasma membrane via cytochrome b558 subunits. Their contents are readily released; however they lack the ability to generate reactive oxygen molecules without the contents of the azurophilic granules, specifically myeloperoxidase (Klebanoff & Clark 1978; Pryzwansky *et al.* 1979).

The clinical importance of proper neutrophil function can be seen in a variety of hereditary disease states such as acute myelogenous leukaemia, congenital dysgranulopoietic neutropenia or Chediak–Higashi syndrome (Bainton 1975; Bainton *et al.* 1977). In congenital dysgranulopoietic neutropenia there is a defective synthesis and degradation of azurophilic granules, an absence or marked deficiency of specific granules and autophagia. Patients with this disease suffer severe life-threatening infections. In Chediak–Higashi syndrome, a rare autosomal recessive disease, there is a presence of abnormally large inclusions within the neutrophil, which appear to be abnormal azurophilic granules (Davis & Douglas 1971; Ohashi *et al.* 1992). These patients demonstrate an increased susceptibility to infection.

Eosinophils

Eosinophils are a type of leucocyte identifiable by its bilobed nuclei and large eosinophilic granules. The large granules in the eosinophil contain peroxidase; however, this peroxidase is chemically different than the peroxidase found in neutrophils (Bujak & Root 1974). Eosinophil peroxidase appears to have no role in the bactericidal activity of eosinophils. The granules also contain a variety of proteins including major basic protein (MBP), an eosinophil cationic protein, which does appear to be cytotoxic to either parasites or mammalian cells. MBP is also responsible for the induction of histamine release by basophils and mast cells (Peretz et al. 1994). There are four known inherited abnormalities of eosinophils. An absence of eosinophil peroxidase, an autosomal recessive trait, usually results in no clinically detectable symptoms (Wright & Gallin 1979; Pouliot et al. 1997). Chediak–Higashi syndrome manifests with large abnormal granules, seen in the eosinophil as well (Davis & Douglas 1971). A third type of abnormality was found in an individual family. It appears to be inherited in an autosomal recessive fashion. Their eosinophils demonstrated large grey inclusion bodies; however, they manifested without any clinical abnormality (Tisdale 1997). The fourth abnormality is an absence of specific granules seen in both neutrophils as well as eosinophils, presenting with repeated infections (Roos et al. 1996).

Platelets

Platelets, with their lack of a nucleus, may appear to be simple in nature but they serve a pivotal role in the regulation of haemostasis, thrombosis and inflammation. Platelet formation is accomplished by the fragmentation of megakaryocyte cytoplasm. In the circulatory system, platelets appear to be passive, smooth discs. However, they maintain the ability to recognize a site of injury, adhere to this site and serve in the activation and propagation of thrombus, as well as mediate the inflammatory pathway. Their lifespan is from 7 to 10 days and in a healthy individual their count can range from 150 000 to 440 000/µl. Platelets contain a circumferential band of microtubules, which serve to maintain the discoid shape, as well as an abundance of both actin and myosin within the platelet. These microtubules are responsible for the change in shape and spicule formation seen in platelets following activation.

Platelets are noted to have granules containing histamine, serotonin and TxA_2, amongst other proteins. It is unclear whether these mediators are developed within the megakaryocyte and are transferred to the platelet via the fragmentation process or whether they are absorbed from the plasma. Regardless, these factors, when released, serve to instigate and propagate many physiological reactions associated with platelet function.

Haemostasis is the culmination of three interactive systems including vascular endothelium, blood platelets and plasma proteins of both the intrinsic and extrinsic coagulation pathways. This process serves to arrest the loss of blood from vessels that have been mechanically traumatized, for example in muscular sprains, strains and fractures. When discontinuity of a vessel occurs, a series of responses termed primary haemostasis ensues. Following trauma, the vessel wall quickly retracts and platelets immediately adhere to the subendothelial collagen. Adherence to the vessel wall prompts platelet activation, which leads to propagation of the thrombus. This is continued until occlusion of the traumatized vessel occurs. The initial adherence is mediated by von Willebrand factor found in the plasma as well as von Willebrand factor released from activated platelet and endothelial cells. Following adhesion and activation (i.e. granule release), P-selectin, a platelet granule membrane glycoprotein, translocates to the cellular surface (Berman et al. 1986; McEver 1991; Frenette & Wagner 1997). This glycoprotein mediates the adhesion of leucocytes such as monocytes and neutrophils. Activation of the platelet eicosanoid pathway occurs, leading to the formation of arachidonic acid (Serhan et al. 1996; Sarraf et al. 1997). Arachidonic acid is released where it is immediately converted to PGH_2. This is then converted to TxA_2, a potent vasoconstrictor (O'Rourke et al. 1997). The activated platelet undergoes a change in shape with the formation of spicules. This change allows more effective binding between platelets as well as increased binding to factor X and activation of factor VII of the extrinsic coagulation cascade.

The platelet not only serves an important role in the regulation of the coagulation cascade, but serves as an important source of vasoactive mediators as well. Following vascular injury, activation of the coagulation cascade or exposure to the basement membrane stimulates platelets to release a variety of factors. These factors include serotonin, TxA_2 and histamine. Serotonin and histamine are generally released from cytoplasmic granules and serve as an immediate stimulant to increase vascular permeability. Thromboxane A_2, an arachidonic acid derivative formed by the breakdown of membrane phospholipids, serves as a stimulant to secondary clot formation as well as the aforementioned function of smooth muscle vasoconstriction. Interestingly, the absence of platelets appears to induce an increased state of vascular permeability. The mechanism of this is unclear, but in patients who are thrombocytopenic, spontaneous cutaneous as well mucosal bleeds are frequent.

T-lymphocytes

T-cells are vitally important in the normal functioning of the human immune system. In the human body, T-cells develop in the thymus. Utilizing the CD4 and CD8 receptor molecules expressed on the surface of T-cells, they can be divided into four subsets (Sprent & Webb 1987; Fink & Bevan 1995). These include CD4+/CD8+, CD4+/CD8–, CD4–/CD8+ and CD4–/CD8–. Both CD4- and CD8-negative T-cells make up about 2% of the total thymocytes. Their function remains unknown; however, they do seem to serve as precursors to the remaining subsets. T-cells are unique—they must display maximal reactivity to an infinite number of antigens but remain complacent in the face of self-antigens. In order to facilitate this, intrathymic precursors undergo a complex process of both positive and negative selection based on their reactivity to self-peptides bound to major histocompatibility complex (MHC) molecules.

Positive selection occurs in the cortical region of the thymus. Since MHC complexes are highly polymorphic, each individual must create a population of T-cells that are capable of recognizing these molecules and reacting to them if they are bound to an antigen (Sprent & Webb 1995). The double positive cells are exposed to self–MHC complexes and those precursors to circulating T-cells that display the ability to recognize these complexes are retained. The cells that are unable to recognize these cells are allowed to die *in situ* (Strang *et al.* 1988). The cells that demonstrate an overly aggressive nature to MHC molecules are removed via a process termed negative selection, leaving only the physiologically reactive T-cell progeny to survive in the post-thymic environment. In contrast to the cortical location of positive selection, it is unclear where the process of negative selection occurs. There is evidence that supports both a cortical and medullary localization of these events (Snijdewint 1993; Neiman 1997). T-cell importance in the acute inflammatory phase has not been well documented although its absence has been shown to decrease the strength of healing collagen, while prolonged activation has been implicated in the formation of excessive scar tissue.

B-lymphocytes

B-cell lymphocytes are derived from the bone marrow in humans. They are a key element in immune responses to foreign antigens. There are two types of B-cell immune responses to antigens: T-cell independent- and T-cell-dependent responses. T-cell-independent responses are accomplished by the binding of an antigen, leading to cross-linking of the B-cell receptors. This stimulates proliferation and differentiation of B-cells into antibody-secreting plasma cells (Nossal 1994; Doody *et al.* 1996). The majority of immune responses to antigens, however, are T-cell dependent. In this process, the B-cells present antigens to T-cells in order to beseech their assistance. After being presented an antigen, the B-cell will either pinocytose or endocytose it via receptors on the cellular membrane. In the B-cell, the antigen is processed and broken down into peptides, which are then presented by the cell's MHC molecules to antigen-specific T-cells. Following recognition of the peptide–MHC complex by the T-cell, a complex interaction occurs between the T-cell and B-cell. This interaction requires cell-to-cell contact and involves multiple receptors and ligands on both cells (Oliver & Essner 1975; Mitchell *et al.* 1995). Signals within this interaction are critical in the development of further immune responses, such as immunoglobulin isotype class switching and the generation of memory B-cells.

In the athlete, the amount of B-lymphocytes as well as T-lymphocytes appears to be decreased during and immediately following vigorous exercise. Some researchers have speculated that an increased incidence of upper respiratory tract infections seen in high-level endurance athletes is a result of this decrease in lymphocytes (Neiman 1997). The decrease in numbers is most probably related to the secretion of exercise-induced hormones such at cortisol (Neiman 1997). Although B-lymphocytes have been implicated in such phenomenon as exercise-induced asthma and upper airway disease in the athlete, their role in the acute phase of injury remains elusive. Considering the complex interactions seen between both plasma and cellular mechanisms of inflammation, one may speculate that B-lymphocytes serve an active role in the generation and/or regulation of the inflammatory response. Further studies are needed, however, to define the exact nature of their involvement.

Natural killer cells

Natural killer (NK) cells represent a discrete subset of the lymphoid population, differing from T-cells and B-cells in that they do not express or rearrange known receptors for antigens. NK cells can account for up to 20% of circulating lymphocytes. NK cells appear to provide a first line of defence against tumour cells and viral infections (Tracey & Smith 1978). They are characterized by the expression of two distinct membrane proteins, the CD56 receptor and the CD16 receptor. CD16 is a low affinity receptor for the Fc portion of immunoglobulin G, whereas CD56, which is analogous to the neural cell adhesion molecule (NCAM) (Tracey & Smith 1978). These cells were found to propagate cytolytic cell destruction in the absence of deliberate immunization and in the absence of MHC complexes. The recognition of these foreign cells seems to be mediated by the absence of MHC class 1 molecule (Ljunggren & Karre 1985; Sprent 1993). The presence of such molecules appears to serve as an inhibitory stimulus to the NK cells. Activation of NK cells not only results in their cytolytic activity, but also stimulates the release of cytokines that can exert a regulatory role in the immune response and inflammation (Trinchieri 1989; Bellone et al. 1993).

The complement system

The complement system is partially responsible for the recognition and destruction of pathogens and altered host cells. In this respect it is a highly complex system that plays an imperative role in both the innate immune system as well as a primed immune system ready to react against a pathological insult. The complement system possesses the ability to directly recognize and eliminate pathogens or damaged host cells. The mechanisms by which this is accomplished will be considered below.

The complement system is made up of more than 30 plasma and cell membrane proteins. When activated by a pathogen or injury, a precisely regulated series of interactions, not only within the complement proteins but also with the pathogen and cell membranes, initiates a series of reactions that can be divided into three stages. The first is the recognition and initiation of one of the two complement-activating pathways (classic pathway and alternate pathway.) The second is C3 binding and amplification; the third and final phase is the membrane attack pathway. The process of activation of the classic pathway involves recognition of the inflammatory agent by the first component of complement (C1). The C1 component consists of three distinct proteins: C1q, C1r and C1s. The C1q protein attaches itself to the Fc component of the instigating immunoglobulin. C1r and C1s are activated with this binding and in turn react with C4 and C2 forming two products, an anaphylatoxin C4a and C3 convertase (C4b and C2a). Cs3 convertase cleaves the C3 molecule forming C3a and C3b (a second anaphylatoxin). The resulting complex binds to the C5 molecule initiating hydrolysis of this molecule forming C5a and C5b. C5b will attach itself to target cell membranes and acts to facilitate binding of C6, C7 and C8 as well as initiating the polymerization of multiple C9 molecules. This forms a macromolecule known as the membrane

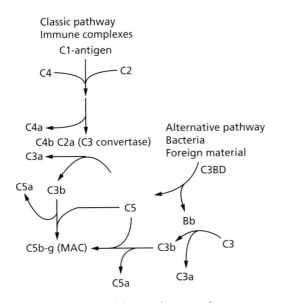

Fig. 2.4 Illustration of the complement pathway demonstrating both the classic and alternative pathways. Note the formation of the membrane attack complex (MAC, C5b) as well as the formation of anaphylaxins C4a, C3a and C5a.

with the release of histamine, PAF and serotonin. These mediators serve to further increase vascular permeability. The anaphylatoxins appear to mediate the smooth muscle contraction seen in bronchial spasm. This is accomplished by one of two pathways, the degranulation of the mast cell or a second pathway utilizing an arachidonic acid derivative. C5a also serves an important role as a chemotactic agent for leucocytes. With the initiation of the complement system, local production of C5a serves to recruit neutrophils and monocytes to sites of tissue injury. This cleavage component also has the ability to stimulate neutrophil degranulation and superoxide anion production (Jose *et al.* 1981).

Mechanical trauma to tissues such as fractures, muscular strains or sprains leads to the exposure of the basement membranes, which in turn activates factor XII (Hageman factor). This activated Hageman factor not only cleaves plasminogen and prekallikrein, generating plasmin and kallikrein, respectively, but also has the capability of activating the alternative complement pathway. Plasmin maintains the capability to induce increased vascular permeability as well as utilizing the anaphylatoxins C3a and C5a to induce changes in microvascular permeability. In this way, acute traumatic injuries utilize the complement system to mediate acute changes in vascular permeability as well as to initiate the inflammatory response.

The complement system is regulated by several mechanisms including: (i) the spontaneous decay of active complexes or cleavage products; (ii) the inactivation of specific components by proteolysis; and (iii) the binding of active components by plasma proteins. Factor I, a plasma protein, is responsible for the down-regulation of both C3b and C4b (Liszewski & Atkinson 1993). A second plasma protein, C1 esterase inhibitor, serves to regulate the activation of the classic pathway by binding to both C1r and C1s making them inactive (Liszewski & Atkinson 1993). Serum carboxylase N can inactivate the anaphylatoxins C4a, C3a and C5a. Factor H is another plasma protein, which binds to the C3b protein, making it more susceptible to cleavage by factor I.

attack complex (Fig. 2.4). Following the assembly of the membrane attack complex on the cell membrane of the target cell, small cylindrical holes are formed within the membrane leading to cell lysis (Cooper 1985; Muller-Eberhard 1986).

Cell products, bacteria or foreign material may also activate the alternative pathway. In this pathway, C3 binds with two plasma proteins, factor B and factor D, with a resultant product Bb catalysing the conversion of C3 to C3a and C3b. With the presence of Bb, C3b functions in an amplification reaction stimulating C3 convertase to form more C3a and C3b. C5 convertase is formed with the generation of C5a and C5b. The membrane attack complex is then formed as in the classic pathway.

When the classic pathway is utilized, the formation of anaphylatoxins (C3a, C4a and C5a) is an important step. Each of these molecules is capable of causing smooth muscle contraction as well as increasing vascular permeability. C3a and C5a also possess the ability to activate mast cells and basophils leading to their degranulation,

Table 2.4 Patterns of disease in complement-deficient patients.

Deficient component	Disease
C1q, C1r, C1s, C4, C2	SLE, autoimmune diseases and recurrent pyogenic infections
C3, factor H, factor I	Recurrent pyogenic infections and immune complex diseases
C5, C6, C7, C8	Recurrent neisserial infections
C1 inhibitor	Hereditary angioedema
CR3, CR4	Severe immunodeficiency, leucocyte disfunction and recurrent infections

SLE, systemic lupus erythematosus.

The importance of the complement system can be seen by examining patients with congenital deficiencies. The absence of any of the classic complement pathway (CCP), components results in systemic lupus erythematosus (SLE) (Liszewski *et al.* 1989). In addition to SLE, the absence of C3, factor H and factor I appear to make an individual more susceptible to repeated pyogenic infections by strains of *Staphylococcus, Streptococcus,* pneumococcus and other organisms (Morgan & Walport 1991). Whereas impaired CCP activation leads to autoimmune disease, immune complex disease and repeated infections, uncontrolled CCP activation occurs in the absence of regulatory proteins. It appears that an unregulated CCP is involved in the pathogenesis of hereditary angioedema (Table 2.4) (Storkus *et al.* 1987; Davis 1988).

Response to injury

Numerous changes occur within the human body after the onset of an inflammatory state. These changes are not only localized to the site of the pathology but also involve numerous organ systems. The acute phase response represents a state in which the body modifies its normal internal environment to appropriately respond to an inciting pathology. Cytokine-induced changes in plasma protein synthesis, the neuroendocrine and haematological systems, metabolic processes, and non-protein plasma components mediate these local as well as distant changes.

The initial response to tissue injury occurs primarily in the vasculature, namely the capillaries and postcapillary venules. Normal vascular anatomy consists of a layer of endothelium connected by tight junctions and a basement membrane composed of type IV collagen, glycosaminoglycans and glycoproteins. This vascular anatomy serves to preserve the normal relationship between the tissue and the circulating plasma and cellular components, which is one of mutual exclusion. After tissue injury, an initial rapid step is activation of the endothelial cells. The endothelium, when activated, has the ability to change its surface properties and become adhesive for both platelets and leucocytes. Shortly after acute trauma, the endothelium expresses an adhesion protein, P-selectin. This protein binds both polymorphonuclear leucocytes and monocytes; it is this binding or tethering that accounts for the rolling of leucocytes along the endothelium. The activated endothelium also stimulates the production of PAF. The synthesized PAF is directed towards the surface of the endothelial cell, but is not released. This localization of PAF to the surface induces tight binding of the leucocytes with their subsequent emigration, and also primes them for degranulation. PAF has also been implicated in the activation of passing platelets by the bound leucocytes. The platelets, once activated, release mediators such as TxA_2, serotonin and histamine, leading to the formation of gap junctions in the endothelium and thus facilitating leucocyte migration (Fig. 2.5). The formation of gap junctions leads to a disruption of endothelial continuity and exposing of the basement membrane, which in turn further activates platelets. This leads to a self-propagating cycle which is vital in the repair of damaged tissue.

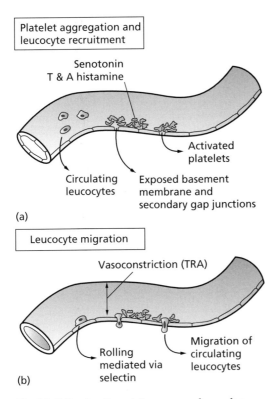

Fig. 2.5 Following tissue injury, exposed vascular collagen stimulates platelet aggregation and activation (a). Activation stimulates the release of mediators leading to gap junction formation as well as leucocyte aggregation to the site of injury, with subsequent migration into the tissues (b).

The response of the vasculature to injury is not only one of increased permeability, but also one of dynamic vasodilatation and vasoconstriction. At sites of injury, vasoactive mediators, both cellular and plasma derived, bind to specific receptors located on the endothelial cells as well as the vasculature smooth muscle, propagating either vasoconstriction or dilatation. The effects of vasodilatation and constriction have variable effects on the tissue, depending on their site of action. Vasodilatation of the arterioles leads to increased blood flow to a tissue, i.e. increased oedema, whereas constriction leads to decreased blood flow, i.e. decreased oedema. Conversely, dilatation of venules decreases capillary hydrostatic pressure leading to decreased oedema formation, whereas constriction leads to increased hydrostatic pressure in the capillaries and subsequent increased tissue oedema.

The postcapillary venule appears to be the primary site of endothelial changes for many of the vasoactive mediators. As mentioned above, during the time immediately following an injury, a complex cascade of biochemical events is initiated, leading to cell contraction, loss of tight junctions and formation of endothelial gaps. This series of events leads to increased vascular permeability with the subsequent extravasation of intravascular fluids into the injured tissue. This process is dynamic and reversible with maximal permeability occurring within 10–30 min after injury. Normal vascular anatomy is regained usually within an hour.

Several modalities have been demonstrated to alter the course of inflammation, both in the acute and chronic setting. Non-steroidal anti-inflammatory drugs (NSAIDs) serve as membrane stabilizers, thus dampening the effects of the arachidonic acid cascade. The use of NSAIDs has not been proven to speed wound healing and in fact has proved to be of minimal benefit in the treatment of acute injuries. Corticosteroids act early in the inflammatory cascade by blocking the release of arachidonic acid. There have been no clinical studies that demonstrate the oral use of corticosteroids in acute sports trauma to be beneficial in the recovery of an athlete. Corticosteroid injection therapy, on the other hand, has been implied in animal models to be advantageous to wound healing, but no conclusive data have been obtained. Injection of corticosteroids should be limited in acute macrotrauma secondary to its catabolic effect, and injections around tendinous and ligamentous structures must be weighed carefully secondary to the deleterious effects on those structures. Physical modalities such as thermotherapy and cryotherapy have been used in the treatment of acute inflammation. Thermotherapy, or heat application, has been shown to relieve the secondary symptoms of inflammation such as muscle spasm. Cryotherapy appears to reduce the local tissue temperature and local blood flow. This serves to decrease the subsequent

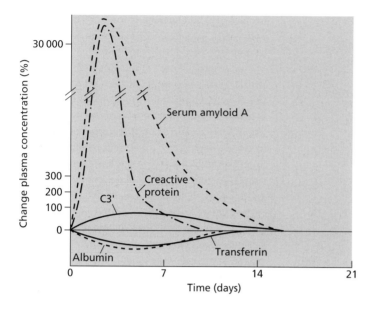

Fig. 2.6 Changes seen in serum concentrations of acute phase proteins during the inflammatory response. (Modified from Kushner 1993.)

oedema and may alter secondary necrotic effects of the initial trauma.

Acute phase proteins are defined as plasma proteins whose amount of production is either increased or decreased by a factor of 25% in the face of an inflammatory stimulus (Izumi *et al.* 1994). Some of the well-known human plasma proteins include ceruloplasmin, the complement components C3 and C4, C-reactive protein (CRP) and serum amyloid (Kushner 1982; McCarty 1982). These proteins are termed positive acute phase proteins in that their production is markedly increased. CRP and serum amyloid is usually present in plasma in trace amounts. After an inflammatory insult their concentration may increase 1000-fold (Fig. 2.6) (McCarty 1982). The synthesis of negative acute phase proteins is by definition decreased by at least 25%. Long recognized negative acute phase proteins include transferin and albumin. The functions of these acute phase proteins are as varied as the proteins themselves. Some, such as complement proteins, are essential in the elimination of foreign pathogens; the functions of other proteins, such as CRP, remain elusive, but do provide us with an adequate marker of the inflammatory status.

Neuroendocrine changes seen in the acute phase response include fever, somnolence, anorexia and altered synthesis of endocrine hormones including corticotrophin-releasing hormone (CRH), glucagon, insulin, adrenal catecholamines, growth hormone, adrenocorticotrophic hormone (ACTH), thyroid-stimulating hormone, aldosterone and vasopressin (Chrousos 1995; Boelen *et al.* 1997). For the most part, these changes in the neuro-endocrine system do not appear to be functional, rather unwanted collateral effects of the mediators of inflammation. Fever has been discussed in the previous section on prostaglandins, but in addition to the effect of PGE on the stimulation of fever, it appears that the cytokine, IL-6, stimulates the induction of fever via its effects on the thermoregulatory centre (Dinarello 1997). The production of IL-6 occurs in the endothelium of hypothalamic organs and is a response to IL-1α and TNF-α, common proinflammatory mediators (Lucino & Wong 1996).

Not only the inflammatory process, but also the stress experienced by the body, affects the neuro-endocrine system. The endocrine abnormalities experienced by the body are the result of a complex interaction between inflammation-associated cytokines—predominantly the hypothalamic–pituitary–adrenal axis (Chrousos 1995). Common hormone increases are seen in insulin, glucagons, cortisol and ACTH, as well as others (Patel &

Neuberger 1993). IL-1, IL-6 and TNF-α appear to be amongst the most potent stimulators of the hypothalamic–pituitary–adrenal axis by stimulating the production of CRH and arginine vasopressin, with a consequent increased production of ACTH and cortisol. The sympathetic and adrenomedullary systems respond to both pro-inflammatory mediators as well as to endocrine changes, with the secretion of neurotransmitters. These further lead to alterations in the neuro-endocrine environment associated with the acute phase response.

Lethargy, anorexia and somnolence appear to be common findings during the acute phase response. In experimental models IL-1 and TNF-α both induce a somnogenic effect on rabbits when injected into their cerebral ventricles (Surh & Sprent 1994). IL-1 has been demonstrated within the central nervous system of humans and appears to play a central role in the somnogenic response in them as well (Surh & Sprent 1994; Leon *et al.* 1997). Several cytokines are implicated in the pathogenesis of anorexia. In animal models, IL-1-induced secretion of IL-6 appears to stimulate an anorexic state; however, clinical trials to support these findings are lacking in humans (Zeidler *et al.* 1992; Fattori *et al.* 1994; Leon *et al.* 1996). Other animal studies have implicated local production of TNF-α as well as IL-1α-induced secretion of leptin (an acute phase reactant) as a stimulant to anorexia (Zeidler *et al.* 1992; Ryan 1997). In truth, as with most types of inflammatory reactions, its causes are most likely multifactorial and remain unclear.

Anaemia of chronic inflammation appears to be secondary to a decreased production of red blood cell progenitors, as well as a decrease in erythropoietin synthesis (Means 1995). Both of these appear to be mediated somewhat by inflammatory cytokines. Some of these cytokines decrease the response of the red blood cell progenitors to erythropoietin, whereas others decrease the synthesis of erythropoietin (Faquin *et al.* 1992). The major component may be the decreased production of erythropoietin, since studies have shown that anaemia secondary to chronic inflammation can be overcome with the administration of erythropoietin alone (Zabucchi *et al.* 1992).

Metabolic changes seen in the face of chronic inflammation include the loss of body mass and altered lipid metabolism. As with neuroendocrine changes, these are probably an untoward effect of circulating cytokines rather than a desired response. Decreases in the amount of skeletal muscle, fat tissue and bone mass result from the effects of numerous cytokines including IL-1, IL-6, TNF-α and interferon gamma (IFN-γ) (Espat *et al.* 1995; Takahashi *et al.* 1996). IL-1 and IL-6 appear to be the primary cytokines responsible for the loss of skeletal muscle, which is a result of decreased protein synthesis as well as increased muscle proteolysis (Cannon 1995). Alterations in lipid metabolism results in the loss of fat tissue and decreases in circulating high-density lipoproteins, as well as increases in serum triglycerides, very low-density lipoproteins and low-density lipoproteins (Liao & Floren 1993; Feingold *et al.* 1994; Banka *et al.* 1995). Unlike the cytokines responsible for muscle degradation, the cytokines responsible for the altered lipid metabolism remain elusive. Studies have demonstrated that chronic injections of IL-6 in Rhesus monkeys appear to induce a state of hypocholesterolaemia, but the correlation to human lipid metabolism remains unclear. Immunosuppression has also been implicated as an acute phase phenomenon (Ettinger *et al.* 1995).

The onset of an inflammatory process is accompanied by numerous physiological reactions at sites distant from the initial insult. The acute phase response to injury represents a complex interaction of numerous organ systems. These interactions appear to be mediated by inflammation-associated cytokines and influenced by modulators of cytokine function as well as endocrine hormones and other circulating factors. Although these changes are frequently seen in association with one another, it is common to have variable responses to inflammation on an individual basis.

The process of tissue repair

When faced with inflammation, the body is forced to initiate the reparative process. The re-establishment of physiologically functional tissue is imperative for the return to activity levels similar to the preinjured state. A coordinated process of cell migration and proliferation directed by specific biochemical mediators facilitates this repair of damaged tissue. This process utilizes various aspects of the humeral and cellular defence mechanisms to alleviate the inciting pathology.

Following an injury in which the vasculature is disrupted, the process of tissue repair begins immediately. As mentioned above, platelet adherence to the exposed collagen stimulates activation with the subsequent release of mediators such as serotonin, histamine and TxA$_2$, among others. Once the acute haemorrhage is controlled by the activated platelet and clotting pathways, the migration of inflammatory cells into the region of damage begins.

In the immediate postinjury period, neutrophils predominate the immigrating leucocytes. They can be detected within 1 h after injury and peak in approximately 24–48 h. Recruitment of these cells is mediated by the process of rolling (via selectins), adhesion (via integrin) and migration through the endothelium (Menger & Vollmar 1996). Immigration into the site of injury is stimulated by complement components (C5) as well as factors released by the activated platelets (Marder *et al.* 1985).

The function of these neutrophils is to clear the wound of fibrin as well as the initiation of inflammation via the release of proinflammatory cytokines (Grinnell & Zhu 1994). As mentioned earlier, the regulation of cytokines is primarily at the transcription level. Messenger RNA of TNF-α is apparent at the site of injury within 12 h, peaking at 72 h. This increase in mRNA may last for up to 5 days after the injury (Feiken *et al.* 1995).

As the number of neutrophils begins to decrease, a concomitant rise in the number of macrophages is seen. This increase in macrophages seems to peak in 5–7 days. The recruitment of these circulating macrophages to the site of injury is secondary to factors released by both platelets and neutrophils (Cromack *et al.* 1990; Ham *et al.* 1991). These macrophages serve as a major source of growth factors and cytokines that recruit and activate additional macrophages and

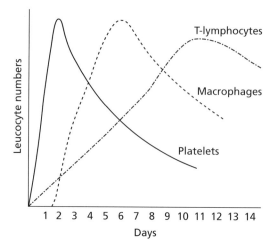

Fig. 2.7 Following an injury to biological tissue, migration of characteristic leucocytes into the damaged tissue follows a consistent pattern. The length of their presence depends on the amount of trauma.

fibroblasts. Macrophages function in debridement of the pathology, recruitment of other inflammatory cells, cell proliferation, and regrowth of peripheral nerves (Leibovitch & Ross 1975; Platt *et al.* 1996; Fritsch *et al.* 1997).

T-lymphocytes have been shown to be present at sites of injury from the first hour postinjury and peaking between 7 and 14 days later (Fig. 2.7) (Martin & Muir 1990). Their function is not clearly understood, although their absence has been shown to lead to decreased wound strength and lower amounts of collagen deposition. Conversely, prolonged activation of T-cells appears to lead to excessive fibrosis as seen in keloid formation (Borgognoni *et al.* 1995). This can be logically expanded to areas of chronic inflammation, where increased amounts of fibrosis are seen, presumably secondary to prolonged T-cell activation (Peters *et al.* 1986).

Following the recruitment of leucocytes and fibroblasts, a tissue termed granulation tissue is formed. This tissue was initially termed granulation tissue secondary to the granular appearance of the newly forming blood vessels. Granulation tissue develops from connective tissue surrounding the site of injury as well as the recently immigrated leucocytes, fibroblasts and myofibroblasts. Over a period of time, this granulation tissue is gradually replaced with more organized collagen, which remodels to eventually form organized scar tissue.

Conclusions

Although inflammation is often thought of as an unwanted effect of trauma or overtraining, it represents a physiological state of repair that's purpose is to return the individual to a state of functional recovery. The development of an inflammatory reaction is multifaceted, utilizing many of the body's systems to mediate its purpose. Complex interactions between cellular and plasma-derived components serve to initiate, propagate and regulate the inflammatory response.

Shortly after a physiological insult in which disruption of the vasculature occurs, platelets aggregate to the site of injury. Via interactions between the platelets, exposed collagen and endothelial cells, factors are secreted which serve to propagate numerous functions. Vasoconstriction at the site of injury initially serves to decrease the blood flow, thus minimalizing the amount of blood loss at the site of injury. Gap junctions are formed within the endothelium to facilitate the transendothelial migration of circulating leucocytes in order to gain access to the site of pathology. The local secretion of cytokines and chemokines, which serve as chemotractants, assists the accumulation of leucocytes at the site of injury. Depending on the type of pathological insult, the type and amounts of cytokines, as well as other stimulators of cellular migration (complement proteins, antigen–antibody complexes), vary. It is the variability of these signals, which dictate the type of cellular components recruited to the site of injury.

Regardless of the cellular mediators, the ultimate goal is the same—removal of diseased tissue with the subsequent regeneration of tissue, functionally equivalent to the prediseased state. Depending on the type and length of the insult, variable amounts of newly generated tissue will be deposited. This newly formed tissue usually takes the form of collagen with the physiological and histological appearance of fibrosis. If the pathological insult is small, the ratio of fibrosis to normal tissue remains small and the functionality of the original tissue is left intact. In instances of prolonged pathological insult, the ratio of fibrosis to normal tissue is elevated, thus compromising the host tissue function. It is for this reason that the athlete as well as the physician attempt to minimize the amount of inflammation.

References

Akira, S., Taga, T. & Kishimoto, T. (1993) Interleukin 6 in biology and medicine. *Advances in Immunology* **54**, 1–78.

Arrang, J.M., Garbarg, M. & Schwartz, J.C. (1983) Highly potent and selective ligands for histamine H3-receptors. *Nature* **302**, 832–837.

Bacon, K.B. & Schall, T.J. (1996) Chemokines and mediators of allergic inflammation. *International Archives of Allergy and Immunology* **109**, 97–109.

Bainton, D.F. (1975) Abnormal neutrophils in acute myelogenous leukemia: identification of subpopulations based on analysis of azurophil and specific granules. *Blood Cells* **1**, 191–199.

Bainton, D.F. (1980) The cells of inflammation: a general view. In: *The Cell Biology of Inflammation*, Vol. 2. (Weissman, G., ed.). Elsevier/North-Holland, New York: 1–25.

Bainton, D.F., Friedlander, L.M. & Shohet, S.B. (1977) Abnormalities in granule formation in acute myelogenous leukemia. *Blood* **49**, 693–704.

Banka, C.L., Yuan, T., de Beer, M.C., Kindy, M., Curtiss, L.K. & de Beer, F.C. (1995) Serum amyloid A (SAA): influence on HDL-mediated cellular cholesterol efflux. *Journal of Lipid Research* **36**, 1058–1065.

Bell, M.D., Lopez-Gonzalez, R., Lawson, L.F. *et al.* (1994) Upregulation of the macrophage scavenger receptor in response to different forms of injury in the CNS. *Journal of Neurocytology* **23**, 605–613.

Bellone, G., Valiante, N.M., Viale, O., Ciccone, E., Moretta, L. & Trinchieri, G. (1993) Regulation of hematopoiesis *in vitro* by alloreactive natural killer cell clones. *Journal of Experimental Medicine* **77**, 1117–1122.

Bemelmans, M.H.A., Van Tits, L.J.H. & Buuman, W.A. (1996) Tumor necrosis factor: function release and clearance. *Critical Reviews in Immunology* **16**, 1–11.

Berman, C.L., Yeo, E.L., Wencel-Drake, J.D., Furie, B.C., Ginsberg, M.H. & Furie, B. (1986) A platelet alpha granule membrane protein that is associated with plasma membrane after activation: characterization and subcellular localization of platelet activation-dependent granule-external membrane protein. *Journal of Clinical Investigations* **78**, 130–137.

Betz, M. & Fox, B.S. (1991) Prostaglandin E2 inhibits production of Th1 lymphokines but not of Th2 lymphokines. *Journal of Immunology* **146**, 108–113.

Black, J.W., Duncan, W.A.M., Durant, C.J., Ganellin, C.R. & Parsons, E.M. (1972) Definition and antagonism of histamine H2-receptors. *Nature* **236**, 385–390.

Boelen, A., Platvoetterschiphorst, M.C. & Wiersinga, W.M. (1997) Immunoneutralization of interleukin-1, tumor necrosis factor, interleukin-6 or interferon does not prevent the LPS-induced sick euthyroid syndrome in mice. *Journal of Endocrinology* **153**, 115–122.

Borgognoni, L., Pimpinelli, N., Martini, L., Brandani, P. & Reali, U.M. (1995) Immuno-histologic features of normal and pathological scars—possible clues to the pathogenesis. *European Journal of Dermatology* **5**, 407–412.

Borregaard, N. (1996) Current concepts about neutrophil granule physiology. *Current Opinions in Hematology* **3**, 11–20.

Borregaard, N., Christensen, L., Bejerrum, O.W., Bigens, H.S. & Clemensen, I. (1990) Identification of a highly mobilizable subset of human neutrophil intracellular vesicles that contain tetranectin and latent alkaline phosphatase. *Journal of Clinical Investigations* **85**, 408–416.

Borregaard, N. & Cowland, B.J. (1997) Granules of the human neutrophilic polymorphonuclear leukocyte. *Blood* **89**, 3503–3521.

Borregaard, N., Lollike, K., Kjeldsen, L. *et al.* (1993) Human neutrophil granules and secretory vesicles. *European Journal of Haematology* **51**, 187–198.

Bretz, U. & Baggiolini, M. (1974) Biochemical and morphological characterization of azurophil and specific granules of human neutrophilic polymorphonuclear leukocytes. *Journal of Cell Biology* **63**, 251–269.

Bryant, W.M. (1977) Wound healing. *Clinic Symptoms* **29**, 1–36.

Bujak, J.S. & Root, R.K. (1974) The role of peroxidase in the bactericidal activity of human blood eosinophils. *Blood* **43**, 727–736.

Cannon, J.G. (1995) Cytokines in aging and muscle homeostasis. *Journal of Gerontology. Series A: Biological Sciences and Medical Sciences* **50**, 120–123.

Chrousos, G.P. (1995) The hypothalamic–pituitary–adrenal axis and immune mediated inflammation. *New England Journal of Medicine* **332**, 1351–1362.

Cooper, N.R. (1985) The classical complement pathway: activation and regulation of the first complement component. *Advances in Immunology* **37**, 151–207.

Cramer, E.M. & Breton-Gorius, J. (1987) Ultrastructural localization of lysozyme in human neutrophils by immunogold. *Journal of Leukocyte Biology* **41**, 242–247.

Cromack, D.T., Porrasreyes, B. & Mustoe, T.A. (1990) Current concepts in wound healing growth factor and macrophage interaction. *Journal of Trauma* **30**, S129–S133.

Davis III, A.E. (1988) C1 inhibitor and hereditary angioneurotic edema. *Annual Review of Immunology* **6**, 595–628.

Davis, W.C. & Douglas, S.D. (1971) Defective granule formation and function in the Chediak–Higashi syndrome in man and animals. *Seminars in Hematology* **9**, 431–450.

Dinarello, C.A. (1996) Biologic basis for interleukin 1 in disease. *Blood* **87**, 2095–2147.

Dinarello, C.A. (1997) Cytokines as endogenous pyrogens. In: *Fever: Basic Mechanisms and Management*, 2nd edn (Mackowiak, P.A., ed.). Lippincott-Raven, Philadelphia: 87–116.

Doody, G.M., Dempsey, P.W. & Fearon, D.T. (1996) Activation of B lymphocytes: integrating signals from CD19, CD22 and FcγRIIb1. *Current Opinions in Immunology* **8**, 378–382.

Espat, N.J., Moldawer, L.L. & Copeland III, E.M. (1995) Cytokine mediated alterations in host metabolism prevent nutritional repletion in cachectic cancer patients. *Journal of Surgical Oncology* **58**, 77–82.

Ettinger, W.H.J., Sun, W.H., Binkley, N., Kouba, E. & Ershler, W. (1995) Interleukin 6 causes hypocholesterolemia in middle-aged and old rhesus monkeys. *Journal of Gerontology* **50**, M137–M140.

Fantone, J.C., Kunkel, S.L., Ward, P.A. & Zurier, R.B. (1980) Suppression by prostaglandin E1 of vascular permeability by vasoactive inflammatory mediators. *Journal of Immunology* **125**, 2591–2596.

Faquin, W.C., Schneider, T.J. & Goldberg, M.A. (1992) Effect of inflammatory cytokines on hypoxia induced erythropoietin production. *Blood* **79**, 1987–1994.

Fattori, E., Cappelletti, M., Costa, P. *et al.* (1994) Defective inflammatory response in interleukin 6 deficient mice. *Journal of Experimental Medicine* **180**, 1243–1250.

Feiken, E., Romer, J., Eriksen, J. & Lund, L.R. (1995) Neutrophils express tumor necrosis factor-alpha during mouse skin wound healing. *Journal of Investigative Dermatology* **105**, 120–123.

Feingold, K.R., Marshall, M., Gulli, R., Moser, A.H. & Grunfeld, C. (1994) Effect of endotoxin and cytokines on lipoprotein lipase activity in mice. *Arteriosclerosis and Thrombosis* **14**, 1866–1872.

Feldberg, W. & Saxena, P.N. (1971) Fever produced by prostaglandin E1. *Journal of Physiology* **217**, 547–556.

Feng, Y., Broder, C.C., Kennedy, P.E. & Berger, E.A. (1996) HIV-1 entry cofactor: functional cDNA cloning of a seven transmembrane, G protein-coupled receptor. *Science* **272**, 872–877.

Ferreira, S.H., Nakamura, M. & Abreu Castro, M.S. (1978) The hyperalgesic effects of prostacyclin and PGE2. *Prostaglandins* **16**, 31–38.

Fink, P.J. & Bevan, M.J. (1995) Positive selection of thymocytes. *Advances in Immunology* **59**, 99–133.

Frenette, P.S. & Wagner, D.D. (1997) Insights into selectin function from knockout mice. *Thrombosis and Haemostasis* **78**, 60–64.

Fritsch, C., Simon Assman, P., Kedinger, M. & Evans, G.S. (1997) Cytokines modulate fibroblast phenotype and epithelial stroma interactions in rat intestine. *Gastroenterology* **112**, 826–838.

Gamble, J.G. (1988) *The Musculoskeletal System: Physiologic Basics*. Raven Press, New York.

Goldblatt, M.W. (1933) A depressor substance in seminal fluid. *Journal of the Society of Chemical Industry* **52**, 1056–1057.

Goodwin, J.S., Bankhurst, A.D. & Messner, R.P. (1977) Suppression of human T-cell mitogenesis by prostaglandin. *Journal of Experimental Medicine* **146**, 1719–1725.

Grinnell, F. & Zhu, M.F. (1994) Identification of neutrophil elastase as the proteinase in burn wound fluid responsible for degradation of fibronectin. *Journal of Investigative Dermatology* **103**, 155–161.

Ham, J.M., Kunkel, S.L., Dibb, C.R., Standiford, T.J., Rolfe, M.W. & Strieter, R.M. (1991) Chemotactic cytokine (IL-8 and MCP-1) gene-expression by human whole blood. *Immunological Investigations* **20**, 387–394.

Izumi, S., Hughes, R.D., Langley, P.G., Pernambuco, J.R.B. & Williams, R. (1994) Extent of the acute phase response in fulminant hepatic failure. *Gut* **35**, 982–986.

Jain, J., Loh, C. & Rao, A. (1995) Transcription regulation of the IL2 gene. *Current Opinions in Immunology* **7**, 333–342.

Jose, P.J., Forrest, M.J. & Williams, T.J. (1981) Human C5a des arg increases vascular permeability. *Journal of Immunology* **127**, 2376–2380.

Kjelsen, L., Bainton, D.F., Sengelov, H. & Borregaard, N. (1993) Structural and functional heterogeneity among peroxidase-negative granules in human neutrophils: identification of a distinct gelatinase-containing granule subset by combined immunocytochemistry and subcellular fractionation. *Blood* **82** (10), 3183–3191.

Klebanoff, S.J. & Clark, F.A. (eds) (1978) *The Neutrophil: Function and Clinical Disorders*. North-Holland, New York.

Kunkel, S.L., Thrall, R.S., Kunkel, R.G., McCormixk, J.R., Ward, P.A. & Zurier, R.B. (1979) Suppression of immune complex vasculitis in rats by prostaglandin. *Journal of Clinical Investigations* **64**, 1525–1529.

Kunkel, S.L., Wiggings, R.C., Chensue, S.W. & Larrick, J. (1986) Regulation of macrophage tumor necrosis factor production by prostaglandin E2. *Biochemical and Biophysical Research Communications* **137**, 404–409.

Kurzok, R. & Lieb, C. (1931) Biochemical studies of human semen: action of semen on the uterus. *Proceedings of the Society of Experimental Biology* **28**, 268–272.

Kushner, I. (1982) The phenomenon of the acute phase response. *Annals of NY Academy of Science* **389**, 39–48.

Leibovitch, S.J. & Ross, R. (1975) The role of the macrophage in wound repair. A study with hydrocortisone and anti-macrophage serum. *American Journal of Pathology* **78**, 71–91.

Leon, L.R., Conn, C.A., Glaccum, M. & Kluger, M.J. (1996) IL1 type I receptor mediates acute phase response to turpentine, but not lipopolysaccharide, in mice. *American Journal of Physiology* **271**, R1668–R1675.

Leon, L.R., Kozak, W., Peschon, J. & Kluger, M.J. (1997) Exacerbated febrile responses to LPS, but not turpentine, in TNF double receptor-knock-out mice. *American Journal of Physiology* **272**, R563–R569.

Liao, W. & Floren, C. (1993) Hyperlipidemic response to endotoxin: a part of the host-defence mechanism. *Scandinavian Journal of Infectious Diseases* **25**, 675–682.

Liszewski, M.K. & Atkinson, J.P. (1993) The complement system. In: *Fundamental Immunology* (Paul, W.E., ed.). Raven Press, New York: 917–939.

Liszewski, M.K., Kahl, L.E. & Atkinson, J.P. (1989) The functional role of complement genes in systemic lupus erythematosus and Sjogren's syndrome. *Current Opinions in Rheumatology* **1**, 347–352.

Livesey, S.A., Buesher, E.S., Drannig, G.L., Harrison, D.S., Linner, J.G. & Choivetti, R. (1989) Human neutrophil granule heterogeneity: immunolocalization studies using cryofixed, dried and embedded specimens. *Scanning Microscopy* **3**, 231–240.

Ljunggren, H.G. & Karre, K. (1985) Host resistance directed selectively against H-2 deficient lymphoma variants: analysis of the mechanism. *Journal of Experimental Medicine* **162**, 1745–1759.

Lucino, J. & Wong, M. (1996) Interleukin 1b and fever. *Natural Medicine* **2**, 1314–1315.

Marder, S.R., Chenoweth, D.E., Goldstein, I.M. & Perez, H.D. (1985) Chemotactic responses of human peripheral blood monocytes of the complement-derived peptide C5a. *Journal of Immunology* **134**, 3325–3331.

Martin, C.W. & Muir, I.F.K. (1990) The role of lymphocytes in wound healing. *British Journal of Plastic Surgery* **43**, 655–662.

Martinez-Hernandez, A. (1988) Repair, degeneration, and fibrosis. In: *Pathology* (Rubin, E. & Farber, J.L., eds). JB Lippencott, Philadelphia: 68–95.

McCarty, M. (1982) Historical perspective on C-reactive protein. *Annals of NY Academy of Science* **389**, 1–10.

McDonald, P.P., Pouliot, M., Borgeat, P. & McColl, S.R. (1993) Induction by chemokines of lipid mediator synthesis in granulocyte–macrophage colony-stimulating factor treated human neutrophils. *Journal of Immunology* **151**, 6399–6409.

McEver, R.P. (1991) Leukocyte interactons mediated by selectins. *Thrombosis and Haemostasis* **66**, 80–87.

Means, R.T. (1995) Pathogenesis of the anemia of chronic disease: a cytokine-mediated anemia. *Stem Cells* **13**, 32–37.

Menger, M.D. & Vollmar, B. (1996) Adhesion molecules as determinants of disease from molecular biology to surgical research. *British Journal of Surgery* **83**, 588–601.

Milton, A.S. & Wendlandt, S. (1971) Effects on body temperature of prostaglandins of the A, E and F series on injection into the third ventricle of unanaesthetized cats and rabbits. *Journal of Physiology* **218**, 325–336.

Mitchell, R.N., Barnes, K.A., Grupp, S.A. *et al.* (1995) Intracellular targeting of antigens internalized by membrane immunoglobulin in B lymphocytes. *Journal of Experimental Medicine* **181**, 1705–1714.

Mnich, S.J., Veenhuizen, A.W., Monahan, J.B. *et al.* (1995) Characterizations of a monoclonal antibody that neutralizes the activity of prostaglandin E2. *Journal of Immunology* **155**, 4437–4444.

Moncada, S., Vane, J. & Ferreira, S.H. (1973) Prostaglandins, aspirin-like drugs and the odema of inflammation. *Nature* **246**, 217–219.

Morgan, B.P. & Walport, M.J. (1991) Complement deficiency and disease. *Immunology Today* **12**, 301–306.

Muller-Eberhard, H.J. (1986) The membrane attack complex of complement. *Annual Review of Immunology* **4**, 503–528.

Murakami, M., Matsumoto, R., Austen, K.F. & Arm, J.P. (1994) Prostaglandin endoperoxide synthase 1 and 2 couple to different transmembrane stimuli to generate prostaglandin D2 in mouse bone marrow-derived mast cells. *Journal of Biological Chemistry* **269**, 22269–22275.

Mutasa, H.C. (1989) Combination of diaminobenzidine staining and immunogold labeling: a novel technical approach to identify lysozyme in human neutrophil cells. *European Journal of Cell Biology* **49**, 319–325.

Neiman, D.C. (1997) Immune response to heavy exertion. *Journal of Applied Physiology* **82**, 1385–1394.

Nossal, G.J.V. (1994) Negative selection of lymphocytes. *Cell* **76**, 229–239.

Ohashi, K., Ruan, K.-H., Kulmacz, R.J., Wu, K.K. & Wang, L.H. (1992) Primary structure of human thromboxane synthase determined from the cDNA sequence. *Journal of Biological Chemistry* **267**, 789–793.

Oliver, C. & Essner, E. (1975) Formation of anomalous lysosomes in monocytes, neutrophils, and eosinophils from bone marrow of mice with Chediak–Higashi syndrome. *Journal of Laboratory Investigations* **32**, 17–27.

O'Rourke, L., Tooze, R. & Fearon, D.T. (1997) Co-receptors of B-lymphocytes. *Current Opinions in Immunology* **9**, 324–329.

Patel, K.J. & Neuberger, M.S. (1993) Antigen presentation by the B cell antigen receptor is driven by the alpha/beta sheath and occurs independently of its cytoplasmic tyrosines. *Cell* **74**, 939–946.

Path, G., Bornstein, S.R., Spathschwalbe, E. & Scherbaum, W.A. (1996) Direct effects of interleukin 6 on human adrenal cells. *Endocrine Research* **22**, 867–873.

Peretz, R., Shaft, D., Yaari, A. & Nir, E. (1994) Distinct intracellular lysozyme content in normal granulocytes and monocytes: a quantitative immunoperoxidase and ultrastructural immunogold study. *Journal of Histochemistry and Cytochemistry* **42**, 1471–1477.

Peters, M.S., Rodriquez, M. & Gleich, G.J. (1986) Localization of human eosinophil granule major basic protein, eosinophil cationic protein, and eosinophil-derived neurotoxin by immunoelectron microscopy. *Laboratory Investigations* **54**, 656–662.

Peterson, J.M., Barbul, A., Breslin, R.J., Wasserkrug, H.L. & Efron, G. (1987) Significance of T-lymphocytes in wound healing. *Surgery* **102**, 300–305.

Platt, N., Suzuki, H., Kurihara, Y., Kodama, T. & Gordon, S. (1996) Role for the class A macrophage scavenger receptor in the phagocytosis of apoptotic thymocytes. *Proceedings of the National Academy of Sciences of the USA* **93**, 12456–12460.

Plemons, J.M., Dill, R.E., Rees, T.D., Dyer, B.J., Ng, M.G. & Iacopino, A.M. (1996) PDGF-β producing cells and PDGF-β gene expression in normal gingival and cyclosporine-A-induced gingival overgrowth. *Journal of Periodontology* **67**, 264–270.

Poranova, J.P., Zhang, Y. & Anderson, G.D. (1996) Selective neutralization of prostaglandin E2 blocks inflammation, hyperalgesia, and interleukin 6 production *in vivo*. *Journal of Experimental Medicine* **184**, 883–891.

Pouliot, M., Baillargeon, J., Lee, J.C., Cleland, L.G. & James, M.J. (1997) Inhibition of prostaglandin endoperoxide synthase-2 expression in stimulated human monocytes by inhibitors of p38 mitogen-activated protein kinase. *Journal of Immunology* **158**, 4930–4937.

Presentey, B. (1984) Ultrastructure of human eosinophils genetically lacking peroxidase. *Acta Haematologica (Basel)* **71**, 331–340.

Pryzwansky, K.B., MacRae, E.K., Spitznagel, J.K. & Cooney, M.H. (1979) Early degranulation of human neutrophils: immunocytochemical studies of surface and intracellular phagocytic events. *Cell* **18**, 1025–1033.

Roos, D., De Boer, M., Kuribayashi, K. *et al.* (1996) Mutations in the X-linked and autosomal recessive forms of chronic granulomatous disease. *Journal of the American Society of Hematology* **87**, 1663–1681.

Rosenberg, H.F. & Gallin, J.I. (1993) Neutrophil-specific granule deficiency includes eosinophils. *Blood* **82**, 268–273.

Ryan, J.J. (1997) Interleukin 4 and its receptor: essential mediators of the inflammatory response. *Journal of Allergy and Clinical Immunology* **99**, 1–5.

Sarraf, P., Frederich, R.C., Turner, E.M. *et al.* (1997) Multiple cytokines and acute inflammation raise mouse leptin levels: potential role in inflammatory anorexia. *Journal of Experimental Medicine* **185**, 171–175.

Serhan, C.N. (1997) Lipoxins and novel aspirin-triggered 15-epi-lipoxins (ATL): a jungle of cell–cell interactions or a therapeutic opportunity? *Prostaglandins* **53**, 107–137.

Serhan, C.N., Haeggstrom, J.Z. & Leslie, C.C. (1996) Lipid mediator networks in cell signaling: update and impact of cytokines. *FASEB Journal* **10**, 1147–1158.

Shaw, J., Meerovitch, K., Bleackley, R.C. & Paetkau, V. (1988) Mechanisms regulating the level of IL 2 in T-lymphocytes. *Journal of Immunology* **140**, 2243–2248.

Snijdewint, F.G.M. (1993) Prostaglandin E2 differentially modulates cytokine secretion profiles of human T helper lymphocytes. *Journal of Immunology* **150**, 5321–5329.

Sprent, J. (1993) T lymphocytes and the thymus. In: *Fundamental Immunology*, Vol. 3 (Paul, W.E., ed.). Raven Press, New York: 75–110.

Sprent, J. & Webb, S.R. (1987) Function and specificity of T cell subsets in the mouse. *Advances in Immunology* **54**, 39–133.

Sprent, J. & Webb, S.R. (1995) Intrathymic and extrathymic clonal deletion of T cells. *Current Opinions in Immunology* **7**, 196–205.

Storkus, W.J., Howell, D.N., Salter, R.D., Dawson, J.R. & Cresswell, P. (1987) NK susceptibility varies inversely with target cell class I HLA antigen expression. *Journal of Immunology* **138**, 1657–1659.

Strang, C.J., Cholin, S., Spragg, J. *et al.* (1988) Angioedema induced by a peptide derived from complement component C2. *Journal of Experimental Medicine* **168**, 1685–1698.

Surh, C.D. & Sprent, J. (1994) T-cell apoptosis detected *in situ* during positive and negative selection in the thymus. *Nature* **372**, 100–103.

Takahashi, S., Kapas, L., Fang, J.D., Seyer, J.M., Wang, Y. & Krueger, J.M. (1996) An interleukin-1 receptor fragment inhibits spontaneous sleep and muramyl dipeptide-induced sleep in rabbits. *American Journal of Physiology* **271**, R101–R108.

Tisdale, M.J. (1997) Cancer cachexia: metabolic alterations and clinical manifestations. *Nutrition* **13**, 1–7.

Tracey, R. & Smith, H. (1978) An inherited anomaly of human eosinophils and basophils. *Blood Cells* **4**, 291–298.

Trinchieri, G. (1989) Biology of natural killer cells. *Advances in Immunology* **47**, 187–376.

Trinchieri, G. (1995) Natural killer cells wear different hats. effector cells of innate resistance and regulatory cells of adoptive immunity and hematopoiesis. *Seminars in Imunology* **7**, 83–88.

van der Pouw, C.T., Kraan, T.C., Boeije, L.C., Smeenk, R.J., Wijdenes, J. & Aarden, L.A. (1995) Prostaglandin E2 is a potent inhibitor of human interleukin 12 production. *Journal of Experimental Medicine* **181**, 775–779.

Von Euler, U.S. (1935) Uber die spezifische blutdrucksenkende substanz des menschlichen prostata- und samenblasensekretes. *Klinische Wochnschrift* **14**, 1182–1183.

Von Euler, U.S. (1934) Zur kenntnis der pharmakologishen wirkungen von nativsekreten und extrakten mannlicher accessorischer geschlechtsdrusen. *Naunyn Schmiedebergsarch Experimental Pathology* **175**, 78–84.

Wedmore, C.V. & Williams, T.J. (1981) Control of vascular permeability by polymorphonuclear leukocytes in inflammation. *Nature* **289**, 646–650.

Wheeldon, A. & Vardey, C.J. (1993) Characterization of the inhibitory prostanoid receptors on human neutrophils. *British Journal of Pharmacology* **108**, 1051–1054.

Williams, T.J. & Morley, J. (1973) Prostaglandins as potentiators of increased vascular permeability in inflammation. *Nature* **246**, 215–217.

Wright, D.G., Bralove, D.A. & Gallin, J.I. (1977) The differential mobilization of human neutrophil granules: effects of phorbol myristate acetate and inophore A23187. *American Journal of Pathology* **87**, 273–284.

Wright, D.G. & Gallin, J.I. (1979) Secretory responses of human neutrophils: exocytosis of specific (secondary) granules by human neutrophils during adherence *in vitro* and during exudation *in vivo*. *Journal of Immunology* **123**, 285–294.

Zabucchi, G., Soranzo, M.R., Menegazzi, R. *et al.* (1992) Eosinophil peroxidase deficiency: morphological and immunocytochemical studies of the eosinophil-specific granules. *Blood* **80**, 2903–2910.

Zeidler, C., Kanz, L., Hurkuck, F. *et al.* (1992) *In vivo* effects of interleukin 6 on thrombopoiesis in healthy and irradiated primates. *Blood* **80**, 2740–2745.

PART 2

BASIC SCIENCE OF TISSUE HEALING AND REPAIR

Chapter 3

Skeletal Muscle Regeneration After Injury: Cellular and Molecular Events

ANDRÉ-XAVIER BIGARD AND EMMANUELLE FINK

Introduction

Muscle damage is frequently observed after sports injuries. The ability of skeletal muscle to regenerate after injury is one of its major characteristics and myofibres are repeatedly damaged and repaired during adult life. At the anatomical level, injuries are commonly divided into shearing injuries, in which both myofibres and framework are torn, and injuries *in situ*, in which only myofibres are damaged, such as after repeated eccentric contractions. Shearing injuries result mainly from direct trauma to skeletal muscle or strain injuries, while *in situ* injuries follow exhaustive exercise, the application of local anaesthetics or are caused by diseases. The treatment and prognosis of muscle injuries vary widely according to the severity and extent of the trauma, but regardless of the origin of the injury, skeletal muscle will regenerate.

In response to injury, skeletal muscle regenerates following two types of regeneration. Epimorphic regeneration is mainly found in amphibians and gives rise to an entire new limb after amputation (Carlson 1970). In contrast to amphibians, skeletal muscle regenerates in mammals utilizing the remnants of the original myofibre complex. Here we review and discuss some important cellular events which follow muscle damage in mammals, and epimorphic regeneration will not be treated further. Muscle regeneration has been broadly divided into two types: continuous and discontinuous regenera-

tion (Hudgson & Field 1973). Discontinuous regeneration, of embryonic type, is characterized by the formation of newly regenerated myofibres from myoblastic cells. In contrast, continuous regeneration, of budding type, results in the outgrowth from the end of the section of a partially damaged myofibre. Continuous regeneration is less understood and will not be treated in this review.

Before describing the several phases of the healing process, it is important to summarize some aspects of the structure of satellite cells which represent stem cells providing myoblasts for regeneration. We will pay particular attention to the molecular events of activation and differentiation of satellite cells, and their clinical relevance now and in the future.

Structure of adult skeletal muscle

Muscle fibres are enveloped by the basal lamina. Between the basal lamina and the sarcolemma of the myofibres, are the satellite cells (Fig. 3.1). These unspecialized mononucleated cells, which were first described by Mauro (1961) in frog muscle, are known to have myogenic potential and to mediate the postnatal growth of skeletal muscle (Rosenblatt *et al.* 1994; Schultz 1996). In addition to their role in muscle hypertrophy and postnatal growth, there is now a large body of evidence indicating that satellite cells function as stem cells that provide myoblasts for muscle regeneration in adults. The exact origin of satellite

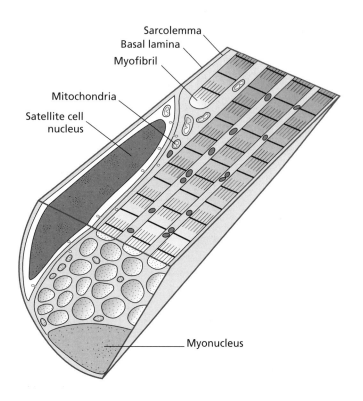

Sarcolemma
Basal lamina
Myofibril

Mitochondria

Satellite cell
nucleus

Myonucleus

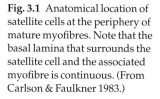

Fig. 3.1 Anatomical location of satellite cells at the periphery of mature myofibres. Note that the basal lamina that surrounds the satellite cell and the associated myofibre is continuous. (From Carlson & Faulkner 1983.)

cells has not been clearly identified. However, it seems that these myogenic cells stem from early myoblasts that were not incorporated in the developing syncitia, and remained in the surface of all fibres (Schultz 1989). Satellite cells adjacent to mature myofibres do not express specific markers of committed myoblasts such as early-acting myogenic regulatory factors (MRFs), Myf-5 and MyoD, growth factors, or other known markers of terminal differentiation. This finding is consistent with the hypothesis that satellite cells are stem cells with an identity distinct from that of myoblasts. The microenvironment of satellite cells, available growth factors and MRFs play a pivotal role for the generation of committed myoblasts.

There is now available evidence that satellite cells are divided into subclasses based on the fibre type in which they lie. Moreover, there is also evidence that satellite cells form a heterogeneous population based on their profile of gene expression (Cornelison & Wold 1997). It has been demonstrated that satellite cells have intrinsic properties dependent on their muscle origin, and independent of environmental cues (Dolenc *et al.* 1994; Martelly *et al.* 2000). Satellite cells from either slow or fast muscles present significant differences on the expression of several protein families such as metabolic enzymes, hormonal receptors or capacity to express MRFs. These differences could have consequences on the capacity of slow and fast muscles to regenerate after injury.

Satellite cells are normally in a non-proliferative, quiescent state, but are activated in response to muscle injury (Schultz *et al.* 1985; Grounds 1998). Multiple rounds of proliferation of these stem cells occur after their activation, giving rise to myogenic precursor cells (Grounds & Yablonka-Reuveni 1993). The number of quiescent satellite cells is dependent on age and muscle fibre type. Skeletal muscle in young animals contains a higher concentration of satellite cells than in adults (Schultz 1989).

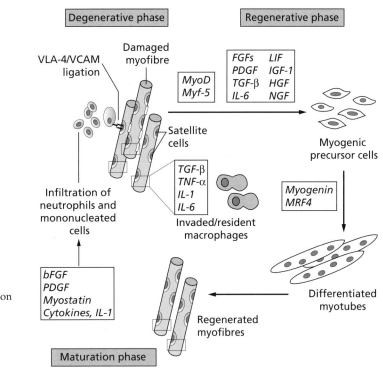

Fig. 3.2 Schematic representation of the cellular and molecular events involved in satellite cell activation following myofibre injury, giving rise to regenerated fibres.

The percentage of satellite cells within muscles decreases with age, and more rapidly from birth through sexual maturity than in adults. The decrease in the percentage of satellite cells with ageing is the result of an increase in myonuclei in both oxidative and glycolytic myofibres, and a decrease in total number of satellite cells. On the other hand, the satellite cell density is higher in oxidative than in glycolytic tissue, at both whole muscle and single fibre levels (Gibson & Schultz 1982, 1983). This heterogeneity in satellite cell content between muscle fibre types has been related to an increase in satellite cell density with the proximity of capillaries and motor neurone junctions. While the population of satellite cells decreases with age, their number remains relatively constant over repeated cycles of degeneration–regeneration. This finding highlights the inherent capacity of these stem cells for self-renewal (Gibson & Schultz 1983). At least three models have been suggested to account for the self-renewal of satellite cells, involving either early-acting MRFs, an asymmetrical satellite cell division and/or the de-differentiation of committed myogenic precursor cells (Seale & Rudnicki 2000).

Skeletal muscle injury is generally followed by a series of processes included in three phases: a degenerative phase, a regenerative phase and a maturation phase (Fig. 3.2) (Plaghki 1985). Many experimental results suggest that basic mechanisms underlying the cellular responses to acute trauma are well conserved regardless of the type of initial injury. Although the sequence of cellular responses of injured muscle regeneration is roughly constant and well determined, the time-course of muscle regeneration processes are tightly related to the types of muscle injury (Carlson 1973). Using drastic experimental models, it has been shown that the regenerative process takes place earlier after *in situ* injuries without destruction of the basement membrane, than after denervation/devascularization of muscle (Lefaucheur & Sebille 1995).

The degenerative phase

First phase of the degenerative process

This is also known as non-inflammatory or intrinsic degeneration, and follows the initial damage of the muscle fibres. An extensive disruption of the structural components of the muscle is first observed at the site of injury. The extent of anatomical damage of the muscle tissue varies significantly according to the nature of the injury and its severity. With regard to exercise-induced muscle injury, many morphological studies showed that the Z-discs are the most vulnerable structures (Fridén & Lieber 2001). Other intracellular anomalies have been reported according to the severity of the injuring process, and damage of the sarcolemma, T-tubules and the cytoskeletal system are commonly observed after exercise-induced muscle injuries. More severe trauma, including strains, contusions, prolonged ischaemia and muscle lacerations are associated with the crush and tear of myofibres, and often the death of nearly all myonuclei (Fig. 3.3).

The early responses to initial damage consist of catabolic events that result in autolysis of the damaged muscular components. A loss of intracellular calcium homeostasis has been shown to activate calcium-dependent proteases referred to as calpains (Armstrong et al. 1991). Such enzymes are able to cleave myosin, α-actinin, vinculin and many other contractile filament components and metabolic proteins in the muscle cell. Calpain activation appears thus to be a key occurrence of damaged muscle autolysis. Most of these alterations become prominent 4–8 h after initial injury. Satellite cells, which are dormant under the basement membrane of myofibres, withstand the initial damage and its early consequences, and then enter into a cycle of activation–proliferation.

Second phase of muscle degeneration

This phase is also called extrinsic or inflammatory degeneration, and involves the removal of

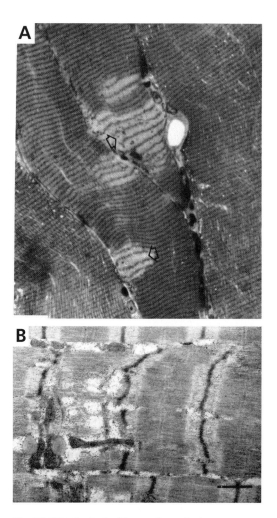

Fig. 3.3 Histological evidence of muscle damage. (A) Longitudinal section of the median head of the triceps brachii muscle immediately after running downhill, stained with toluidine blue O. Note the widened I-bands (arrows). The scale bar represents 25 μm (from Armstrong et al. 1983). (B) Transmission electron micrograph showing sarcomeric dissolution and Z-line streaming in skeletal muscle after eccentric contractions. The scale bar represents 1 μm (from Warren et al. 1993).

all traces of the originally damaged myofibres. This phase of muscle repair includes phagocytosis, which is secondary to an inflammatory cell response, and is dependent on the presence of invading macrophages (Fig. 3.2).

NEUTROPHILS AND
MONONUCLEATED CELLS

Neutrophils and mononucleated cells accumulate at muscle injury sites. Neutrophils respond early to muscle injury. The neutrophil population increases significantly within 1–6 h and declines 9–12 h after damage (Orimo *et al.* 1991). In certain cases this rapid increase in the neutrophil population endures for a few days (Fielding *et al.* 1993). This early increase in the number of inflammatory cells may result either from chemotaxis of specific cells to the site of muscle damage and/or from mitogenesis of inflammatory cells initially present in skeletal muscle near the myofibres. There is experimental evidence that chemotaxis is the primary mechanism by which the number of inflammatory cells increases in injured muscle (Bintliff & Walker 1960).

The exact nature of the substances acting as chemoattractants for inflammatory cells remains a matter of debate (Tidball 1995). Several molecules released from injured muscles have been viewed as active substances for leading inflammatory cells from the circulatory system to the injury site (Table 3.1) (Chen & Quinn 1992). Basic fibroblast growth factor (bFGF or FGF-2) may be released through membrane lesions, but while it is capable of attracting myogenic cells, there is no experimental evidence to support a role in attracting inflammatory cells after injury. It is

thus unlikely that bFGF is a key chemoattractive stimulus for inflammatory cells. In contrast, platelet-derived growth factor (PDGF), released from injured muscle, is known as a mitogen and chemoattractant for inflammatory cells. However, its low concentration in myofibres and short half-life make uncertain its role as a chemoattractant to mediate the inflammatory response to muscle injury (Bowen-Pope *et al.* 1984). Myostatin, a new muscle-specific growth-inhibiting factor, has been recently suggested to act as a chemoattractant for phagocytes and inflammatory cells (Kirk *et al.* 2000). The specific role played by many other soluble factors such as cytokines as chemoattractants in damaged muscle remains unknown to date. Additional data suggest that the early activation of resident macrophages or fibroblasts could initiate the release of other chemoattractant substances, leading to the translocation of inflammatory cells within injured muscle. Once resident macrophages and/or fibroblasts are activated by chemoattractant substances, these later inflammatory cells could initiate chemotaxis of additional cells by a wound hormone unidentified to date.

The inflammatory response to muscle injury is initiated by the local proteolysis of extracellular matrix molecules. Fibroblasts probably play a significant role in degrading extracellular matrix molecules, mainly by an increase in collagenase expression. PDGF and cytokines

Table 3.1 The main effects of several growth factors and cytokines on chemotaxis, proliferation and differentiation of satellite cells.

Growth factor or cytokine	Basic effects on muscle		
	Chemotaxis	Proliferation	Differentiation
bFGF	+/−	++	−−
PDGF	+	++	−−
IL-1	+ (lymphocytes)		
IL-6		++	
LIF		++	
IGF-I, IGF-II		++	++
TGF-β	+	+/−	−−
TNF-α	+	−	−−
NGF	+	+	+

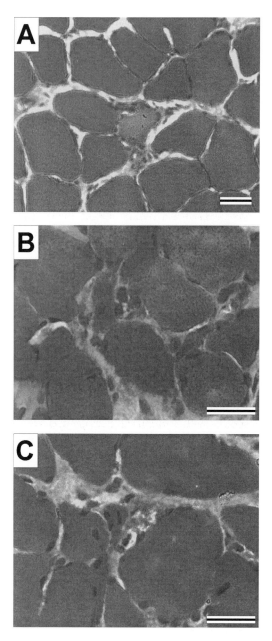

Fig. 3.4 Light microscopy cross-sections of skeletal muscle from a rat 48 h after a bout of prolonged downhill exercise (H&E staining). Details of the muscle show: (A) a degenerative myofibre with altered cytoplasm and infiltration of mononuclear cells, representative of an early stage of development; (B) a myofibre invaded by mononuclear cells; and (C) a small-sized regenerative fibre with internalized nuclei. The scale bars represent 50 μm.

detected in injured muscle, such as interleukin-1 (IL-1), may stimulate collagenase secretion by fibroblasts and thus contribute to the proteolysis of extracellular matrix molecules (Dayer *et al.* 1986).

POLYMORPHONUCLEAR LYMPHOCYTES
AND MACROPHAGES

Polymorphonuclear lymphocytes and macrophages migrate to sites of tissue damage within a few hours of the injury (Fig. 3.4). Macrophages constitute the major type of invading cell during the inflammatory response to muscle injury. They are the predominant inflammatory cell type 1 day postinjury, and more than 50% of inflammatory cells are macrophages following exercise-induced injury (Round *et al.* 1987). Many investigations have confirmed the marked increase in macrophages within damaged muscle and emphasized the major importance of these cells in muscle inflammation. Distinct subclasses of macrophages are involved in the development of muscle inflammation. Macrophages normally present in the circulatory system increase significantly early after injury, while macrophages normally resident in muscle tissue increase thereafter (St Pierre & Tidball 1994). It is thus likely that macrophages increase in damaged tissue both by emigration from the circulatory system (mainly by chemotaxis) and also by cell division of resident tissue macrophages.

Functional role of inflammatory cells in damaged muscle

Neutrophils rapidly invade the injury site and are associated with early promotion of the inflammatory response. They are involved in the release of cytokines or soluble factors that can attract and activate additional inflammatory cells. As discussed above, fibroblasts are candidates as mediators of the chemotaxis of inflammatory cells, but above all can cause proteolysis of extracellular matrix proteins, one of the early stages of inflammation. Two pivotal roles for macrophages have been proposed based on observations that myogenesis is markedly impaired in the absence of macrophage infiltration (Lescaudron *et al.* 1999).

PHAGOCYTIC ROLE OF MACROPHAGES

Macrophages and inflammatory cells play a prominent role in removing all traces of the damaged myofibres and consensus has been reached in considering that the phagocytic role of these inflammatory cells is their most prominent function during the recovery from muscle injury. This response of inflammatory cells is an important component of the successful repair of injured muscle. Treatment with non-steroidal anti-inflammatory drugs (NSAIDs) is known to impair the recovery of damaged muscles. It has been shown that rats treated with NSAIDs exhibit a slower muscle regeneration than animals receiving placebo (Almekinders & Gilbert 1986). The impaired recovery in muscles of treated rats is mainly attributed to a less phagocytic activity in damaged muscle, a slow down in the removal of cellular debris and a decrease in the synthesis of cytokines involved in successful muscle repair. These data clearly demonstrate that macrophages and neutrophils are directly involved in the process of muscle repair, and inhibiting the early activation and infiltration of inflammatory cells affects muscle fibre repair. As a consequence, the early treatment with NSAIDs after muscle trauma has a bad prognosis. Other situations where phagocytosis by macrophages is impaired, such as ageing, affect the success of muscle regeneration (Zacks & Sheff 1982).

Macrophage populations comprise distinct subclasses of cells. Macrophages, including the ED1 antigen, which are associated with lysosomal membranes, also called ED1+ macrophages, are present at high concentrations in areas that contain necrotic fibres. They have been shown to have a high phagocytic activity and to remove cellular debris in injured tissue (Honda *et al.* 1990; McLennan 1993). This specialized subpopulation of macrophages declines in muscle after the phagocytic stage is completed.

MACROPHAGES AND THE SECRETION OF GROWTH FACTORS AND CYTOKINES

The success of muscle regeneration also relies on functions other than phagocytosis that may be mediated by macrophages. Although restricted in number, resident macrophages could provide growth factors and cytokines important for the early development of the inflammatory response in damaged muscle, such as transforming growth factor beta (TGF-β), IL-1, IL-6 and tumour necrosis factor alpha (TNF-α) (Rappolee & Werb 1992). TNF-α is known to induce skeletal muscle protein breakdown, angiogenesis and the production of components of inflammation. IL-1 is expected to exert important influences on the development of inflammation. This cytokine is a mitogen and chemoattractant for fibroblasts, T-lymphocytes and B-lymphocytes, and increases the cytotoxicity of macrophages. IL-1 also induces the expression of other inflammatory cytokines such as IL-6 and interferons. The postexercise increase in serum and muscle IL-1 is rapid, and suggests a post-translational control of the secretion of this inflammatory cytokine (Tidball 1995). The early response of IL-1 to muscle damage appears to be mainly attributable to an increase in its production by each activated cell, rather than by a proliferation of inflammatory cells.

Taken together, these findings show that besides their role in phagocytosis, non-muscle cells such as macrophages may play pivotal and essential roles in mediating muscle repair. The first invading subpopulation of macrophages phagocytoses tissue debris, while together with neutrophils the macrophages are involved in the early inflammatory response, mainly through the secretion of soluble factors such as cytokines and local growth factors.

Skeletal muscle regeneration

The regeneration of myofibres begins after phagocytosis of cellular debris. The first step of regeneration includes the activation of satellite cells from their relatively dormant state, giving rise to myogenic precursor cells (Fig. 3.2). Thereafter, they proliferate, differentiate into myoblasts, and fuse to form multinucleated myotubes that then differentiate into myofibres. Myoblasts are myogenic precursor cells expressing myogenic markers. This later step of regeneration leads to mature fibres comprising adult isoforms of the several families of proteins, consistent with the expected muscle phenotype (Plaghki 1985). The activation of satellite cells and their differentiation into myoblasts does not begin until the necrotic debris within the regenerating basal lamina cylinders have been removed by macrophages (Hurme et al. 1991). Most myoblasts giving rise to new myofibres arise from local satellite cells lying underneath the basal lamina. Although this problem has not been entirely settled, there appears to be little recruitment of satellite cells from adjacent muscles and, in most cases, repair of a muscle is the responsibility of the intrinsic satellite cell population of the damaged muscle (Schultz et al. 1986).

Activation of satellite cells

After injury, the satellite cells take several hours to be mobilized. Several non-selective markers are used to characterize the proliferating satellite cell pool, such as the incorporation of ^{3}H-thymidine or bromodeoxyuridine. Autoradiographic studies demonstrated that satellite cells were labelled by ^{3}H-thymidine 15–20 h after crush injury (Schultz et al. 1985). Activated satellite cells were not detected in damaged muscle before phagocytosis of the necrotic debris by macrophages had begun. This finding clearly demonstrates that the removal of the necrotic muscle debris by macrophages seems to be a prerequisite for the activation and proliferation of satellite cells.

Diverse mechanisms have been assumed to be involved in the activation of satellite cells, including events of the inflammatory response and the release of growth factors.

LEUCOCYTE–SATELLITE CELL
INTERACTIONS DURING REGENERATION

Quiescent satellite cells express a cell-surface adhesion molecule called vascular cell adhesion molecule 1 (VCAM-1). The integrin receptor of VCAM-1, called very late antigen 4 (VLA-4), is present in leucocytes infiltrating muscle early after injury. Cell–cell interactions of infiltrating VLA-4(+) leucocytes and satellite cells, mediated by VCAM-1/VLA-4 ligation, mediates the recruitment of leucocytes to muscle after injury and focuses the invading leucocytes specifically to the sites of regeneration (Jesse et al. 1998). Infiltrating leucocytes may also initiate a series of molecular events implicated in muscle regeneration. On the other hand, the activation of satellite cells seems to be dependent on factors either synthesized and secreted by macrophages, or released from the necrotic tissue by phagocytes (Hurme & Kalimo 1992). These soluble factors have not been clearly identified but could be growth factors released either by neutrophils or invading macrophages. Several cytokines and growth factors have been shown to play key roles in the activation and proliferation of satellite cells (Table 3.1) (Husmann et al. 1996).

GROWTH FACTOR AND CYTOKINE
RESPONSES DURING MYOFIBRE
REGENERATION

Fibroblast growth factors

The actions of FGFs on muscle precursor cell activation have been extensively studied (Sheehan & Allen 1999). FGFs exist as nine different isoforms but only FGF-1, -2, -4, -6 and -9 are active on satellite cells. In normal skeletal muscle, FGFs are stored in the extracellular matrix and are bound to proteoheparan sulphates. After muscle injury, FGFs are released, and high levels of both mRNA and protein have been reported in proliferating satellite cells before the formation of myotubes. High concentrations of FGF-1 have been previously correlated with a high level of myoblast proliferation in damaged muscles of dystrophin-deficient mice that display persistent cycles of myofibre degeneration–regeneration (Dimario & Strohman 1988).

It is thus very likely that FGFs contribute to the proliferation of satellite cells and are involved in the chemotaxis of further muscle precursor cells. The main action of FGFs is the activation of muscle precursor cell proliferation to provide enough cells to allow regeneration to take place. Studies using mouse knockout models show the ability of redundant FGF family members to compensate for one another to preserve the role of these growth factors on satellite cell proliferation under pathological conditions.

Moreover, the availability of basic FGF, also called FGF-2, is of importance for capillary growth during muscle regeneration—a key factor for the success of muscle repair. Another member of the FGF family, FGF-5, might be important for the reinnervation process, when the presence of nerve is important for recovering the expected contractile and metabolic phenotype. Even bFGF can interact with other growth factors to stimulate the secretion of nerve growth factor (NGF) and contribute to the survival of neurones (Unsicker *et al.* 1992).

Collectively, FGFs are mainly involved in the activation and proliferation of satellite cells, in order to provide and activate stem cells to allow regeneration to occur. The exact mechanisms by which FGFs push satellite cells towards proliferation remain unknown, but it could be hypothesized that FGFs promote satellite cell activation, at least partly, by inhibiting the differentiation of myoblasts into myotubes. This effect of FGFs could be mainly related through inhibition of the expression of insulin-like growth factor II (IGF-II) (Rosenthal *et al.* 1991) or MyoD, one of the mammalian MRFs (Vaidya *et al.* 1989). As a consequence, other factors must either repress FGF production and/or strongly promote the differentiation of myoblasts, later during recovery, in order to minimize the repressing activity of FGFs on the differentiation of muscle precursor cells into myoblasts.

During the period of satellite cell proliferation, the expression of FGF receptor 1 (FGF-R1) increases, and the decrease in FGF-R1 expression is associated with a concomitant increase in satellite cell differentiation.

Platelet-derived growth factor

PDGF is first released from degranulated platelets, and later by activated macrophages and vessels in damaged muscle. This growth factor is chemotactic for adult muscle precursor cells and shows a highly stimulating effect on the proliferation of satellite cells (Ross *et al.* 1986). Moreover, together with FGFs, PDGF exerts a strong inhibition of the terminal differentiation of satellite cells into myoblasts.

TRANSFORMING GROWTH FACTOR BETA

Like PDGF, TGF-β is released from degranulating platelets after injury. This growth factor is chemotactic for macrophages and leucocytes, contributes to the synthesis of proteins of the extracellular matrix, and plays a pivotal role in angiogenesis. Many of the biological effects of TGF-β concern the reorganization of the extracellular matrix, particularly the reconstruction of the basement membrane surrounding the regenerating myofibres. Those effects are mediated by the production of: (i) extracellular matrix proteases; (ii) protease inhibitors such as plasminogen activator inhibitor 1 (Laiho *et al.* 1986); and (iii) extracellular matrix components. TGF-β plays an important role in regulating repair after muscle injury and it has been suggested that excessive TGF-β-induced deposition of the extracellular matrix can lead to fibrosis (Border & Ruoslahti 1992). TGF-β regulates a subset of genes that encode growth factors and their receptors, and this finding could help to explain the varied cellular responses to TGF-β (Nielsen-Hamilton 1990). As for FGFs, TGF-β can be stored in an inactive form in the extracellular matrix and thus both are available for direct action after injury, without the need for new synthesis before their local action. Moreover, this growth factor exerts a control on satellite cells by inhibiting their proliferation and terminal differentiation, mainly by silencing the transcriptional activation of the MyoD family members (Allen & Boxhorn 1989).

Other cytokines

Other cytokines such as IL-6 and leukaemia inhibitory factor (LIF) have been shown to stimulate the proliferation of myogenic precursor cells *in vitro* (Kurek *et al.* 1996). LIF is markedly increased very early after muscle injury, probably prior to infiltration of immune cells. The activating effect of LIF on the proliferation of myogenic precursor cells is additive to those of other growth factors such as bFGF and TGF-β, which suggests different mechanisms of action (Husmann *et al.* 1996). LIF has been shown to be produced by both damaged muscle fibres and resident non-muscle cells such as leucocytes and macrophages (Kurek *et al.* 1996).

IL-6 appears later in damaged muscle, between 12 and 24 h after injury. This cytokine, together with LIF, is one of the putative growth factors secreted by macrophages, which accounts for the role of these infiltrating monocytes on the proliferation of myogenic precursor cells (Cantini *et al.* 1994). As discussed above, there is clear evidence that besides their scavenger role, macrophages play a pivotal role in the activation and proliferation of satellite cells and myogenic precursor cells during muscle regeneration. Moreover, IL-6 promotes the degradation of necrotic tissue and induces apoptosis of macrophages following muscle injury (Cantini & Carraro 1996).

Insulin-like growth factors

Another group of growth factors, IGF-I and IGF-II, also called somatomedins, has been shown to be mitogenic for satellite cells and myoblasts (Florini *et al.* 1996). Besides these effects on the proliferation of myogenic cells, IGF-II also shows a marked stimulating effect on myoblast differentiation.

Other growth factors

Many other growth factors are already known to play a role in the regulation of skeletal muscle regeneration. Heparine-affine regulatory peptide, ciliary neurotrophic factor, NGF and hepatocyte growth factor (HGF) can interact with the most potent growth factors discussed above, to contribute in the activation of satellite cells, their proliferation and the reconstruction of the basement membrane and extracellular matrix (Husmann *et al.* 1996). HGF and its receptor c-Met have been localized in satellite cells and adjacent myofibres, and their expression has been related to the extent of muscle injury (Hawke & Garry 2001). Furthermore, HGF has been involved in the activation of satellite cells, as well as in the inhibition of myoblast differentiation, mainly by an inhibition of the expression of myogenic regulatory factors. Clearly, the efficiency of muscle regeneration is related to the fine growth factor interactions and to their role in the expression of myogenic regulators and extracellular matrix components.

Furthermore, differentiation of myogenic precursor cells has been shown to be regulated by a family of regulatory factors that can interact with certain of the growth factors mentioned above. The molecular mechanisms involved in the control of the differentiation of myogenic precursor cells and the role of MRFs should be examined.

Differentiation of myogenic precursor cells

GROWTH FACTORS AND MUSCLE CELL DIFFERENTIATION

Most growth factors involved in the activation and proliferation of satellite cells inhibit their differentiation into myoblasts, except for IGFs which exert a stimulating effect on the differentiation and fusion of myogenic cells (Table 3.1). It has been shown that IGF-I exerts less activation of myoblast differentiation than IGF-II, but taken together these growth factors play a key role at the onset of differentiation (Husmann *et al.* 1996). Some experimental evidence suggests that IGF-I acts first by stimulating muscle precursor cell proliferation, subsequently activating muscle cell differentiation. As specified above, several local growth factors inhibit muscle cell differentiation; this is the case for FGFs and it has been suggested that this inhibitory effect is related to a down-regulation of the IGF-II gene. It appears that a strong interaction exists between several growth factors such as FGFs, IGF-I and IGF-II.

MRFS AND MUSCLE CELL DIFFERENTIATION

Myogenic regulatory factors, members of the basic helix–loop–helix family (bHLH), are expressed in the embryo during development. These molecular factors activate the myogenic programme in embryonic precursor cells, thus initiating muscle differentiation. This family of myogenic factors, which includes MyoD, Myf5, MRF4 and myogenin, forms dimers with ubiquitous proteins. The heterodimeric complexes are transcription factors that bind to the E-box consensus DNA sequence that is found in the regulatory region of many muscle-specific genes. Studies support a role for MyoD and Myf5 in the determination of the myogenic cell fate and the formation of myoblasts, while myogenin and MRF4 appear to act later on muscle differentiation (Hawke & Garry 2001). Thus, these myogenic factors play a pivotal role in the commitment and differentiation of embryonic myoblasts during development (Seale & Rudnicki 2000).

The MRF expression programme during regeneration is similar to that observed during embryonic development. Not detected in quiescent satellite cells, MyoD is expressed very early, within 12 h after muscle injury, prior to molecular markers of cell proliferation (Mendler et al. 1998; Seale & Rudnicki 2000). The expression of MyoD mRNA has been strongly related to the proliferation of satellite cells and the beginning of regeneration (Olson & Klein 1994). Satellite cells entering the cell cycle express first either mainly MyoD or more seldom Myf5, followed by the coexpression of these two factors. The expression of these two early acting factors is shown to have a similar time course in regenerating slow and fast muscle. Following proliferation, myogenin and MRF4 are expressed in cells during their differentiation and expression of muscle-specific proteins. However, the expression of these late-acting MRFs changes in a different way in regenerating fast and slow muscles (Mendler et al. 1998). Levels of myogenin and MRF4 mRNA decrease transiently in slow muscle, while mRNA levels remain relatively constant in fast-twitch muscles.

MRF mRNA is lacking in quiescent satellite cells and this finding is consistent with the hypothesis that these cells represent stem cells, distinct from myoblasts, that give rise to myogenic cells after the beginning of their proliferative phase. In summary, an up-regulation of MyoD and Myf5 appears to be required for satellite cells to enter the proliferative phase, while MRF4 and myogenin appear later to participate to the regulation of their differentiation into myoblasts.

Skeletal muscle maturation

The differentiation of myogenic precursor cells is characterized by the capability for myoblasts to synthesize muscle-specific proteins. Differentiated myoblasts then migrate side by side, loose their membranes and fuse to form multinucleated myotubes. The fusion of myoblasts to form myotubes is associated with the expression of muscle-specific proteins. Striking changes of gene expression occur with the fusion of myoblasts, and genes encoding muscle-specific proteins are turned on.

The presence of specific proteins in the tissue is required to produce a viable cellular structure and/or to play a tissue-specific role accounting for the properties of a system. Thus, skeletal muscle can be approached from a molecular viewpoint, particularly the contractile proteins which account for the mechanical function and performance. Several families of proteins present a high degree of molecular variability, due to the existence of multiple isoforms. Some of the proteins accounting for the contractile and metabolic properties exist as adult mature and developmental immature isoforms.

Skeletal muscle is characterized by the existence of numerous types of fibres and a highly organized arrangement, resulting in a variety of functional capabilities. A high molecular variety of myofibrillar and enzymatic proteins, due to the existence of multiple isoforms, accounts for this myofibre diversity. Three isozymic systems are particularly relevant to the functional heterogeneity of myofibre types: myosin and especially the isoforms of myosin heavy chain (MHC), the creatine kinase (CK) isozymes and the lactate dehydrogenase (LDH) isozymes.

Myosin transition in regenerating skeletal muscle

One of the most informative methods of delineating muscle fibre types is based on the examination of specific myosin profiles. Myosin is the most essential part of the contractile machinery and contributes to the functional diversity of myofibres. A strong correlation has been shown between myosin isoforms, contractile properties and physiological measurements of myofibres (Schiaffino & Reggiani 1996). The myosin isoform composition is thus a molecular marker for different muscle fibres, for the physiological state of muscle tissue, and for the maturation state of regenerated muscle.

It is a well-known fact, that muscle regeneration recapitulates the embryonic development of skeletal muscle fibres. The new myogenesis that takes place in regenerating muscles has been related to the myogenesis which occurs during normal development. The major steps of regeneration closely recapitulate those of normal ontogenesis, and these two types of myogenesis display many similar morphological and biochemical features (Swynghedauw 1986). However, the transition from the immature to adult isoforms is more precocious in regenerating than in developing muscles (d'Albis et al. 1988).

The sarcomeric myosin molecule is a hexamer, consisting of two MHCs, two essential or alkali myosin light chains (MLCs) and two regulatory or phosphorylable MLCs. MHCs account for about 85% of the myosin molecule. This subunit has been found to be both highly conserved in structural terms and highly polymorphic (i.e. present as numerous isoforms). Two developmental isoforms have been described in rat and human skeletal muscle: MHC-emb, predominant in embryonic stages, and MHC-neo, predominant in perinatal stages (Whalen et al. 1981). Rat skeletal muscles contain three major fast MHC isoforms, called MHC-IIa, MHC-IIx and MHC-IIb, and one slow isoform, called MHC-β/

slow, that is present in slow fibres (Schiaffino & Reggiani 1996).

MHC EXPRESSION DURING DEVELOPMENT

Muscle development is characterized by the asynchronous differentiation of successive fibre generations—into at least primary and secondary generations of myofibres in rats. These sequential events have been mainly described in rats and mice, since in these species a more complete picture of MHC isoform expression is available. At early stages of embryonic development, all fibres express high levels of MHC-emb and low levels of MHC-neo and MHC-β/slow. By days 16–17, MHC-β/slow and MHC-neo are segregated in different myofibres, and fibre-type diversification is then detectable (Condon et al. 1990). At this stage of muscle development, primary generation fibres express either MHC-emb and MHC-β/slow, or MHC-neo and MHC-emb. Secondary generation fibres express mainly MHC-neo.

The major phase of myofibre maturation occurs during the perinatal period, with the appearance of the adult fast MHC isoforms and the emergence of the definitive fibre types. Myofibres expressing MHC-emb and MHC-neo undergo a further diversification process during the postnatal week in rats. They give rise to one of the four major fibre-type phenotypes, characterized by the expression of at least one of the four adult MHC isoforms (Schiaffino & Reggiani 1996). These adult MHC isoforms are initially coexpressed with MHC-emb and/or MHC-neo, which progressively disappear during the first month of life. The MHC isoform profile of myofibres is not definitively established during the early postnatal period but undergoes further changes with ageing.

MHC ISOFORM TRANSITIONS IN REGENERATING MUSCLES

New myofibres formed after muscle injury transiently express developmental myosin isoforms before switching to adult isoforms. Immature types of myosin are synthesized before a normal adult pattern is achieved (Sartore *et al.* 1982; Whalen *et al.* 1990). However, embryonic and neonatal isoforms disappear faster during regeneration than during normal myogenesis (d'Albis *et al.* 1988). Moreover, both fast- and slow-twitch regenerating muscles show the same transition, first toward a predominantly fast-type isoform profile, and secondly toward a slow-type profile for slow-twitch muscles.

It is not clear to date if satellite cells are programmed to express specific myosin isoforms. Some data suggest that satellite cells are not predetermined with respect to the type of adult myosins which will accumulate in the fibres they form (Whalen *et al.* 1990). This finding supports the notion that the programme expressed by satellite cells is not strictly determined and could be influenced by several factors, including the presence of nerve. More recent data clearly point to intrinsic differences between satellite cells from fast and slow muscles (Düsterhöft & Pette 1993; Dolenc *et al.* 1994; Martelly *et al.* 2000).

Two major controlling influences play a role in determining the specific adult myosin type that ultimately appears in mammalian muscle fibres. Continuous innervation is an important factor for the maintenance of slow myosin expression during regeneration in rats (d'Albis *et al.* 1988; Whalen *et al.* 1990). Innervation plays a clear role in determining which adult myosin isoform will accumulate in regenerated muscle. Slow myosin is expressed in regenerated slow-twitch muscles only in the presence of slow nerves. In contrast, a switching of myosin from embryonic and neonatal MHC isoforms toward fast, and not slow, isoforms was observed in regenerated slow muscle in the absence of nerve, suggesting the existence of a 'default programme' of MHC expression (Buttler-Browne *et al.* 1982).

Thyroid hormone levels also contribute to the control of MHC isoform transitions during regeneration. Hypothyroidism has been shown to inhibit the replacement of neonatal myosin by adult fast myosin isoforms during regeneration; conversely, hyperthyroidism induces a precocious induction of fast myosin expression (d'Albis *et al.* 1987). It is thus clear that the presence of motor nerves and the thyroid hormone status play determinant roles in myosin isoform expression, with potential consequences on muscle function.

Members of the bHLH family of transcriptional regulators probably play a role in the expression of the MHC isoforms during regeneration. The E-box sequence, specific to the heterodimers made up of MRFs and E-proteins (see above), has been found in the regulatory regions of several genes encoding for phenotypic proteins, including fast MLCs and type I and type IIb MHCs (Talmadge 2000). The primary function of MRFs is to initiate the expression of muscle-specific proteins during development and regeneration. Moreover, it has been suggested that myogenin and MyoD could play a role in determining the slow and fast phenotype, based on the distribution of these two factors in slow and fast myofibres, respectively (Hughes *et al.* 1993).

Creatine kinase in regenerating skeletal muscle

The enzyme CK has been involved in the maintenance of the intracellular energy supply of cells with intermittently high and fluctuating energy requirements, such as skeletal muscle. It has been suggested that CK, which catalyses the reversible reaction:

$$\text{Phosphocreatine}^{2-} + \text{MgADP}^- + \text{H}^+ \leftrightarrow \text{Creatine} + \text{MgATP}^{2-},$$

fulfils different roles in fast- and slow-twitch muscles. This enzyme exists as multiple isoforms; cytosolic isoforms of CK are heterodimeric associations of two types of monomer subunits, known as M, muscle, and B, brain (MM-, MB- and BB-CK). The MM-CK isozyme is bound to myofilaments and rephosphorylates ADP produced by myosin ATPase, contributing to maintain a locally high ATP : ADP ratio during periods of muscle contractions. Moreover, two additional CK isozymes have been detected in mitochondria, either specific for striated muscle, called mi_a-CK, or ubiquitous, mi_b-CK. These isozymes play pivotal roles in high oxidative muscles by favouring phosphocreatine resynthesis from oxidative phosphorylation (Ventura-Clapier *et al.* 1994). The activity and pattern of this enzyme is of functional relevance since resistance to fatigue is partly related to the ability of skeletal muscle to sustain ATP levels through increased oxidative metabolism.

During myogenesis, there is a progressive increase in the total activity of CK, as well as a shift from BB- to MM-CK isozyme. The onset of the expression of the M-subunit of CK and the increase in the specific activity of the MM-CK isozyme have been correlated with the development of functional muscle. Moreover, the M-CK promoter is under the control of MyoD, one of the most early MRFs, and the expression of the M-subunit is associated with that of other muscle-specific protein isoforms encoded by genes having an E-box sequence in their regulatory regions. The developmental pattern of expression of the various isozymes has been studied in the heart, where this multienzyme system appears to be essential for the adaptation to increased metabolic demand (Hoerter *et al.* 1994). However, little is known about the expression of mi-CK during the development of slow oxidative skeletal muscle.

Skeletal muscle degeneration using bupivacain is associated with a marked decrease in the total activity of CK (Plaghki 1985), and an increase in the specific activity of the BB-CK isozyme. The CK isozyme composition recovers a pattern similar to that of control muscle 10 days after initial injury (Sadeh *et al.* 1984). The specific activity of mi-CK isozyme, linked to the site of production of energy, is similar in control and regenerated skeletal muscle 8 weeks after infiltration with a myotoxin (Bigard *et al.* 2000). However, the time-course of expression of mi-CK during regeneration remains to be examined. This issue is of importance in slow oxidative muscles because mi-CK located in the inner mitochondrial membranes couples ATP synthesized during oxidative phosphorylation with creatine formed during muscle metabolism to produce phosphocreatine.

Lactate dehydrogenase activity in regenerating skeletal muscle

Lactate dehydrogenase exists in multiple molecular forms as a tetrameric association of two types of monomer subunits, known as H (heart) and M (muscle), which may be combined in five different ways and result in five isozymes. A correlation between the LDH isozyme pattern and the anaerobic/aerobic glycolysis capacity of muscle has been suggested. Heart contains a predominantly H type of LDH subunit, while fast glycolytic muscle contains the M type. The LDH isozyme pattern of slow oxidative skeletal muscles is roughly mixed with equal specific activities of H- and M-subunits.

During the fetal development, there a shift from the H toward the M-subunit, while the specific activity of the M-subunit increases during postnatal development (Plaghki 1985). A marked decrease in the total activity of LDH has been reported early after muscle injury. Thereafter, the activity of total LDH increases from the fusion of precursor myogenic cells to myotubes. As for the expression of MHC isoforms, regeneration recapitulates the events that normally occur during myogenesis, and the pattern of LDH isoforms shifts from a predominance of H-subunits toward M-subunits in regenerated slow muscles. Regenerated fast skeletal muscles recovered a LDH isoform pattern similar to that expected by 2 months after initial injury (Bigard *et al.* 2000).

Practical consequences for muscle healing

Treatment of muscle injuries varies widely depending on the nature and severity of the trauma. Besides the classic treatment of injured muscle, different biological approaches can be used to enhance muscle healing. Recent advances in knowledge of the mechanisms of muscle degeneration and regeneration after injury highlight the functional importance of the inflammatory response and support the therapeutic potential of several growth factors to improve muscle healing. On the other hand, the physical activity pattern is an environmental factor known to affect muscle growth and maturation during the early phases of regeneration. Therefore, it is of clinical interest to determine the specific effects of exercise on muscle healing.

Initial inflammatory response to muscle injury

As discussed above, the injured muscle first undergoes necrosis and is infiltrated by macrophages and neutrophils. Inflammatory cells are important components of the successful repair of injured muscle. The early use of NSAIDs, which inhibit the function of macrophages and neutrophils, leads to a slower muscle regeneration than in untreated animals (Almekinders & Gilbert 1986). The impaired recovery in the muscles of treated animals was attributed to both the slow removal of cellular debris and the decrease in synthesis and release of soluble factors important for the activation of regenerative processes by macrophages. Because the early response of inflammatory cells to muscle injury is a determining factor in directing muscle repair, there is an argument for not using anti-inflammatory drugs during this period. It appears especially important to respect the inflammatory response to acute muscle injury, with the aim of protecting the macrophage invasion, first to remove cellular debris and second to promote the involvement of activated macrophages in muscle fibre

regeneration by producing specific soluble factors. Whether the rest, ice, compression and/or elevation components of the principal therapy affect the inflammatory response to acute muscle injury has not been determined to date. Immobilization after muscle injury has been shown to limit the amount of connective tissue, but it is likely that this beneficial effect is not directly related to the inflammatory response.

Growth factors and muscle healing

The activation of satellite cells, and their proliferation, differentiation into myoblasts and fusion to form myotubes and myofibres are under the control of many soluble factors such as growth factors (see above). Many growth factors interact to control the involvement of inflammatory and satellite cells in the healing process, and to regulate the reorganization of the basement membrane and the extracellular matrix. Several studies have previously shown that individual or combined growth factors play specific roles during regeneration and therefore are able to improve muscle healing. The number and the mean diameter of regenerating fibres increased in muscles receiving serial and direct injections of bFGF and IGF-I in comparison with non-treated muscles, reflecting improved healing (Fig. 3.5) (Kasemkijwattana *et al.* 2000; Menetrey *et al.* 2000). At 1 month, and in contrast with non-treated muscles, regenerating myofibres were uniformly

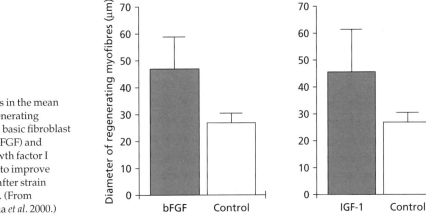

Fig. 3.5 Changes in the mean diameter of regenerating myofibres when basic fibroblast growth factor (bFGF) and insulin-like growth factor I (IGF-I) are used to improve muscle healing after strain injury ($P < 0.05$). (From Kasemkijwattana *et al.* 2000.)

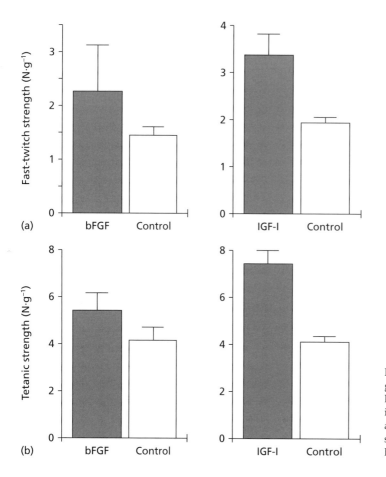

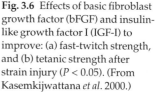

Fig. 3.6 Effects of basic fibroblast growth factor (bFGF) and insulin-like growth factor I (IGF-I) to improve: (a) fast-twitch strength, and (b) tetanic strength after strain injury ($P < 0.05$). (From Kasemkijwattana *et al.* 2000.)

located in the deep and superficial parts of the muscle treated with bFGF and IGF-I, their mean diameter was similar to the surrounding normal fibres, and many of their nuclei were already peripherally located. Moreover, the development of fibroblastic tissue was also reduced in treated muscles, suggesting that muscle healing was accelerated in these muscles when compared with non-treated muscles. A significant improvement in fast-twitch and tetanic strength was observed 15 days after injury in muscles treated with growth factors (bFGF and IGF-I) when compared with sham injected injured muscles (Fig. 3.6). Taken together, these studies demonstrated that selected growth factors properly applied and injected within injured muscle are able to enhance muscle healing after injury.

However, it is unlikely that a treating physician or a patient will accept repeated intramuscular injections or implanted perfusion pumps, particularly with the infection risk. Thus, other approaches have be considered to achieve a sustained expression of exogenous genes to skeletal muscle, such as myoblast transplantation or gene therapy based on viral and non-viral vectors. The application of these emerging technologies to deliver sustained expression of growth factors in the injured muscle has been previously examined (Kasemkijwattana *et al.* 1998). In this study, the ability of recombinant adeno-associated virus to mediate direct and *ex vivo* the transfer of a marker gene (β-galactosidase) within the contused injured muscle, suggested that this biological approach could be able to deliver an efficient and persistent

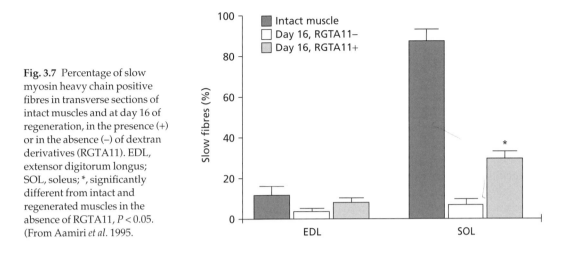

Fig. 3.7 Percentage of slow myosin heavy chain positive fibres in transverse sections of intact muscles and at day 16 of regeneration, in the presence (+) or in the absence (–) of dextran derivatives (RGTA11). EDL, extensor digitorum longus; SOL, soleus; *, significantly different from intact and regenerated muscles in the absence of RGTA11, $P < 0.05$. (From Aamiri *et al.* 1995.

expression of selected growth factors. It is likely that the development of those vectors carrying selected growth factors and the delivery of growth factors, using such new technologies, represent potential strategies in improving muscle healing that will be available for humans in the near future.

Heparin sulphate proteoglycans and muscle repair

Growth factors such as FGFs and TGF-β are transmitted to the cell either by one tyrosine kinase receptor or by binding to low-affinity heparan sulphate proteoglycans located on the cell surface and in the extracellular matrix. As for other growth factors, the interaction between them and the heparan sulphate components of the extracellular matrix might play a pivotal role in regeneration. Selected dextran derivatives have been shown to mimic some properties of heparin and heparan sulphate to stabilize and protect heparin-binding growth factors such as FGFs and TGF-β. A single injection of a dextran derivative was found to improve the regenerative process in a fast skeletal muscle after a crush injury (Gautron *et al.* 1995). Besides clear positive effects on the histological structure of regenerated muscle, dextran derivatives were shown to accelerate the shift from the neonatal to adult MHC isoforms (Aamiri *et al.* 1995). Crushed slow

muscle that had regenerated in the presence of dextran derivatives showed a fourfold increase in the number of slow fibres, in comparison with muscle regenerating in the absence of dextran derivatives (Fig. 3.7). It is thus likely that dextran derivatives act by protecting and favouring the effects of heparin-binding growth factors (FGFs and TGF-β) involved in the process of muscle regeneration. This family of polymers may therefore open a new therapeutic approach to accelerate skeletal muscle repair after injury.

Physical exercise and muscle regeneration

To determine the impact of physical exercise and contractile activity on muscle regeneration requires the use of animal models. A decreased mechanical load after the removal of weight-bearing activity impairs the rate and degree of growth and maturation during regeneration (Esser & White 1995). The degree of restoration to control adult protein concentration values of regenerating muscle is markedly altered by decreased mechanical load. Even the timing of transitional expression of MHC isoforms is delayed in unweighted regenerating muscles (Esser & White 1995; Bigard *et al.* 1997). There are thus experimental data suggesting that growth and maturation are impaired by a decreased mechanical load on regenerating muscles. On the other hand, increased mechanical load by ablation of synergistic muscles enhances the growth of regenerated muscle but not maturation (Esser & White 1995). While ablation of synergistic muscles is a model of chronic mechanical overload, it is of interest to evaluate the specific influence of the metabolic component by examining the response of regenerating muscle to running exercise. The growth of damaged muscle and its oxidative capacity are improved by run conditioning. On the other hand, the response of the MHC composition to endurance training has been shown to be more marked in regenerated muscle, at least for fast MHC isoforms (Bigard *et al.* 1996). Taken together, these results clearly demonstrate that the removal of contractile activity and mechanical load have deleterious effects on muscle growth and maturation. It is thus suggested that muscular activity plays a key role in the recovery of damaged skeletal muscle.

Conclusions

Although studies using laboratory animals amply demonstrate that skeletal muscle can regenerate after injury, our knowledge of muscle regeneration in humans is fragmentary and is still growing to date. The treatment and prognostics of muscle injury vary widely according to the severity and the extent of the trauma, more particularly according to the presence of nerve and vascularization. Satellite cells, normally in a quiescent state, are stem cells activated in response to muscle injury, giving rise to myogenic cells, myotubes and new myofibres. In addition, nonmuscle cells also play complex and essential roles in regulating the muscle repair response, in removing cellular debris, in activating the proliferation of myogenic cells, and in initiating structural changes in myofibres and extracellular matrix. The time-course changes in the expression of muscle-specific proteins, such as MHC, CK and LDH, should be considered during muscle regeneration, to control the recovery of the functional properties of skeletal muscle.

Many different growth factors interact simultaneously and sequentially with satellite cells to trigger muscle-specific gene products. Most of these growth factors stimulate the proliferation of satellite cells and concomitantly inhibit their differentiation and fusion, except for IGFs, which promote the differentiation of the myogenic precursor cells. TGF-β also plays an important role in muscle regeneration in promoting the reorganization of the basement membrane and extracellular matrix components. The interaction of those growth factors during muscle regeneration requires further investigation. A better understanding of growth factor interactions and their role in the expression of myogenic regulators and extracellular matrix components is needed to identify specific growth factors or cytokines able to improve skeletal muscle repair. Exercise resting with increased contractile activity but without mechanical overload is good advice in promoting efficient muscle healing after damage. On the other hand, the improvement of muscle healing after injury may be enhanced by the development of new technologies, such as gene therapy, that may be able to deliver target proteins to the damaged muscle without systemic side effects.

References

Aamiri, A., Butler-Browne, G.S., Martelly, I., Barritault, D. & Gautron, J. (1995) Influence of a dextran derivative on myosin heavy chain expression during rat skeletal muscle regeneration. *Neuroscience Letters* **201**, 243–246.

Allen, R.E. & Boxhorn, L.A. (1989) Regulation of skeletal muscle satellite cell proliferation by transforming growth factor β, insulin-like growth factor-I and fibroblast growth factor. *Journal of Cellular Physiology* **138**, 311–315.

Almekinders, L.C. & Gilbert, J.A. (1986) Healing of experimental muscle strains and the effects of nonsteroidal inflammatory medicine. *American Journal of Sports Medicine* **14**, 303–308.

Armstrong, R.B., Ogilvie, R.W. & Schwane, J.A. (1983) Eccentric exercise-induced injury to skeletal muscle. *Journal of Applied Physiology* **54**, 80–93.

Armstrong, R.B., Warren, G.L. & Warren, J.A. (1991) Mechanisms of exercise-induced muscle fibre injury. *Sports Medicine* **12**, 184–207.

Bigard, A.X., Janmot, C., Merino, D., Lienhard, F., Guezennec, C.Y. & d'Albis, A. (1996) Endurance training affects myosin heavy chain phenotype in regenerating fast-twitch muscle. *Journal of Applied Physiology* **81**, 1658–1665.

Bigard, A.X., Serrurier, B., Merino, D., Lienhard, F., Berthelot, M. & Guezennec, C.Y. (1997) Myosin heavy chain composition of regenerated soleus muscles during hindlimb suspension. *Acta Physiologica Scandinavica* **161**, 23–30.

Bigard, A.X., Mateo, P., Sanchez, H., Serrurier, B. & Ventura-Clapier, R. (2000) Lack of coordinated changes in metabolic enzymes and myosin heavy chain isoforms in regenerated muscles of trained rats. *Journal of Muscle Research and Cell Motility* **21**, 269–278.

Bintliff, S. & Walker, B.E. (1960) Radioautographic study of skeletal muscle regeneration. *American Journal of Anatomy* **106**, 233–245.

Border, W.A. & Ruoslahti, E. (1992) Transforming growth factor β: the dark side of tissue repair. *Journal of Clinical Investigation* **90**, 1–7.

Bowen-Pope, D.F., Malpass, T.W., Foster, D.M. & Ross, R. (1984) Platelet-derived growth factor *in vivo*: levels, activity, and rate of clearance. *Blood* **64**, 458–469.

Buttler-Browne, G.S., Bugaiski, L.B., Cuenoud, S., Schwartz, K. & Whalen, R.G. (1982) Denervation of newborn rat muscles does not block the appearance of adult fast myosin heavy chain. *Nature* **299**, 830–833.

Cantini, M. & Carraro, F. (1996) Control of cell proliferation by macrophage–myoblast interactions. *Basics of Applied Myology* **6**, 485–489.

Cantini, M., Massimino, M.L., Bruson, A., Catani, C., Libera, L.D. & Carraro, U. (1994) Macrophages regulate proliferation and differentiation of satellite cells. *Biochemical and Biophysical Research Communications* **202**, 1688–1696.

Carlson, B.M. (1970) Relationship between the tissue and epimorphic regeneration of muscle. *American Zoologist* **10**, 175–186.

Carlson, B.M. (1973) The regeneration of skeletal muscle—a review. *American Journal of Anatomy* **137**, 119–150.

Carlson, B.M. & Faulkner, J.A. (1983) The regeneration of skeletal muscle fibers following injury: a review. *Medicine and Science in Sports and Exercise* **15**, 187–198.

Chen, G. & Quinn, L.S. (1992) Partial characterization of skeletal myoblast mitogens in mouse crushed muscle extract. *Journal of Cellular Physiology* **153**, 563–574.

Condon, K., Silberstein, L., Blau, H.M. & Thompson, W.J. (1990) Development of muscle fiber types in the prenatal rat hindlimb. *Developmental Biology* **138**, 256–274.

Cornelison, D.D. & Wold, B.J. (1997) Single-cell analysis of regulatory gene expression in quiescent and activated mouse skeletal muscle satellite cells. *Developmental Biology* **191**, 270–283.

d'Albis, A., Weiman, J., Mira, J.C., Janmot, C. & Couteaux, R. (1987) Regulatory role of thyroid hormone in myogenesis. Analysis of myosin isoforms during muscle regeneration. *Compte-Rendu de l'Academie des Sciences, Paris* **305**, 697–702.

d'Albis, A., Couteaux, R., Janmot, C., Roulet, A. & Mira, J.C. (1988) Regeneration after cardiotoxin injury of innervated and dennervated slow and fast muscles of mammals. Myosin isoform analysis. *European Journal of Biochemistry* **174**, 103–110.

Dayer, J.M., De Rochemonteix, B., Burrus, B., Demczuk, S. & Dinarello, C.A. (1986) Human recombinant interleukin 1 stimulates collagenase and prostaglandin E$_2$ production by human synovial cells. *Journal of Clinical Investigation* **77**, 645–648.

Dimario, J. & Strohman, R.C. (1988) Satellite cells from dystrophic mouse muscle are stimulated by fibroblast growth factors *in vitro*. *Differentiation* **39**, 42–49.

Dolenc, I., Crne-Finderle, N., Erzen, I. & Sketelj, J. (1994) Satellite cells in slow and fast rat muscles differ in respect to acetylcholinesterase regulation mechanisms they convey to their descendant myofibers during regeneration. *Journal of Neuroscience Research* **37**, 236–246.

Düsterhoft, S. & Pette, D. (1993) Satellite cells from slow rat muscle express slow myosin under appropriate culture conditions. *Differentiation* **53**, 25–33.

Esser, K.A. & White, T.P. (1995) Mechanical load affects growth and maturation of skeletal muscle grafts. *Journal of Applied Physiology* **78**, 30–37.

Fielding, R.A., Manfredi, T.J., Ding, W., Fiatarone, M.A., Evans, W.J. & Cannon, J.G. (1993) Acute phase response in exercise. III. Neutrophil and IL-1β accumulation in skeletal muscle. *American Journal of Physiology* **265**, R166–R172.

Florini, J.R., Ewton, D.Z. & Coolican, S.A. (1996) Growth hormone and the insulin-like growth factor system in myogenesis. *Endocrinology Reviews* **17**, 481–517.

Fridén, J. & Lieber, R.L. (2001) Eccentric exercise-induced injuries to contractile and cytoskeletal muscle fibre components. *Acta Physiologica Scandinavica* **171**, 321–326.

Gautron, J., Kedzia, C., Husmann, I. & Barritault, D. (1995) Acceleration of the regeneration of skeletal muscles in adult rats by dextran derivatives. *Compte-Rendu de l'Academie des Sciences, Paris* **318**, 671–676.

Gibson, M.C. & Schultz, E. (1982) The distribution of satellite cells and their relationship to specific fiber types in soleus and extensor digitorum longus muscles. *Anatomical Record* **202**, 329–337.

Gibson, M.C. & Schultz, E. (1983) Age-related differences in absolute numbers of skeletal muscle satellite cells. *Muscle and Nerve* **6**, 574–580.

Grounds, M.D. (1998) Age-associated changes in the response of skeletal muscle cells to exercise and regeneration. *Annals of the New York Academy of Sciences* **854**, 78–91.

Grounds, M.D. & Yablonka-Reuveni, Z. (1993) Molecular and cell biology of skeletal muscle regeneration. *Molecular and Cell Biology of Human Diseases Series* **3**, 210–256.

Hawke, T.J. & Garry, D.J. (2001) Myogenic satellite cells: physiology to molecular biology. *Journal of Applied Physiology* **91**, 534–551.

Hoerter, J.A., Ventura-Clapier, R. & Kuznetsov, A. (1994) Compartmentation of creatine kinases during perinatal development of mammalian heart. *Molecular and Cellular Biochemistry* **133/134**, 277–286.

Honda, H., Kimura, H. & Rostami, A. (1990) Demonstration and phenotypic characterization of resident macrophages in rat skeletal muscle. *Immunology* **70**, 272–277.

Hudgson, P. & Field, E.J. (1973) Regeneration of muscle. In: *The Structure and Function of Muscle* (Bourne, G.H., ed.). Academic Press, New York: 312–359.

Hughes, S.M., Taylor, J.M., Tapscott, S.J., Gurley, C.M., Carter, W.J. & Peterson, C.A. (1993) Selective accumulation of MyoD and myogenin in fast and slow adult skeletal muscle is controlled by innervation and hormones. *Development* **118**, 1137–1147.

Hurme, T. & Kalimo, H. (1992) Activation of myogenic precursor cells after muscle injury. *Medicine and Science in Sports and Exercise* **24**, 197–205.

Hurme, T., Kalimo, H., Lehto, M. & Järvinen, M. (1991) Healing of skeletal muscle injury. An ultrastructural and immunohistochemical study. *Medicine and Science in Sports and Exercise* **23**, 801–810.

Husmann, I., Soulet, L., Gautron, J., Martelly, I. & Barritault, D. (1996) Growth factors in skeletal muscle regeneration. *Cytokine and Growth Factors Reviews* **7**, 249–258.

Jesse, T.L., LaChance, R., Iademarco, M.F. & Dean, D.C. (1998) Interferon regulatory factor-2 is a transcriptional activator in muscle where it regulates expression of vascular cell adhesion molecule-1. *Journal of Cellular Biology* **140**, 1265–1276.

Kasemkijwattana, C., Menetrey, J., Somogyi, G. *et al.* (1998) Development of approaches to improve healing following muscle contusion. *Cell Transplant* **7**, 585–598.

Kasemkijwattana, C., Menetrey, J., Bosch, P. *et al.* (2000) Use of growth factors to improve muscle healing after strain injury. *Clinical Orthopaedics and Related Research* **370**, 272–285.

Kirk, S., Oldham, J., Kambadur, R., Sharma, M., Dobbie, P. & Bass, J. (2000) Myostatin regulation during skeletal muscle regeneration. *Journal of Cellular Physiology* **184**, 356–363.

Kurek, J.B., Nouri, S., Kannourakis, G., Murphy, M. & Austin, L. (1996) Leukemia inhibitory factor and interleukin-6 are produced by diseased and regenerating skeletal muscle. *Muscle and Nerve* **19**, 1291–1301.

Laiho, M., Saksela, O., Andreasen, P.A. & Keski-Oja, J. (1986) Enhanced production and extracellular deposition of the endothelial-type plasminogen activator inhibitor in cultured human lung fibroblasts by transforming growth factor-β. *Journal of Cellular Biology* **103**, 2403–2410.

Lefaucheur, J.P. & Sebille, A. (1995) The cellular events of injured muscle regeneration depend on the nature of the injury. *Neuromuscular Disorders* **5**, 501–509.

Lescaudron, L., Peltekian, E., Fontaine-Perus, J. *et al.* (1999) Blood borne macrophages are essential for the triggering of muscle regeneration following muscle transplant. *Neuromuscular Disorders* **9**, 72–80.

Martelly, I., Soulet, L., Bonnavaud, S., Cebrian, J., Gautron, J. & Barritault, D. (2000) Differential expression of FGF receptors and of myogenic regulatory factors in primary cultures of satellite cells originating from fast (EDL) and slow (soleus) twitch rat muscles. *Cellular and Molecular Biology* **46**, 1239–1248.

Mauro, A. (1961) Satellite cells of skeletal muscle fibres. *Journal of Biophysics, Biochemistry and Cytology* **9**, 493–495.

McLennan, I.S. (1993) Resident macrophages (ED2 and ED3-positive) do not phagocytose degenerating rat skeletal muscle fibres. *Cellular Tissue Research* **272**, 193–196.

Mendler, L., Zádor, E., Dux, L. & Wuytack, F. (1998) mRNA levels of myogenic regulatory factors in rat slow and fast muscles regenerating from notoxin-induced necrosis. *Neuromuscular Disorders* **8**, 533–541.

Menetrey, J., Kasemkijwattana, C., Day, C.S. *et al.* (2000) Growth factors improve muscle healing *in vivo*. *Journal of Bone and Joint Surgery* **82B**, 131–137.

Nielsen-Hamilton, M. (1990) Transforming growth factor-beta and its actions on cellular growth and differentiation. *Current Topics in Developmental Biology* **24**, 95–136.

Olson, E.N. & Klein, W.H. (1994) bHLH factors in muscle development: dead lines and commitments, what to leave in and what to leave out. *Genes Development* **8**, 1–8.

Orimo, S., Hiyamuta, E., Arahata, K. & Sugita, H. (1991) Analysis of inflammatory cells and complement C3 in bupivacaine-induced myonecrosis. *Muscle and Nerve* **14**, 515–520.

Plaghki, L. (1985) Regeneration et myogenese du muscle strie. *Journal of Physiology (Paris)* **80**, 51–110.

Rappolee, D.A. & Werb, Z. (1992) Macrophage-derived growth factors. *Current Topics in Microbiology and Immunology* **181**, 87–140.

Rosenblatt, J.D., Yong, D. & Parry, D.J. (1994) Satellite cell activity is required for hypertrophy of overloaded adult rat muscle. *Muscle and Nerve* **17**, 608–613.

Rosenthal, S.M., Brown, E.J., Brunetti, A. & Goldfine, I.D. (1991) Fibroblast growth factor inhibits insulin-like growth factor-II (IGF-II) gene expression and increases IGF-I receptor abundance in BC3H-1 muscle cells. *Molecular Endocrinology* **5**, 678–684.

Ross, R., Raines, E.W. & Bowen-Pope, D.F. (1986) The biology of platelet-derived growth factor. *Cell* **46**, 156–169.

Round, J.M., Jones, D.A. & Cambridge, G. (1987) Cellular infiltrates in human skeletal muscle: exercise induced damage as a model for inflammatory muscle disease? *Journal of Neurology Science* **82**, 1–11.

Sadeh, M., Stern, L.Z., Czyzewski, K., Finley, P.R. & Russell, D.H. (1984) Alterations in creatine kinase, ornithine decarboxylase, and transglutaminase during muscle regeneration. *Life Science* **34**, 483–488.

Sartore, S., Gorza, L. & Schiaffino, S. (1982) Fetal myosin heavy chains in regenerating muscle. *Nature* **298**, 294–296.

Schiaffino, S. & Reggiani, C. (1996) Molecular diversity of myofibrillar proteins: gene regulation and functional significance. *Physiological Reviews* **70**, 371–423.

Schultz, E. (1989) Satellite cell behavior during skeletal muscle growth and regeneration. *Medicine and Science in Sports and Exercise* **21**, S181–S186.

Schultz, E. (1996) Satellite cell proliferative compartments in growing skeletal muscles. *Developmental Biology* **175**, 84–94.

Schultz, E., Jaryszak, D.L. & Valliere, C.R. (1985) Response of satellite cells to focal skeletal muscle injury. *Muscle and Nerve* **8**, 217–222.

Schultz, E., Jaryszak, D.L., Gibson, M.C. & Albright, D.J. (1986) Absence of exogenous satellite cell contribution to regeneration of frozen skeletal muscle. *Journal of Muscle Research and Cell Motility* **7**, 361–367.

Seale, P. & Rudnicki, M.A. (2000) A new look at the origin, function, and 'stem-cell' status of muscle satellite cells. *Developmental Biology* **218**, 115–124.

Sheehan, S.M. & Allen, R.E. (1999) Skeletal muscle satellite cell proliferation in response to members of the fibroblast growth factor family and hepatocyte growth factor. *Journal of Cell Physiology* **181**, 499–506.

St Pierre, B.A. & Tidball, J.G. (1994) Differential response of macrophage subpopulations to soleus muscle reloading after rat hindlimb suspension. *Journal of Applied Physiology* **77**, 290–297.

Swynghedauw, B. (1986) Developmental and functional adaptation of contractile proteins in cardiac and skeletal muscles. *Physiological Reviews* **66**, 710–771.

Talmadge, R.J. (2000) Myosin heavy chain isoform expression following reduced neuromuscular activity: potential regulatory mechanisms. *Muscle and Nerve* **23**, 661–679.

Tidball, J.G. (1995) Inflammatory cell response to acute muscle injury. *Medicine and Science in Sports and Exercise* **27**, 1022–1032.

Unsicker, K., Reichert-Preibsch, H. & Wewetzer, K. (1992) Stimulation of neuron survival by basic FGF and CNTF is a direct effect and not mediated by non-neuronal cells: evidence from single cell cultures. *Developmental Brain Research* **62**, 285–288.

Vaidya, T.B., Rhodes, S.J., Taparowsky, E.J. & Konieczny, S.F. (1989) Fibroblast growth factor and transforming growth factor beta repress transcription of the myogenic regulatory gene MyoD1. *Molecular and Cellular Biology* **9**, 3576–3579.

Ventura-Clapier, R., Veksler, V. & Hoerter, J.A. (1994) Myofibrillar creatine kinase and cardiac contraction. *Molecular and Cellular Biochemistry* **133**, 125–144.

Warren, G.L., Hayes, D.A., Lowe, D.A. & Sesosia, S. (1993) Mechanical factors in the initiation of eccentric contraction-induced injury in rat soleus muscle. *Journal of Physiology (London)* **464**, 457–475.

Whalen, R.G., Sell, S.M., Butler-Browne, G.S., Schwartz, K., Bouveret, P. & Pinset-Härström, I. (1981) Three myosin heavy-chain isozymes appear sequentially in rat muscle development. *Nature* **292**, 805–809.

Zacks, S.I. & Sheff, M.F. (1982) Age-related impeded regeneration of mouse minced anterior tibial muscle. *Muscle and Nerve* **5**, 152–161.

Chapter 4

Tissue Healing and Repair:
Tendons and Ligaments

BARRY W. OAKES

Introduction

This chapter will briefly review recent basic scientific information on the structure and biomechanics of tendons and ligaments, discuss mechanisms of injury to ligaments/tendons and their repair response, and attempt to relate this to practical clinical patient rehabilitation management. Several recent, excellent reviews are available in this area: Benjamin *et al.* (1986, 1995), Daniel *et al.* (1990), Kannus *et al.* (1992a, 1992b), Jackson *et al.* (1993), Archambault *et al.* (1995), Benjamin and Ralphs (1995), Viidik (1996), Frank and Jackson (1997), Jozsa and Kannus (1997), Frank (1999), Frank *et al.* (1999), Rodeo and Izawa (1999) and Woo *et al.* (2000).

Structure and biomechanics of ligaments and tendons

There are subtle differences between ligament and tendon morphology (Amiel *et al.* 1983) but for the sake of this discussion they will be treated as very similar tissues.

The fibroblasts of mature tendons lie in longitudinal rows and are flat, very elongated cells squeezed laterally between the collagen fibrils. Recently McNeilly and associates (1996) have demonstrated elegantly (using confocal microscopy coupled with fluorescent dye cellular labelling techniques) that tendon fibroblasts communicate with one another via an extensive three-dimensional network of long cell processes and gap junctions ramifying between the collagen

matrix (Fig. 4.1). This new information indicates the possibility of intercellular 'talk' between cells similar to that of osteocytes and hence that these tendon cells may be able to sense and coordinate a response to mechanical load or lack of load.

Mature adult ligament and tendon are composed of large diameter type I collagen fibrils (150 nm or more in diameter) tightly packed together in a rope-like configuration with a small amount of type III collagen dispersed in an aqueous gel containing small amounts of

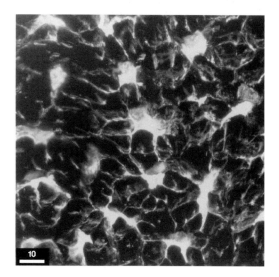

Fig. 4.1 Confocal microscope image of fluorescent membrane-labelled cryosections of a rat digital flexor tendon. The cell bodies are brightly fluorescent and show a network of fluorescent lateral cell processes meeting those of adjacent cells. (From McNeilly *et al.* 1996, with permission from *Journal of Anatomy*).

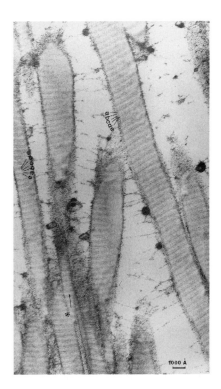

Fig. 4.2 Adult rat ACL collagen fixed with ruthenium red after treatment with elastase at pH 8.8. for 12 h. There is typical regular banding periodicity (labelled) and linking filaments probably hyaluronate, which link the fibrils between the c and d bands. The fibre marked with the asterisk appears to be dividing into a smaller fibril. Proteoglycan granules are attached to the fibrils in the region of the c and d bands. (Magnification × 98 000.)

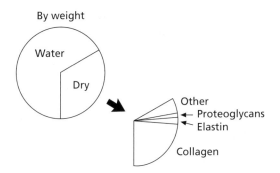

Fig. 4.3 Approximate amounts of main tendon/ligament components by weight. Collagen forms the main protein component of the dry weight with smaller amounts of elastin and proteoglycans.

proteoglycan and elastic fibres. (Figs 4.2 and 4.3). The outstanding feature of both these unique load-bearing tissues is the collagen 'crimp', which is a planar wave pattern found extending in phase across the width of all ligaments and tendons (Fig. 4.4) (Diamant *et al.* 1972). This collagen 'crimp' appears to be built into the tertiary structure of the collagen molecule and is probably maintained *in vivo* by inter- and intramolecular collagen cross-links as well as a strategically placed elastic fibre network. The 'crimp' may help to attenuate muscle loading forces at the tendoperiosteal junction as well as at the musculotendinous junction.

Viidik (1996) has recently reviewed the basic biomechanics of ligaments and tendons and the reader is referred to this text for a more detailed examination of structure–function relationships. The basic function of tendons and ligaments is to transmit force with 'reasonable safety margins' (Viidik 1996). The longitudinal array of collagen fibrils converts externally applied axial loads to internal lateral compression which results in interfibril friction and heat generation. This heat generation may be responsible for central fibroblast death in thick tendons, which has recently been described as exercised-induced hyperthermia (Wilson & Goodship 1994). Peak intratendinous core temperatures in the range of 43–45°C have been recorded in race horse tendons. Temperatures greater than 42.5°C are known to cause fibroblast death *in vitro*.

Also of interest is the notion that the muscle–tendon unit can act as a spring and the tendon can recoil after being eccentrically stretched, for example during the landing phase of a hopping kangaroo. During this landing phase the tendon stretch of the Achilles tendon is stored as elastic energy which is then converted to add extra lift for the animal during the concentric phase of the hop and hence leads to energy conservation (Morgan *et al.* 1978; Proske & Morgan 1987). Indeed, in the slowly hopping wallaby, strain energy storage in tendons and ligaments accounts for 33% of the negative and positive work that is done whilst the feet are on the ground (Ker *et al.* 1986)!

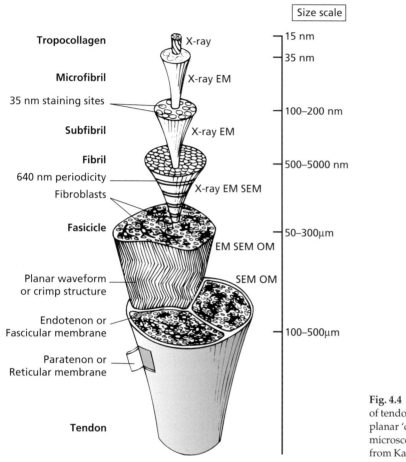

Size scale

Tropocollagen — X-ray ⸻ 15 nm
⸻ 35 nm

Microfibril — X-ray EM

35 nm staining sites ⸻ 100–200 nm

Subfibril — X-ray EM

Fibril — ⸻ 500–5000 nm
640 nm periodicity
Fibroblasts — X-ray EM SEM

Fasicicle — ⸻ 50–300μm

EM SEM OM

Planar waveform — SEM OM
or crimp structure

Endotenon or ⸻ 100–500μm
Fascicular membrane

Paratenon or
Reticular membrane

Tendon

Fig. 4.4 Structural organization of tendon and ligament. Note the planar 'crimp' seen at the light microscopic level. (Adapted from Kastelic *et al.* 1978.)

Ligament and tendon injury can be closely correlated with the load–deformation curve (Butler *et al.* 1979; Oakes 1981). The load–strain curve can be divided into three regions (Fig. 4.5):

1 The 'toe' region or initial concave region represents the normal physiological range of ligament/tendon strain up to about 3–4% of initial length, and is due to the flattening of the collagen 'crimp'. Repeated cycling within this 'toe region' or 'physiological strain range' of 3–4% (which may be up to near 10% in cruciate ligaments due to the intrinsic macrospiral of collagen cruciate fibre bundles) can normally occur without irreversible macroscopic or molecular damage to the tissue.

2 The second part of the load–deformation curve is the linear region where pathological irreversible ligament/tendon elongation occurs due to partial rupture of intermolecular cross-links. As the load is increased further intra- and intermolecular cross-links are disrupted until macroscopic failure is evident clinically. Electron microscopic studies (Viidik & Ekholm 1968) have shown the collagen fibrils are elongated in this phase and the periodicity increases from 67–68 nm to 72 nm and the banding pattern may become disjointed across the fibrils indicating intrafibril damage by molecular slippage under shear strain (Kastelic & Baer 1980). With continued loading into the third region, the banding pattern is completely lost and in immature collagen no free ends are seen ultrastructurally. This suggests that damaged fibrils can still bear

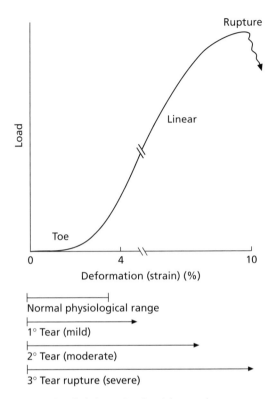

Fig. 4.5 Load–deformation (strain) curve for ligament/tendon and the clinical correlation with the grading of the injury. The 'toe' region of the curve is entirely within the normal physiological range; more than about a 4% strain causes tissue damage.

load and may represent a form of work hardening. In mature tendon, ruptured collagen fibril ends can be observed. Elegant X-ray diffraction and electron microscopic studies, coupled with accurate fast and slow loading studies, of both rat tail and human finger tendons has confirmed that initial damage to the fibril is an intrafibrillar sliding process that occurs only a few milliseconds before macroscopic fibre slippage occurs (Knorzer *et al.* 1986). The early part of the linear region corresponds to mild ligament tears or grade 1 ligament tears (0–50% fibre disruption) and the latter part to grade 2 (50–80% fibre disruption) where there is obvious clinical laxity on stress testing. Grade 1 and 2 injuries always have some pain after the initial trauma, and usually with a grade 2 injury the athlete cannot continue and

this is a rough guide to the clinical severity of the injury.

3 In the third region, if continued loading occurs, the linear part of the curve flattens and then the yield or failure point is reached at 10–20% strain, depending on the ligament/tendon fibre bundle macro-organization. In this region, complete ligament tendon rupture occurs at 'maximal breaking load' and this is the dangerous grade 3 ligament rupture seen on clinical testing. It is 'dangerous' because the athlete has severe momentary pain when the trauma is applied and then little pain, and the athlete (and often inexperienced examiners) erroneously believe the injury is trivial and treat it as such with disastrous consequences.

Tendons and ligaments behave as non-linear elastic materials. Viscous and plastic behaviour become obvious when cyclical loading–unloading protocols are used during laboratory tensile testing. The laboratory testing protocols can be similar to the cyclical loading imposed on tendons and ligaments during running. During such cyclical testing the load–strain curves initially have a large hysteresis loop and as the cycles progress with time this hysteresis loop is lost; this is thought to be due to squeezing of water from the tissue and concurrently aligning the collagen fibrils along the axis of loading. This 'preconditioning' cycling could be thought of as an important part of the warm-up procedure in athletes and is reversible during the non-running period as water and proteoglycans redistribute amongst the non-loaded fibrils. If, whilst cycling testing a specimen of tendon in the laboratory, the cycling is stopped two further protocols can be used. If the stress is kept constant by slowly increasing the strain, a creep phenomenon results. If the strain or deformation is kept constant by increasing the load slowly, stress–relaxation of the tissue occurs (Viidik 1996).

An enormous amount of research has been performed on the biomechanical properties of the human knee ligaments, with the anterior cruciate ligament (ACL) dominating research because of its key role in anteroposterior stability of the knee. Rotational injury to the knee with the foot fixed, as well as hyperextension of the knee, appear to be the two key mechanisms involved in human ACL disruption. Forces of the order of 2000 N are required to disrupt the ACL and are even higher for the posterior cruciate ligament (PCL). Direct falls onto the tibia or collisions with opponents, such that a posterior displacement force of the tibia occurs on the femur, appears to be a common mechanism for PCL injury. Collateral ligament injury involves excessive varus, valgus or rotational forces. The ligament–bone junction with its special fibrocartilage transition zone is a common region of clinical failure. Recent experimental animal studies indicate that ligament mid-substance strain is much lower than at the insertion sites and this appears to be due to a differing collagen-fibre crimp amplitude and angle. This higher strain at the insertion sites, together with ligament insertion geometry, could be an explanation of preferential failure of some ligament insertion sites—especially the femoral attachment of the medial collateral ligament of the knee, which has an almost 90° insertion into the region of the medial femoral epicondyle compared with its tibial periosteal insertion.

Ligament/tendon insertion to bone

Benjamin and his co-workers (Benjamin et al. 1986, 1995; Benjamin & Evans 1990; Evans et al. 1990; Benjamin & Ralphs 1995) have recently studied extensively tendon–bone junctions where the fibrocartilage interface or enthesis exists between the tendon and the bone. The width of this unique fibrocartilage interface, they hypothesize, is dependent upon the relative degree of movement that occurs between the tendon and its bone attachment (Fig. 4.6). They suggest that the enthesis prevents collagen fibre bending and perhaps undergoing shearing, fraying and failure at this special junction region. They have found the thickest fibrocartilage interface in the very mobile Achilles tendon and a lesser thickness of this interface in tendons such as the tibialis anterior posterior and very little in the long flexor tendons (Frowen & Benjamin 1995). It is of interest that they observed longitudinal splits in

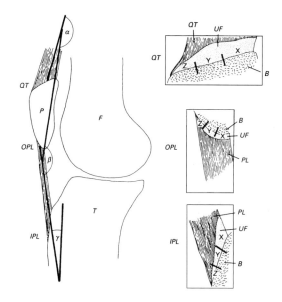

Fig. 4.6 The attachment zones studied are the insertion of the quadriceps (QT), the origin (OPL) and the insertion (IPL) of the patellar ligament. The angles between the long axis of tendon or ligament and bone are α, β and γ. The change in these angles is quite large during knee motion. The subdivision of each attachment site into regions X, Y and Z and the major differences in the quantities and distribution of uncalcified fibrocartilage (UF) are illustrated diagrammatically in the drawings to the right of the figure. B, bone; F, femur; P, patellar ligament; T, tibia. (From Benjamin & Evans 1990, with permission from *Journal of Anatomy*).

the Achilles tendon with some evidence of repair and also transverse tears at the bone–tendon junction that were filled with fat cells and no repair tissue (Rufai et al. 1995), which Frank et al. (1999) recognize as mechanical 'flaws' during tendon repair (see below).

Correlation of collagen fibril size with mechanical properties of tissues

Parry et al. (1978) have completed detailed quantitative morphometric ultrastructural analyses of collagen fibrils from a large number of collagen-containing tissues in various species. They came to a number of conclusions that can be summarized as follows:

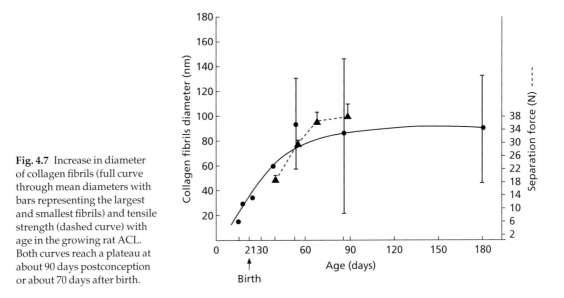

Fig. 4.7 Increase in diameter of collagen fibrils (full curve through mean diameters with bars representing the largest and smallest fibrils) and tensile strength (dashed curve) with age in the growing rat ACL. Both curves reach a plateau at about 90 days postconception or about 70 days after birth.

1 Type 1-orientated tissues, such as ligament and tendon, have a bimodal distribution of collagen fibril diameters at maturity.

2 The ultimate tensile strength and mechanical properties of connective tissues are positively correlated with the mass average diameter of collagen fibrils. In the context of the response of ligaments to exercise they also concluded that the collagen fibril diameter distribution is closely correlated with the magnitude and duration of loading of tissues (Fig. 4.7).

Collagen fibril diameter quantification with age and correlation with ACL tensile strength

Oakes (1988) measured collagen fibrils at various ages of the rat from 14 days fetal to 2-year-old senile adult rats. The mean diameter and the range of fibres from the largest to the smallest for each time interval were plotted against age and are shown in Fig. 4.7. The mean fibril diameter begins to plateau at about 7 weeks after birth. Also plotted on this figure is the separation force required to rupture the ACL in the rat with age. Special grips were used in this study to obviate epiphyseal separation and 70% of the failures occurred within the ACL. It can be seen that the two curves closely coincide, indicating a close correlation between the size of the collagen fibrils and the ultimate tensile strength of the ACL as has been suggested by Parry *et al.* (1978). This rapid increase in collagen fibril size over 6 weeks in the growing rat is not seen during normal ligament tissue repair or remodelling (Matthew *et al.* 1987; Oakes *et al.* 1991).

Work by Shadwick (1986, 1990) has also demonstrated a clear correlation between collagen fibril diameter and the tensile strength of tendons. He determined that the tensile strength of pig flexor tendons was greater than that of extensor tendons and that this greater flexor tendon tensile strength was correlated with a population of larger diameter collagen fibrils not present in the weaker extensor tendons. Also, studies by Oakes *et al.* (1998), using the rabbit patellar tendon, have demonstrated a high correlation between the area-weighted mean collagen fibril diameter (this method adjusts for the varying numbers of large and small fibrils within a tendon) and both modulus ($R = 0.79$) and ultimate tensile strength ($R = 0.63$) (Fig. 4.8).

It should be noted here that the original large collagen fibrils seen in normal tendons and ligaments are *not* replaced after ligament/tendon

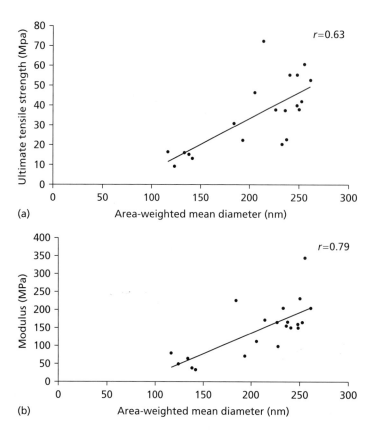

Fig. 4.8 Area-weighted mean collagen fibril diameter (nm) across full width of rabbit patellar tendon versus (a) patellar tendon ultimate tensile strength, and (b) patellar tendon modulus. (a) The good correlation ($r = 0.63$) should be noted and indicates an important relation between mean collagen fibril size and tensile properties of tendons. (b) The excellent correlation ($r = 0.79$) indicates mean fibril diameter and material properties are closely related. (From Oakes *et al.* 1998.)

rupture or injury and this is the probable explanation for the poor material properties of repair scars even 1 year after repair. They are also not replaced when ligament replacements are used as scaffolds, such as for the reconstruction of the knee ACL when autograft or allograft tendons are used. This is a major explanation for the high failure rate of such knee ACL reconstructions, apart from any surgical misadventure (see below for further discussion).

Basic biomechanics of tissue injury

Muscle–tendon–bone injury

The basic causes of intrinsic muscle injury are still not entirely clear, but have been attributed to inadequate muscle length and strength (for example tight hamstrings, especially in adoles-cent boys), muscle fatigue and inadequate muscle skills. It is also clear that most muscle injuries occur in the lower limb and most involve two-joint muscles such as the hamstrings and the rectus femoris, probably because of the complex reflexes involved in simultaneous co-contraction and co-relaxation (Oakes 1984). An excellent review of current knowledge of muscle strain injuries has been published by Garrett (1996). Recently, Hartig and Henderson (1999) have clearly demonstrated that increased hamstring flexibility decreased lower limb overuse injuries in military basic trainees.

Both concentric and eccentric muscle–tendon unit loading can cause muscle–tendon–bone junction injury. The use of eccentric muscle loading to cause increased muscle hypertrophy, as against the use of more conventional concentric loading, has led to the phenomenon of eccentric muscle soreness which is now known to be due in part to muscle sarcomere disruption at the Z-lines (Friden *et al.* 1983). Eccentric muscle–tendon–bone load can generate more force than concentric contractions and may be the mechanism by which the patellar tendon and its attachments lead to tendoperiosteal partial disruptions at both the superior and inferior poles of the patellar. Studies by Chun *et al.* (1989) demonstrated that the inferomedial collagen fibre bundles of the human patellar tendon, when subjected to mechanical analysis, fail at loads which are much less than the lateral fibre bundles. The biological reasons for this are not clear at the moment but it helps to explain the prevalence of inferomedial tenderness, which is such a common cause of anteromedial knee pain or 'jumper's knee'.

The bone–tendon junction or enthesis is one of the commonest sites for tissue injury, as is seen with the classic infrapatellar tendonitis which is so refractory to treatment. Benjamin *et al.* (1986) have suggested that the zone of fibrocartilage at the enthesis minimizes local stress concentrations and appears to be characteristic of tendons and ligaments where there is a great change in angle between the tendon or ligament and bone during movement. It is of interest that the enthesis which gives the most problems in the clinic (the inferior patellar pole and the patellar tendon) is the one with the least thickness of fibrocartilage (see Fig. 4.6). It is possible that a major mechanism of failure at this very mobile enthesis may be collagen fibril shear.

A study by Cooke *et al.* (1997) found that more than one-third of athletes with patellar tendinopathy were unable to return to sport for more than 6 months because of recurrent or persistent pain and eventually required surgery, indicating the difficulty of the reformation of a normal load-bearing enthesis after repeated tension–avulsion injury. Also it was clear from their studies that imaging such as ultrasonograms and magnetic resonance imaging (MRI) scans do not always correlate with the clinical and histopathological findings (Khan *et al.* 1998).

A recent detailed study of chronic patellar tendinopathy treated surgically by either open or arthroscopic patellar tenotomy, revealed that about 40% of subjects could not return to their previous level of sporting activity and that with either form of patellar tenotomy could expect little improvement in symptoms beyond 12 months postoperatively. In this study those patients that achieved postsurgical sporting success appeared to have an 80% chance of having prolonged success. There was no difference in outcomes between the open or arthroscopic procedures (Coleman *et al.* 2000).

Muscle–tendon junction injury

Failure at this junctional region is common. There is an increased muscle cell membrane folding of the terminal end of the last muscle sarcomere that has important mechanical implications for reducing the stress at this critical junctional region. It has been determined that a typical vertebrate fast-twitch cell can generate about 0.33 MPa of stress across the cell. The stress placed on the cell's junctional complex at the muscle–tendon junction by the complex folding of the terminal sarcomeres experiences a maximal stress of 1.5×10^4 Pa, which is much less than 33×10^4 Pa, and this difference may determine whether mechanical failure occurs at this junctional region.

With muscle injury at this junctional site it is probable that the complex sarcomere muscle membrane infolding—to increase the surface area and hence decrease substantially the stress—is probably not reproduced following repair and this may be an explanation for the reccurence of tears at this junction in athletes. A detailed comprehensive review has been published by Noonan and Garrett (1992). Kannus *et al.* (1992a) (Kvist *et al.* 1991) have demonstrated in the rat that type II (fast-twitch) fibres have a more complex folding pattern than the type II (slow-twitch) fibres. The type II fibres have an increase of 30–40% in contact surface area compared to the type I fibres. In this way the larger forces transmitted via the myotendinous junction with type II muscle can be transmitted through this junction without increasing the force applied per surface unit of the junction (Fig. 4.9).

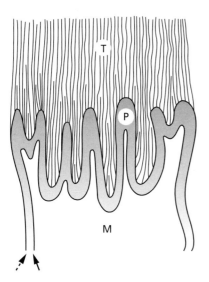

Fig. 4.9 Schematic figure of the ultrastructure of the myotendinous junction. Dotted arrow, lamina lucida of the muscular basement membrane; solid arrow, lamina densa of the muscular basement membrane; M, muscle cell; P, muscle cell processes; T, tendon collagen fibrils. (From Kannus *et al.* 1991, with permission.)

Tendon injury

Tendon injury in sport is common because of the large loads applied. Komi (1987) has measured the high forces generated in the human Achilles tendon with the surgical introduction of a calibrated buckle transducer for short periods of time. Forces of up to 4000 N were recorded in the Achilles tendon with toe running. Thus it is not surprising that with repetitive loadings of these magnitudes microfatigue failure could occur with long-distance running, especially in a tendon of small cross-sectional area (Engstrom *et al.* 1985). Studies by Hasselman *et al.* (1995) indicate that the proximal tendon of the rectus femoris extends well distal into the muscle belly, and tears at this muscle–tendon junction can appear as mid-muscle belly haematomata.

Wilson and Goodship (1994) have demonstrated a rise of the core temperature of the equine superficial digital flexor tendon under galloping conditions to a mean peak temperature of 43.3°C and a maximum of 45.4°C in one animal. They suggest these core temperatures or central tendon hyperthermia are not survivable by tendon fibroblasts and may explain the central lesions seen in the equine superficial digital flexor tendon and also in the human Achilles tendon.

Spontaneous tendon rupture is uncommon in the young athlete and usually occurs in the older sportsman (for example the long head of the biceps brachii) and then is usually associated with degenerative pathology of the collagen fibrils, although the biochemical detail has not been delineated.

Supraspinatus tendon rupture is common with ageing and may be related to a decreased tendon cross-sectional area and also to increased stiffness of the tissue with increased collagen cross-links. This increased 'stiffness' may be further aggravated by matrix changes such as fibrocartilage transformation and frank intratendinous calcification. Recently, Katayose and Magee (2001) have performed an elegant and detailed study of the cross-sectional areas (CSAs) of the normal dominant and non-dominant supraspinatus tendon as a function of age using diagnostic ultrasound with a high level of interobserver reliability. They found that the CSA of the dominant side was significantly larger than the non-dominant side and that the CSA decreased significantly with ageing. They noted that the CSAs of the 70–79-year age group were 82% of those in the 20–29-year age group.

Ligament/tendon repair

There are three main phases of ligament/tendon repair: inflammation, repair (or proliferation) and remodelling (see Figs 4.10–4.14).

Acute inflammation

The gap in the ligament/tendon is filled immediately with erythrocytes and inflammatory cells, especially polymorphonuclear leucocytes. Within 24 h, monocytes and macrophages are the predominant cell and actively engage in phagocytosis of debris and necrotic cells. These are gradually replaced by fibroblasts from either intrinsic or

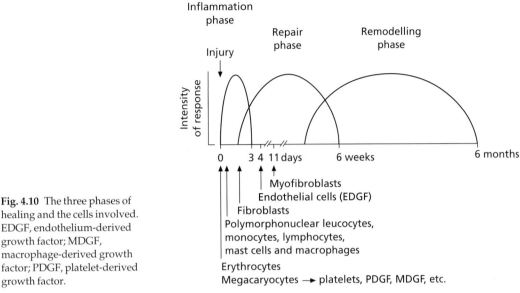

Fig. 4.10 The three phases of healing and the cells involved. EDGF, endothelium-derived growth factor; MDGF, macrophage-derived growth factor; PDGF, platelet-derived growth factor.

extrinsic sources and the initial deposition of the type III collagen scar is commenced. At this stage collagen concentration may be normal or slightly decreased but the total mass of ligament collagen scar is increased. Glycosaminoglycan (GAG) content, water, fibronectin and DNA content are increased (Fig. 4.11).

Proliferation

Fibroblasts predominate in this phase. Water content remains increased and collagen content increases and peaks during this phase (3–6 weeks). Type I collagen now begins to predominate and GAG concentration remains high. The increasing amount of scar collagen and reducible cross-link profile has been correlated with the increasing tensile strength of the ligament matrix. Recent quantitative collagen fibril orientation studies indicate that early mobilization of a ligament at this stage (within the first 3 weeks) may be detrimental to collagen orientation. After this time there is experimental evidence that mobilization increases the tensile strength of the repair and probably enhances this phase and the next phase of remodelling and maturation

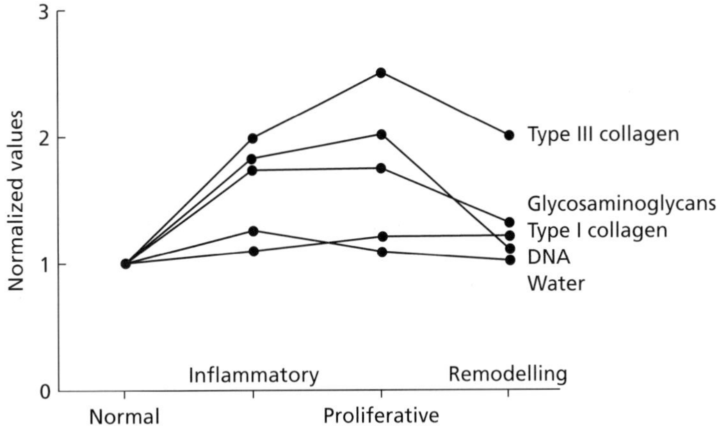

Fig. 4.11 Ligament repair during the phases of healing and the 'normalized' content of type I and III collagen, water, DNA and glycosaminoglycans. (From Andriacchi et al. 1988, with permission.)

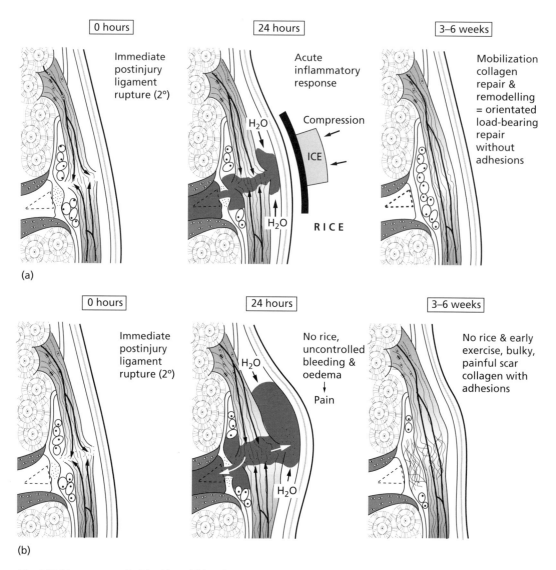

Fig. 4.12 Ligament repair: (a) with and (b) without RICE (rest, ice, compression and elevation) management and early mobilization.

(Figs 4.12 and 4.13) (Vailas *et al.* 1981; Hart & Danhers 1987; Woo *et al.* 1987b).

With this basic biological knowledge there is now a rationale for the use of early controlled mobilization of patients with ligament/tendon trauma. The use of a limited motion cast with an adjustable double-action hinge for the knee joint is now clinically accepted and enhances more rapid repair and remodelling as well as preserving

quadriceps muscle bulk. Patients are now usually mobilized in a limited motion cast for 3–6 weeks rather than the previously empirical time of 6 weeks. An initial range of motion of 20–60° of flexion is used because this places minimal loading on all knee ligaments (Helbing & Burri 1977). The beneficial effects of functional tendon casting versus rigid casting has also been recently demonstrated in a rabbit Achilles tenotomy model

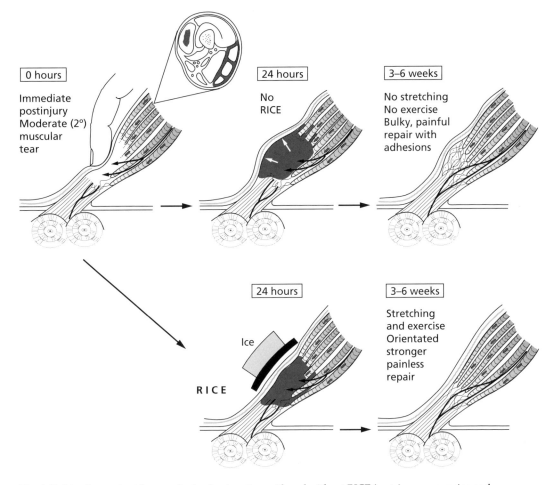

Fig. 4.13 Muscle repair at the muscle–tendon junction with and without RICE (rest, ice, compression and elevation) management and early mobilization.

that demonstrated a 60% increase in tendon collagen and a 20% increase in maximum load and maximum stress compared with control rigid casts when measured 15 days' post-tenotomy (Stehno-Bittel *et al.* 1998). Such basic science studies have led to the earlier mobilization of human Achilles tendons after surgical repair (Mandelbaum *et al.* 1995; Aoki *et al.* 1998; Speck & Klaue 1998).

Remodelling and maturation (6 weeks to 12 months)

During this phase there is a decrease in cell numbers and hence a decreased collagen and GAG synthesis. Water content returns to normal and collagen concentration returns to slightly *below* normal, but total collagen content remains slightly increased. With further remodelling there is a trend for scar parameters to return to normal but the matrix in the ligament scar region continues to mature slowly over months or even years. Scar collagen matrix and adjacent normal matrix may actually shorten the repair region, perhaps by interaction of ligament/tendon myofibroblasts with their surrounding collagen matrix (Danhers *et al.* 1986). Collagen fibril alignment in the longitudinal axis of the ligament occurs even though small-diameter fibrils are involved (Figs 4.14 and 4.15).

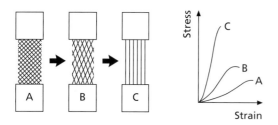

Fig. 4.14 The effect of collagen repair with identical fibrils but different geometry and the corresponding load–strain response to tensile testing. (Adapted from Viidik 1980.)

Occasionally calcium apatite crystals will be deposited in the damaged tissues and the classic site for this to occur is in the rotator cuff supraspinatus tendoperiosteal attachment to the greater tubercule of the humerus.

Achilles tendon and infrapatellar tendon injuries, especially partial tears, present a dilemma for the clinician in that they are often intractable to reasonable short-term management although Stanish *et al.* (1986) claim good clinical results from graded eccentric loading regimes for patellar tendonitis. The author has examined Achilles tendon biopsies of patients with chronic localized tears and more generalized thickened, tender, chronic Achilles tendons. The feature which characterized the pathology ultrastructurally was the persistence of small-diameter collagen fibrils < 100 nm diameter. The large fibrils of the original tendon do not appear to be replaced in the mature adult in either a repairing tendon or ligament (Fig. 4.15) (see below); increasing the collagen fibril diameters (and their alignment) is needed to enhance the repair scar tensile strength.

ACL injuries appear to be unique in that the chondrocyte-like cells in this special ligament apparently have a limited capacity to proliferate and synthesize a new collagen matrix and hence

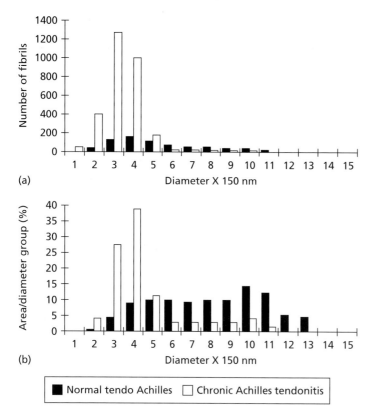

Fig. 4.15 (a) Number of fibrils versus fibril diameter in patients with chronic Achilles tendonitis; (b) expressed as per cent area occupied for each diameter group versus diameter. The preponderance of small-diameter fibrils in 'repairing' chronic Achilles tendonitis should be noted. The large-diameter normal fibrils > 100 nm are not replaced.

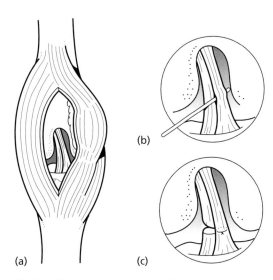

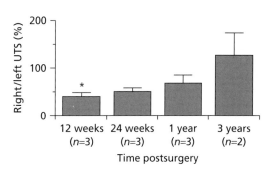

Fig. 4.17 The mean and standard deviations of normalized (right/left ratio) percentage ultimate tensile strength (UTS) for the posterolateral bundles of hemisected ACLs at intervals after surgery. *, significantly different from 3-year results. (From Ng *et al.* 1996b, with permission from *American Journal of Sports Medicine*.)

Fig. 4.16 The operative procedure for a hemitransection injury to the ACL. (a and b) A medial arthrotomy is performed and the patella is displaced laterally; a probe is inserted to separate the anteromedial and posterolateral bundles. (c) The posterolateral bundle is completely severed, leaving the anteromedial bundle intact as an internal splint, and a black silk suture is placed on the anteromedial bundle opposite the cut level as a marker of the incision site. (From Ng *et al.* 1996b, with permission from *American Journal of Sports Medicine*.)

repair appears to be limited. Collagenase release may also affect the effectiveness of the repair process (Amiel *et al.* 1989). However Ng *et al.* (1996a, 1996b) have completed a long-term biomechanical study of the repair of the goat ACL after hemisection injury showing that, contrary to the current orthopaedic dogma, the ACL can heal even after partial tears. To test the healing capacity of the partially torn ACL, ligaments were tested at 12, 24 and 52 weeks and 3 years after surgery (Fig. 4.16). As early as 12 weeks after surgery, a translucent fibrous tissue covered the transected posterolateral bundle. A comparison of anteroposterior laxity between the right and left knees measured at 45 and 90° of flexion showed no significant difference at each time period. Results of Instron testing of the posterolateral bundle revealed that normalized changes in load–relaxation and Young's modulus were also not significantly different at each time

period, but the ultimate tensile strength and stiffness at 3 years were significantly higher than at 12 weeks ($P < 0.05$). Failure started at the repair site for the 12-week group, but at 24 and 52 weeks the failure occurred through the ligament. At 3 years, the posterolateral bundle specimens failed by bony avulsion, indicating the repaired tissue was not the weakest link of the bone–ligament–bone complex.

This study showed that under the favourable biological conditions of the experiment, partial ACL injuries in the goat are capable of adequate mechanical repair. What is more important, the high ultimate tensile strength and stiffness of the 3-year repaired tissue indicate that full structural repair of such an artificial transection injury is possible (Figs 4.16–4.18).

Clinical and ultrastructural observations of Achilles tendon injuries

In this section I will attempt to relate the three phases of healing of soft tissues with that seen in Achilles tendon injuries. Achilles tendon injuries can be classified as described above for ligament injuries, i.e. grades 1–3 with the latter being complete rupture. Several patient histories will be used to illustrate these three phases of healing and attempted repair.

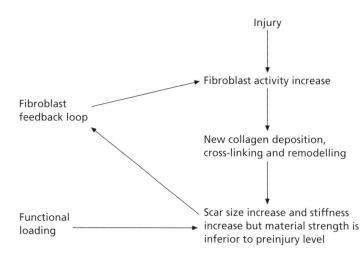

Fig. 4.18 The hypothetical feedback loop mechanism of collagen deposition control during ligament repair. (From Ng *et al.* 1995, with permission from *Journal of Orthopaedic Research.*)

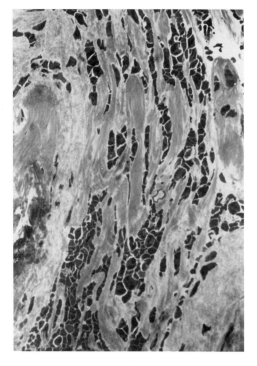

Fig. 4.19 Light micrograph of an acute Achilles tendon rupture at 1 week postinjury, showing red cells extravascular together with many polymorphs and macrophages. (Epon-araldite, Azure A-Methylene blue.)

Grade 3: complete rupture

Australian Rules football rover, aged 26, powering off to avoid an opponent. Clinical signs were a palpable defect in the Achilles tendon as well as a positive Thompson's sign. A biopsy was taken during surgical repair.

With this disastrous injury there is both collagen bundle failure as well as vascular disruption and hence bleeding is a feature of these injuries when seen at early surgical repair. This trauma to the tendon initiates the acute inflammatory phase and hence microscopically there is massive red cell extravasation, fibrin clot formation and collagen fibril disruption. The damaged tendon becomes oedematous and polymorphonuclear monocytes migrate into this area and release their lysosomal contents as well as actively phagocytosing cellular and other debris. Macrophages also move into the rupture site and commence phagocytosis of damaged cells and tissue. This phase lasts 0–72 h or so and is followed by the repair phase (Fig. 4.19).

Grade 2: tear

Australian Rules football ruckman with 6 months' painful thickened Achilles tendon. The operation involved the excision of paratenon and tendon incision to remove damaged, haemorrhagic and

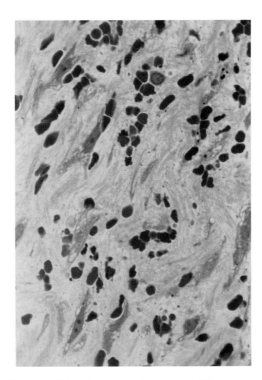

Fig. 4.20 Light micrograph of an acute Achilles tendon grade 2 partial tear after 6 months of pain and swelling. The tendon is oedematous and very cellular and the fibroblasts are dilated with enlarged rough endoplasmic reticular indicative of active collagen synthesis. (Epon-araldite, Azure A, Methylene blue.)

necrotic regions. A biopsy was taken for light and electron microscopy.

Light microscopy demonstrated a thickened paratenon and an oedematous thickened tendon (Fig. 4.20). Ultrastructurally many fibroblasts had dilated rough endoplasmic reticulum and prominent nucleoli indicative of increased collagen synthesis. Apart from the many free red cells, the other feature was the prevalence of many small-diameter collagen fibrils not aligned or closely packed (18–20 nm diameter) in amongst the older, larger, pre-existing fibrils ranging from 80 to 150 nm diameter. Polymorphonuclear monocytes and macrophages were not common at this stage, reflecting perhaps the slowness of repair in this unique tissue.

The biopsy demonstrated the features of the repair phase that follows the acute inflammatory phase and lasts 72 h to 4–6 weeks; but in this patient the repair phase had been perpetuated because of continued activity by the athlete. In other patients where there is less florid tendonitis and the tendon is clinically painful but not obviously enlarged, discrete areas of increased cellularity are seen in the tendon in the form of free red cells, cell debris and viable fibroblasts surrounded by both large- and many small-diameter collagen fibres. These areas are almost 'walled-off' from the densely packed collagen of the rest of the tendon by a fibrin precipitate. These discrete areas are probably due to collagen fibre ruptures or microtears corresponding to the early part of the second region of the load–deformation curve. There is as yet no evidence that the use of massage or deep friction enhances this repair phase (Walker 1984).

Grade 1: injury

Runner, aged 25, with a painful tender lump in the Achilles tendon for 18 months! A biopsy was obtained at open operation.

The lump at operation was firmer than the rest of the tendon and was slightly darker in colour. On light microscopy of the biopsy taken from the nodule, the changes in the collagen bundles were very subtle. There was less regular 'crimping' of the collagen bundles and they were not as tightly packed. However, ultrastructually the cause of this less regular collagen crimp was obvious in that between the large-diameter fibrils were many small-diameter fibrils that were less well orientated longitudinally (Fig. 4.15). These tendons were interpreted as being in the remodelling phase as there were no increased fibroblast numbers in the nodules and no inflammatory cells were observed (Fig. 4.15).

The mechanism of acute complete rupture in young athletes 'powering-off' during sprinting indicates that the gastrocnemius–soleus complex can generate sufficient force to rupture the tendon. However, tendon strength usually exceeds that of its muscle by a factor of two and hence rupture is unusual. The mechanisms involved in partial

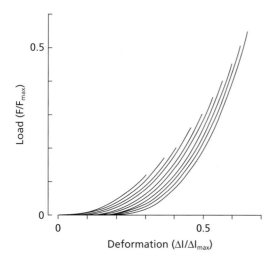

Fig. 4.21 The effect of 'fatigue failure' or 'plasticity' of load–strain curves with repeated loadings of a tendon to successively higher loads (the curve of the next loading is shifted to the right) within the 'toe' region of the curve and before the linear part of the curve. This effect may be operating in chronic human Achilles tendonitis, especially in those athletes with a small cross-sectional area tendon. (Adapted from Viidik 1973.)

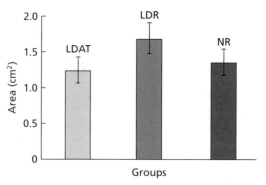

Fig. 4.22 Cross-sectional area (cm²) of human Achilles tendons measured by ultrasound for two running groups matched for age, weight and distance compared with a sedentary control group (NR). The smaller cross-sectional area of the Achilles tendons in the LDAT group ($P < 0.05$) should be noted. LDAT, runners with grade I Achilles tendonitis; LDR, runners without Achilles tendonitis. (Courtesy of Professor A.W. Parker.)

grade 1 and 2 tears in the Achilles tendon are not as obvious. Viidik (1973) has shown that rat tendons *in vitro* undergo increasing deformation or 'plasticity' if cycled to loads of less than one-tenth of its failure load, and that the strain or deformation occurs well before region two or the linear part of the load–strain curve begins (Fig. 4.21). Similar observations have been made both *in vivo* and *in vitro* for rat knee joint ligaments by Weisman *et al.* (1980). It is possible that in distance runners a similar fatigue plasticity and elongation occurs in the tendon and this causes the microruptures and the thickened repair nodules already described.

The notion that some running athletes may not have an Achilles tendon of sufficient CSA to sustain the repetitive tendon loading of distance without injury has been investigated by Engstrom *et al.* (1985). In an elegant study they used ultrasound to measure the CSA of the human Achilles tendon *in vivo* and validated this technique as a reliable method to measure the Achilles tendon

CSA using cadaver Achilles tendons. Two groups of distance athletes with and without grade 1 Achilles tendonitis who were age, weight and distance matched had their Achilles tendon CSA measured using the previously validated ultrasound technique. They demonstrated that athletes with grade 1-type Achilles tendonitis had about a 30% decrease in the CSAs of their Achilles tendons (Fig. 4.22). This indicates that a major mechanism in this type of common injury may simply be fatigue creep failure of Achilles tendon collagen as shown in Fig. 4.21. Komi *et al.* (1987) have developed an *in vivo* buckle transducer which they located around the Achilles tendon in a number of subjects. Direct force measurements were made on several subjects who were involved in slow walking, sprinting, jumping and hopping after calibration of the transducer. During running and jumping forces close to the previous estimated ultimate tensile strength of the tendon were recorded, indicating that fatigue creep in a small cross-sectional tendon is a possible mechanism of injury without the need to invoke other lower limb biomechanical pathology as has been suggested by Clement *et al.* (1984) and Williams (1986).

Use of physical modalities in attempts to increase collagen deposition for enhancing the tensile strength of soft tissue repair: electrical, ultrasound and laserphoto stimulation

The original *in vitro* work of Fitton-Jackson and Bassett (1980), in which fibroblasts were stimulated to increase collagen synthesis under the influence of pulsed magnetic fields, has been in part confirmed by other workers. However, the gains in increased ligament strength have been meagre compared to the dramatic 40% or so reduction in healing times for fresh fractures of the tibia and radius with the use of low-intensity ultrasound applied to fracture healing as originally described in the human by Heckman *et al.* (1994), and recently reviewed by Rubin *et al.* (2001). In fracture repair, ultrasound was demonstrated with substantive data to enhance the three basic stages of the healing process described above. Such observations have been also demonstrated in part in soft tissue repair, but not with the same large increases in matrix deposition (collagen) as for bone deposition. Frank *et al.* (1983a, 1983b) demonstrated accelerated early healing of a rabbit medial collateral ligament (MCL) to which a solid core electromagnet energized the tissues with a square wave of unidirectional current 7 h per day for up to 6 weeks postinjury. An increased tensile strength of almost double the control MCL was observed at 21 days, but at 42 days there was no difference between the treated and control ligaments.

Enwemeka (1989) applied therapeutic ultrasound daily for 5 min for nine treatments to tenotomized rabbit Achilles tendons, and noted significant increases in tensile strength and energy absorption to failure in the early healing phase (10 days' post-tenotomy).

Kesava Reddy *et al.* (1998) applied a combined laser treatment and electrical stimulation to the repairing rabbit Achilles tendon after complete tenotomy over a short 5-day period. No statistical difference was found between the experimental and the control tenotomies in terms of mechanical performance although there was a 32% increase in collagen deposition at the repair site. Previous studies using low-intensity laser did moderately increase the biomechanical load-bearing capacity of healing rabbit Achilles tendons after 14 days of treatment (Enwemeka *et al.* 1990).

Clearly, more long-term studies need to be done in this area to attempt to understand the biological mechanisms involved and also to determine the long-term therapeutic value of such treatments.

Effects of immobilization on the capsule and synovial joints

Akeson *et al.* (1987) reviewed their work and others' work on this important topic. There is articular cartilage atrophy with proteoglycan loss and an associated fibrofatty connective tissue that is synovial derived, which adheres to the articular cartilage. Ligament insertion sites are weakened and the ligament itself has increased compliance with reduced load to failure due to loss of collagen mass, which may occur with only 8–12 weeks' immobilization but may take up to 1 year to recover after mobilization (Amiel *et al.* 1983). Capsular changes include loss of water due to loss of GAGs and hyaluronic acid, leading to joint stiffness. Clearly joint immobilization is to be avoided if possible to prevent the above changes from occurring which take many months to recover (Fig. 4.23). Similarly Steno-Bittel *et al.* (1998) have demonstrated that functional casting of rabbits after an Achilles tendon complete transection and surgical repair in a short-term experiment (15 days); increased collagen deposition (60%) and increased maximum tensile strength (20%) and maximum stress (21%) in the repairing tendon compared to complete Achilles tenotomies and suture repair with classic immobilization of the lower limb with non-functional load bearing.

Thus the thrust in recent years has been to minimize immobilization times and to avoid soft and hard tissue immobilization if practically possible. With wounds to soft tissues and hard tissue injuries, such as fractures to bone, it may be necessary to immobilize these tissues either

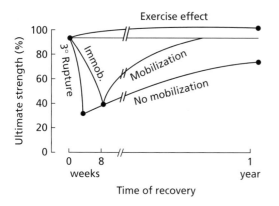

Fig. 4.23 Effects of immobilization, mobilization and exercise on the recovery of ligament ultimate tensile strength. The loss in ligament tensile strength after a relatively short period of immobilization (about 8 weeks) requires many months to recover—with no mobilization it may take up to 1 year. The effect of exercise on ligament ultimate tensile strength is small. (Adapted from Woo *et al.* 1987a.)

externally (or internally with surgery) until healing is well underway. This is so these tissues will have developed enough intrinsic mechanical strength—through neocollagen fibril deposition —so as not to be disrupted by early mobilization and to allow the remodelling phase of the repair process to be enhanced (Vailas *et al.* 1981; see below). Both tensile-bearing soft tissues such as tendon and ligament require regular minimal loading to maintain their intrinsic mechanical tensile strength; they are similar to bone and articular cartilage in this respect (Caterson & Lowther 1978; Rubin & Lanyon 1987).

Effect of immobilization and mobilization on ligament tensile strength

Effect of immobilization

The most important study in this context is that by Noyes *et al.* (1974) using the ACL in monkeys. They demonstrated clearly that 8 weeks of lower limb cast immobilization led to a substantial loss of ligament tensile strength which took 9 months to recover from, even with a reconditioning programme. The predominant mode of failure in these

experiments was ligament failure as opposed to avulsion fracture failure. The latter mode of failure was more predominant in the immobilized group due to resorption of Haversian bone at the ligament attachment; but after 5 months of reconditioning femoral avulsion fractures did not occur. It should be noted that there was no surgery, just simple immobilization.

Another important study with direct implications for clinical practice is that of Amiel *et al.* (1985). Although this work was done in rabbits, in the context of the previous work by Noyes, it is very relevant. The timeframes for the changes in ligament tensile strength are similar and hence are applicable to clinical rehabilitation. These investigators were able to show that 12 weeks of immobilization of the MCL in the growing rabbit led to profound atrophy, such that there was a decrease of approximately 30% in collagen mass as a result of increased collagen degradation. Remarkably most of this atrophy occurred during weeks 9–12 of immobilization. Again, there was no trauma or surgery to the MCL in this study.

Hence it appears from the above two studies that prolonged immobilization, i.e. 6–12 weeks without trauma, can itself lead to profound atrophy of both the collateral and cruciate ligaments of the knee joint and recovery may require at least many months or even a year. This timeframe must be kept in mind when managing patients after prolonged knee immobilization and advising them when they can best return to full competitive sport.

Amiel *et al.* (1985) have also shown that there is a close relationship between joint stiffness induced by immobilization and a decrease of total GAG in the periarticular connective tissues. They demonstrated alleviation of this joint stiffness in a rabbit model using intra-articular hyaluronate.

Apart from the original, classic work of Noyes *et al.* (1974) in which the effects of immobilization on the ACL of the primate were examined, there have been few investigations of the cause of the decreased strength and elastic stiffness of the ACL in response to immobilization. Tipton *et al.* (1970) reported that collagen fibre bundles (viewed with light microscopy) were decreased in number and size in immobilized dogs, suggesting that this was the cause of the decreased CSA seen in immobilized rabbit MCLs (Woo *et al.* 1987a). The explanation for the decreased strength and elastic stiffness in these immobilized ligaments may be found at the collagen fibril level. Binkley and Peat (1986) showed a decrease in the number of small-diameter fibrils after 6 weeks of immobilization in the rat MCL.

Effect of mobilization (exercise)

There have been a large number of studies investigating this area. The literature has been reviewed by Tipton *et al.* (1986) Tipton and Vailas (1989), Butler *et al.* (1979) and Parker and Larsen (1981).

NORMAL LIGAMENTS

The results in experimental animals generally indicate an increase in bone–ligament–bone preparation strength as a response to endurance-type exercise. However, no change in ligament or tendon strength has been recorded by some workers and this may reflect different exercise regimes, methods of testing as well as species differences.

The observations by Tipton *et al.* (1970, 1975), Cabaud *et al.* (1980), Parker and Larsen (1981) and others that ligament strength is dependent on physical activity prompted an ultrastructural investigation as to the mechanism of this increase in tensile strength. Increased collagen content was found in the ligaments of exercised dogs and this correlated with increased CSA and larger fibre bundles. This accounts for the increased ligament tensile strength but whether this increased collagen was due to the deposition of collagen on existing fibres or due to the synthesis of new fibres was not investigated. Larsen and Parker (1982) had already shown that with a 4-week intensive exercise programme in young male Wistar rats, both the ACLs and PCLs showed a significant strength increase ($P < 0.05$).

Oakes *et al.* (1981) and Oakes (1988) quantified the collagen fibril populations in young rat ACLs and PCLs subjected to an intensive 1-month alternating treadmill and swimming exercise programme. This study was performed in an attempt to explain the increased tensile strength found in

these ligaments with the intensive endurance exercise programme and to determine if this could be explained at the level of the collagen fibril, which is the fundamental tensile unit of ligament.

Five 30-day-old pubescent rats were placed on a progressive 4-week exercise programme of alternating days of swimming and treadmill running. At the conclusion of the exercise programme the rats were running 60–80 min at 26 m·min^{-1} on a 10% treadmill gradient and on alternate days swimming 60 min with a 3% body weight attached to their tails. Five caged rats of similar age and commencing body weights were controls. Analysis of ultrathin transverse sections cut through collagen fibrils of the exercised ACLs revealed: (i) a larger number of fibrils per unit area examined (29% increase, $P < 0.05$) compared with the non-exercised caged control ACLs; (ii) a fall in mean fibril diameter from $9.66 \pm 0.3 \text{ nm}$ in the control ACLs to $8.30 \pm 0.3 \text{ nm}$ in the exercised ACLs ($P < 0.05$); and (iii) as a consequence of (i) and (ii) the major CSA of collagen fibrils was found in the 11.25 nm diameter group in the exercised ACLs and in the 15 nm diameter group in the control ACLs. However, total collagen fibril cross-section per unit area examined was approximately the same in both the exercised and the non-exercised control ACLs. Similar changes occurred in the exercised and control PCLs. These results are shown in Figs 4.24–26. In the exercised PCL, collagen per microgram of DNA was almost double that of the control suggesting that the PCL was more loaded with this exercise regime than the ACL. The conclusion from this study is that ACL and PCL fibroblasts deposit tropocollagen as smaller diameter fibrils when subjected to an intense 1 month's intermittent loading (exercise) rather than the expected accretion and increase in size of the pre-existing larger diameter collagen fibrils. Very similar ultrastructural observations have been made for collagen fibrils of exercised mice flexor tendons (Michna 1984).

The mechanism of the change to a smaller diameter collagen fibril population is of interest and may be related to a change in the type of proteoglycans synthesized by ligament fibroblasts in response to the intermittent loading of exercise.

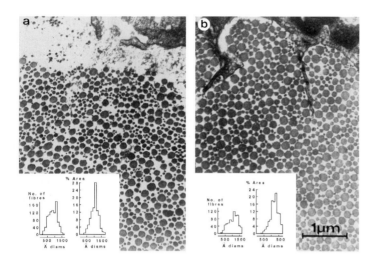

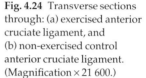

Fig. 4.24 Transverse sections through: (a) exercised anterior cruciate ligament, and (b) non-exercised control anterior cruciate ligament. (Magnification × 21 600.)

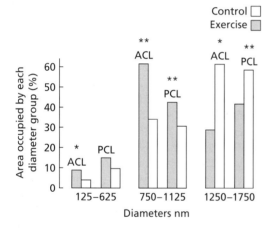

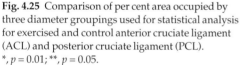

Fig. 4.25 Comparison of per cent area occupied by three diameter groupings used for statistical analysis for exercised and control anterior cruciate ligament (ACL) and posterior cruciate ligament (PCL). *, $p = 0.01$; **, $p = 0.05$.

It is well recognized since the original work of Toole and Lowther (1968) that GAGs have an effect on determining collagen fibril size *in vitro* and this has been confirmed *in vivo* by Parry *et al.* (1982). Merrilees and Flint (1980) demonstrated a change in collagen fibril diameters between the compression and tension regions of the flexor digitorum profundus tendon as it turns 90° around the talus. Amiel *et al.* (1984) have also shown that rabbit cruciate ligaments have more GAGs than the patellar tendon and hence it is likely that GAGs also play an important role in determining collagen fibril populations in cruciate ligaments (see below for further discussion).

SURGICALLY REPAIRED LIGAMENTS

Tipton *et al.* (1970) demonstrated a significant increase in the strength of surgically repaired MCLs of dogs after treadmill exercise training for 6 weeks, after 6 weeks' cast immobilization.

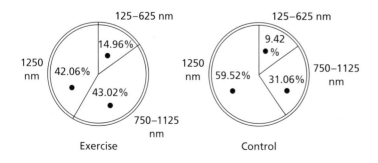

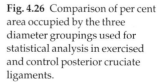

Fig. 4.26 Comparison of per cent area occupied by the three diameter groupings used for statistical analysis in exercised and control posterior cruciate ligaments.

However, they emphasized that at 12 weeks' postsurgery (6 weeks of immobilization and 6 weeks of exercise training) the repair was only approximately 60% that of the normal dogs and results suggested that at least 15–18 weeks of exercise training may be required before a return to 'normal' tensile strength is achieved. Similar observations have been made by Piper and Whiteside (1980), using the MCL of dogs. They observed that mobilized MCL repairs were stronger and stretched out less, i.e. less valgus laxity, than MCL repairs managed by casting and delayed mobilization. This conclusion is supported by the work of Woo *et al*. (1987a, 1987b).

Some insight into the biological mechanisms involved in the repair response with exercise has come from the elegant work of Vailas *et al*. (1981). By using 3H-proline pulse labelling to measure collagen synthesis in rat MCL surgical repairs and coupling this with DNA analyses and tensile testing of repaired ligaments subjected to exercise and non-exercise regimes, they were able to show that treadmill running exercise commencing 2 weeks after surgical repair enhanced the repair and remodelling phase by inducing a more rapid return of cellularity, collagen synthesis and ligament tensile strength to within normal limits. Further, Woo *et al*. (1987b) have demonstrated almost complete return (98%) of structural properties of the transected canine femoral–medial collateral ligament–tibial (FMT) complex at 12 weeks' post-transection without immobilization. Canines immobilized for 6 weeks with the FMT complex tested at 12 weeks, had mean loads to failure of 54% that of the controls. However, the tensile strength of the MCL was only 62% of controls at 48 weeks. This apparent paradox in the non-immobilized dogs was explained by the approximate doubling in CSA of the healing MCL (and hence increased collagen deposition) during the early phases of healing. This repair collagen was most probably small-diameter fibrils and would account for the poor strain performance of the MCL scar collagen and would be similar to the lower curve on Fig. 4.23.

Woo *et al*. (1987a) examined the effects of prolonged immobilization and then mobilization on the rabbit MCL without any surgical inter-vention. Both the structural properties of the FMT complex and the material properties of the MCL were examined. After immobilization, there were significant reductions in the ultimate load and energy-absorbing capabilities of the bone–ligament–bone complex. The MCL became less stiff with immobilization and the femoral and tibial insertion sites showed increased osteoclastic activity, bone resorption and disruption of the normal bone attachment to the MCL. With mobilization, the ultimate load and energy-absorbing capabilities improved but did not return to normal. The stress–strain characteristics of the MCL returned to normal, indicating that the material properties of the collagen in rabbit MCL return relatively quickly after remobilization but that the ligament– bone junction strength return to normal may take many months (see Fig. 4.23).

The detailed biological cellular mechanisms involved in this enhancement and remodelling of the repair are not understood but may involve prostaglandin and cAMP synthesis by fibroblasts subjected to repeated mechanical deformation by exercise.

Amiel *et al*. (1987) have shown that maximal collagen deposition and turnover occurs during the first 3–6 weeks postinjury in the rabbit. Chaudhuri *et al*. (1987) used a Fourier domain directional filtering technique to quantify collagen fibril orientation in repairing ligaments. Results indicated that ligament collagen fibril reorientation does occur in the longitudinal axis of the ligament during remodelling. MacFarlane *et al*. (1989) and Frank *et al*. (1991) have further shown that collagen remodelling of the repairing rabbit MCL appears to be encouraged by early immobilization but after 3 weeks collagen alignment and remodelling appears to be favoured by mobilization.

We have recently completed a study on the repair of the goat ACL. It has almost become an axiom amongst orthopaedic surgeons that the ACL does not repair after injury, even partial injury. This seems to be the case with complete ACL rupture (Grontvedt *et al*. 1996) if there is no continuity in either the synovial membrane ACL sleeve or its contained collagen fibre bundles. However, the repair of partial tears of the ACL (grade 1 and 2) has not been examined carefully in the long term in large animals. To test the healing of the partially torn ACL, we transected the posterolateral bundle of the ACL in 11 adult female goats and tested the ligaments at 12, 24 and 52 weeks and 3 years after surgery as previously described on page 69. Translucent repair tissue was seen filling in the 'wound' region as early as 12 weeks post-hemisection. There was also no difference in the antero-posterior laxity between the hemisected and normal control knees at each time period examined. Load-relaxation and Young's modulus also were not significantly different at each time period; but surprisingly the hemisected-ACL ultimate tensile strength and stiffness at 3 years were significantly higher than at 12 weeks ($p < 0.05$). Also surprising was the fact that at 3 years, the ACL specimens all failed with bone avulsion indicating the repair tissue was very strong and not the weakest link of the bone–ligament–bone complex as one might have expected (see Figs 4.16 and 4.17).

This study emphasizes that under favourable conditions, partial ACL injuries or tears are capable of an adequate tensile strength repair. Perhaps more importantly as far as athletes are concerned the high ultimate tensile strength and stiffness of the 3-year repaired tissue indicates that full structural repair of such an artificial hemi-transection injury model is possible (Ng *et al.* 1996). This work suggests such partial human ACL injuries may be adequately repaired in athletes, (if diagnosed early with MRI examination) which is contrary to current orthopaedic opinion.

With this basic biological knowledge there is now a rationale for the use of early controlled mobilization of patients with ligament trauma. The use of a limited motion cast with an adjustable double-action hinge for the knee joint is now accepted in clinical practice and enhances more rapid repair and remodelling as well as preserving quadriceps muscle bulk and strength. Patients are now usually mobilized early in a limited motion cast for a minimum of 3 weeks with a range of motion from 20 to 60° (Helbing & Burri 1977) rather than the previously empirical time of 6 weeks' immobilization.

Collagen fibril populations in human knee ligaments and grafts

Human ACL autograft quantitative collagen fibril studies

In order to gain some biological insight into collagen repair and remodelling mechanisms within human cruciate ligament grafts, biopsies were obtained from autogenous ACL grafts from patients subsequently requiring arthroscopic

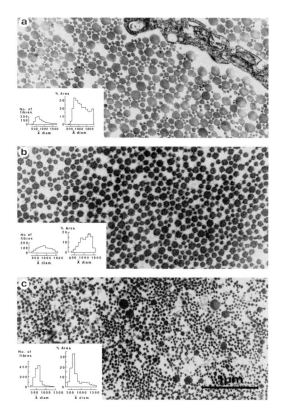

Fig. 4.27 Transverse sections through collagen fibrils of: (a) normal young adult patellar tendon (mean of six biopsies); (b) normal young adult ACL (mean of six biopsies); and (c) Jones' free graft (mean of nine biopsies). (Magnification × 34 100.) The insets show: on the left, the number of fibrils versus diameter; and on the right, per cent area occupied / diameter group. The preponderance of small-diameter fibrils in the graft (c), and large fibrils in the patellar tendon (a), which are not seen in the 'normal' ACL (b), should be noted.

Fig. 4.28 Summary and comparison histograms of collagen fibril profiles for normal tissues used for anterior cruciate ligament (ACL) grafting (patellar tendon [PT, $n = 7$], iliotibial band [ITB, $n = 3$] and semitendinosus [ST, $n = 1$]) with ACL autografts derived from the same tissues expressed as per cent area per diameter group. Large-diameter fibrils > 100 nm are found predominantly in the hamstring (ham.), ST and to a lesser extent in the normal PT. The ITB has a profile not unlike that of the normal ACL. All the autografts— patellar tendon Jones' free ACL grafts (JFG, $n = 39$), hamstring ACL grafts ($n = 9$) and ITB ACL grafts ($n = 15$)—have predominantly small-diameter fibrils. (From Oakes 1993, with permission from Raven Press.)

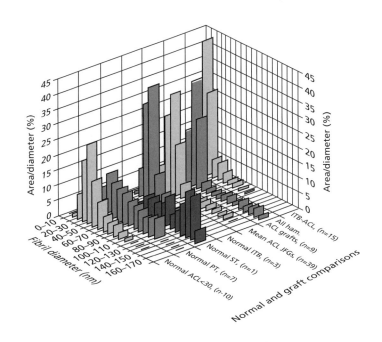

intervention because of stiffness, meniscal and/ or articular cartilage problems or removal of prominent staples used for fixation. Most of the ACL grafts were from the central one-third of the patellar tendon as a free graft ($n = 39$), or in some left attached distally ($n = 8$) and in others the hamstrings ($n = 9$, graft age 10 months to 6 years) or the iliotibial tract was used ($n = 15$, graft age 10 months to 6 years). These biopsies represented approximately 20% of the total free grafts performed over the 3 years of this study. The clinical ACL stability of the biopsy group differed little from the remainder. All had a grade 2–3 pivot shift (jerk) preoperatively (10– 15 mm anterior drawer neutral), eliminated postoperatively in 87% of patients (0.5 mm). Sub-sequent clinical review at 3 years showed an increase in the anterior drawer with a return in 20% of a grade 1 pivot shift.

A total of 39 biopsies have been quantitatively analysed for collagen fibril diameter popula-tions in patients aged 19–42 years. These data were compared with collagen fibril populations obtained from biopsies of cadaver ACLs ($n = 5$)

and also biopsies of ACLs from young (< 30 years, $n = 5$) people who had not sustained a recent ACL injury. Biopsies were also obtained from normal patellar tendons at operation ($n = 7$) (Figs 4.27 and 4.28). Eighteen ACL graft biopsies have been obtained from other surgeons, both nationally and internationally (Oakes *et al.* 1991; Oakes 1993).

The results from the collagen fibril diameter morphometric analysis in all ACL grafts clearly indicated a predominance of small-diameter collagen fibrils (Figs 4.28–4.30). Absence of a 'regular crimping' of collagen fibrils was observed by both light and electron microscopy, as was a less ordered parallel arrangement of fibrils. In most biopsies, capillaries were present and most fibroblasts appeared viable.

Collagen typing of normal human ACL and ACL grafts

Recent biochemical analyses of human patellar tendon autografts *in situ* for 2–10 years indicates a large amount of type III as well as type V col-lagen. This confirmed our suspicion that a large

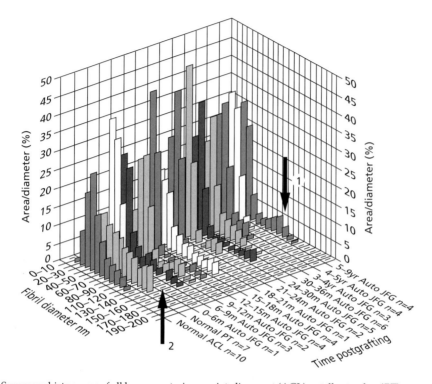

Fig. 4.29 Summary histograms of all human anterior cruciate ligament (ACL) patellar tendon (PT) autografts (*n* = 39) versus time postgrafting compared with normal young ACL (*n* = 10) and normal young PT (*n* = 7) expressed as per cent area per diameter group. The presence of large fibrils (> 100 nm) in the older (5–9-year-old grafts; arrow 1) and the rapid loss of < 100 nm fibrils in the 0–6-month postgraft group (arrow 2), which are present in the donor PT (to the left of arrow 2) should be noted. (From Oakes 1993, with permission from Raven Press.)

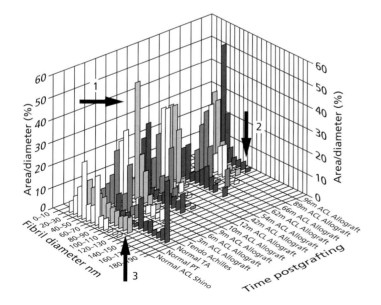

Fig. 4.30 Summary histograms of all human anterior cruciate ligament (ACL) allografts versus time postgrafting compared with normal young ACL, normal patellar tendon (PT), reconstituted tibialis anterior (TA) and Achilles tendons expressed as per cent area per diameter group. The early preponderance of the small fibrils at 3 months postgraft (arrow 1) and their persistence even at 96 months postgraft in the majority of biopsies examined should be noted. Some large fibrils are present (arrow 2) at 96 months, but the majority of the large fibrils present in the donor tissues are removed (to the right of arrow 3). (From Oakes 1993, with permission from Raven Press.)

Table 4.1 Human ACL collagen typing.

	Type I (+/−SD)	Type III (+/−SD)
Normal ACL (N = 10, age 16–40)	71.13 +/− 9.77	28.1 +/− 10.18
Acute ACL rupture (n = 11, age 16–30, < 1-week-old)	65.51 +/− 7.80	33.77 +/− 7.86
Jones' free ACL grafts (n = 9, age 19–27, graft age 9–2yrs)	70.20 +/− 6.75	28.48 +/− 7.02
Iliotibial band ACL grafts (n = 3, age 25–35, graft age 4–10yrs)	60.27 +/− 13.89	39.03 +/− 13.90

amount of collagen in these remodelled grafts at this age may be type III and not type I as is normally found in the patellar tendon and adult ACL (Deacon *et al.* 1991).

We have examined and quantified the types of collagen in the normal ACL and in ACL grafts using quantitative sodium dodecyl sulphate gel densitometry of cyanogen bromide peptides derived from the tissue in question (Chan & Cole 1984). Tissue was obtained from: 10 acute ruptured ACLs (< 1 week old), 10 normal ACLs and nine autogenous patellar tendon grafts (age 3 months to 2 years.).

The normal ACL contained a mean type I collagen content of 71.13 ± 9.77 (SD) and type III content of 28.1 ± 10.18. The acute ACL ruptures had similar type I and III collagen contents as did the patellar tendon grafts (Table 4.1).

The high content of type III collagen in the normal human ACL (28.1%) is surprising and was similar to that found in the patellar tendon autografts and the acute ACL ruptures. This is much higher than that reported by Amiel *et al.* (1984) for normal rabbit ACL. They suggest the high type III content may reflect a wide variety of force vectors that the rabbit ACL is subjected to. These new data may indicate unrecognized or documented previous injury to the 'normal' ACL tissue (Oakes 1993).

Before discussing the biopsy data it is of interest to compare the collagen profiles for the patellar tendon with the normal ACL. It can be seen that the profiles are different in that the dis-

tribution in the patellar tendon is skewed to the right with a small number of large fibrils not present in the normal ACL (Figs 4.27–4.30). Elegant work by Butler *et al.* (1985) has shown that the patellar tendon is significantly stronger than the human ACL, PCL and lateral collateral ligament from the same knee in terms of maximum stress, linear modulus and energy density to maximum strength. The larger fibrils observed in the patellar tendon are not found in the ACL and are an obvious explanation for the stronger biomechanical tensile properties of the normal patellar tendon.

The biopsies from the grafts were obtained from patients with a good to fair rating in terms of a moderate anterior drawer (0–5 mm) and correction of the pivot shift, but both these tests of ACL integrity showed an increasing laxity of the ACL at the 3-year clinical review. The length of time the grafts were *in vivo* prior to biopsy varied from 6 months to 6 years. The collagen fibril population did not alter that much for the older grafts (namely > 3 years), which is not what was hoped for or expected but is in keeping with the observation clinically that the ACL grafts 'stretched out' postoperatively.

The most striking feature of all the biopsies from the autografts, irrespective of whether they were 'free grafts', Jones' grafts, fascia lata, hamstring grafts, and independent of the surgeon, was the invariable prevalence of small-diameter fibrils in amongst a few larger fibrils that probably were the original large-diameter patellar fibrils. The packing of the small fibrils in the grafts was not as tight as is usually observed in the normal patellar tendon (compare Figs 4.27a, c and 4.29, arrows 1 and 2).

It appears from the quantitative collagen fibril observations in this study that the large-diameter fibrils of the original graft are removed and almost entirely replaced by smaller, less well-packed and less well-orientated fibrils than the larger diameter fibrils found in the normal patellar tendon. The smaller diameter fibrils are probably recently synthesized because they are of smaller diameter than those found in the original patellar tendon. Hence the entire collagen matrix of the original patellar tendon is remodelled and replaced with newly synthesized small-diameter collagen fibrils.

Is gentle mechanical loading in the ACL grafts an important stimulus to fibroblast proliferation and collagen deposition? Inadequate mechanical stimulus may occur, especially if grafts are non-isometric and are 'stretched out' by the patient before they have adequate tensile strength. A lax ACL graft may not induce sufficient mechanical loading on graft fibroblasts to alter the GAG or decorin/collagen biosynthesis ratios to favour large-diameter fibril formation. Certainly in this study there was ACL graft laxity which increased postoperatively. This would lend credence to the above notion. However, use of continuous passive motion in grafted primates does not increase the strength of grafts.

Another more likely possibility is that the replacement fibroblasts in the ACL grafts are derived from stem cells from the synovium (and synovial perivascular cells) which are known to synthesize hyaluronate, which in turn favours small-diameter fibril formation (Parry *et al.* 1982). The strong correlation of small-diameter fibrils with a lower tensile strength has been observed by Parry *et al.* (1978) and Shadwick (1990), and the observations in this study would confirm this. Our observations also correlate with the observations of Clancy *et al.* (1981) and Arnoczky *et al.* (1986). The observations by Amiel *et al.* (1989) indicate that collagenase may play a role in the remodelling of ACL tears/grafts.

The conclusion from these ultrastructural observations is that the predominance of small-diameter collagen fibrils (< 7.5 nm) and their poor packing and alignment in *all* the ACL grafts, irrespective of the type of graft (auto- or allograft), their age and the surgeon, may explain the clinical and experimental evidence of a decreased tensile strength in such grafts compared with normal ACL. It appears that in the adult, the replacement fibroblasts in the remodelled ACL graft cannot reform the large-diameter, regularly crimped and tightly packed fibrils seen in the normal ACL, even after 6 years, which was the oldest graft analysed.

The origin of the replacement fibroblasts which remodel the ACL grafts is not known at the moment. It is the author's hunch that they will not come from the actual graft itself although some of these cells may survive due to diffusion. However, the bulk of the stem cells involved in the remodelling process are probably derived from the surrounding synovium and its vasculature.

Beynon *et al.* (1997) mechanically tested a human patellar tendon ACL graft 8 months post-surgery. The stiffness and the ultimate failure load approached that of normal after 8 months of healing and graft remodelling. The antero-posterior (AP) laxity was 1.85 and 1.26 that of the normal knee at 10 and 60° of knee flexion, respectively. This increase in AP laxity (6.3 mm greater than normal) was substantially greater than the 2 mm right-to-left variation in AP laxity seen in subjects with healthy knees. This was also reflected in greater strain values when compared with the normal ACL. Also, energy absorbed to failure was only 53% of the normal ACL. These values of increased strain, increased AP laxity and low energy to failure indicate the poor quality of the remodelled collagen matrix of this ACL and is similar to that of the scar seen in the repairing dog (Woo *et al.* 1987b) and rabbit MCL (Frank *et al.* 1999; see below).

Human ACL allografts

Recent further studies of biopsies obtained from ACL human allografts utilizing fresh frozen Achilles or tibialis anterior tendons, ranging in age from 3 to 54 months, indicated a similar predominance of small-diameter collagen fibrils (Shino *et al.* 1990, 1991, 1995).

Human ACL allograft specimens were studied as above for the autografts with quantitative collagen fibril analyses (Oakes 1993), and were compared with ACL autografts. The allograft specimens were procured at the time of second-look arthroscopy from the superficial region of the mid-zone of ACL grafts after synovial clearage. The grafts used for the ACL reconstruction were usually from fresh frozen allogeneic Achilles or tibialis posterior or anterior tendons and were implanted 3–96 months prior to biopsy.

Thirty-eight patients who had undergone allograft ACL replacement and whose AP stability had been adequately restored were randomly selected. The restored stability of the involved knees was carefully confirmed with both Lachman and pivot shift signs and an objective quantitative knee instability testing apparatus. All of these patients were subjected to second-look arthroscopy as a part of the procedure to remove hardware installed for graft fixation. Thirty-five graft biopsies were obtained from this patient group. Their age ranged from 15 to 37 years at the time of reconstruction.

ACL reconstruction was performed using fresh frozen allografts, 8–9 mm in diameter; part of the Achilles tendon, the tibialis anterior or posterior, peroneal or other thick flexor tendons without any bone attached to their ends were used as an ACL substitute. Postoperatively, the knee was immobilized for 2–5 weeks, then full weight bearing allowed at 2–3 months, jogging recommended at 5–6 months, and full activity allowed at 9–12 months.

The normal tissues used were compared with the normal ACL and the ACL allografts.

NORMAL TISSUES USED FOR ALLOGRAFTS

The reconstituted Achilles tendon demonstrated a large number of fibrils in the 90–140 nm range (40% of total CSA) together with small-diameter fibrils of 30–80 nm. The reconstituted tibialis anterior tendon showed larger diameter fibrils and fewer smaller fibrils than the Achilles tendon.

The large fibrils constituted about 80% of the total fibril CSA. In contrast, the normal ACL had about 85% of its total CSA composed of fibrils < 100 nm, but there were a small number of large fibrils which accounted for about 15% of its total CSA.

ALLOGRAFT RESULTS VERSUS TIME (Fig. 4.30)

By 3 months postoperatively ($n = 2$), there was a predominance of small-diameter fibrils which accounted for > 85% of the total CSA of these biopsies with a 'tail' of larger fibrils making the fibril distribution bimodal in shape. At 6 months ($n = 5$), the fibril distribution was now unimodal with most (*c.* 90%) of the fibril CSA in the < 100 nm diameter group. Fibrils of > 100 nm were obviously fewer than in the 3-month specimens. By 12 months ($n = 12$) almost all the CSA resided in the < 100 nm diameter fibril group and there was almost complete absence of the large > 100 nm fibrils.

This profile persisted in the 13–96-month-old allografts. However, there were two exceptions, where one 12-month-old and one 54-month-old ACL allograft biopsy specimen had significant numbers of large-diameter fibrils in contrast to the earlier observations. In these two specimens the large-diameter fibrils (> 100 nm) accounted for 40% of the total CSA of the collagen fibrils. However, the large-diameter fibrils in these exceptional grafts were smaller in size and had more irregular surfaces than those in the allografts prior to implantation, suggesting perhaps a 'collagenase sculpting' of their exposed surface fibrils.

Parry *et al.* (1978) were the first to describe the bimodal distribution of the collagen fibrils in adult mature tendon collagen that is subjected to high tensile loads. The reconstituted (treated by freezing and thawing) human allografts (Achilles and tibialis tendons) and the normal ACL in this study are also shown to have a bimodal distribution of small- and large-diameter fibrils similar to that described by Parry and colleagues in a large range of other tissues.

Most ACL allograft biopsies also demonstrated a bimodal distribution of large and small fibrils similar to the 'normal reconstituted' tendons up until about 6 months postimplantation. However, after this time the distribution became more unimodal, such that there was an increasing predominance of small-diameter fibrils with a concomitant and progressive loss of the larger 'host tendon' fibrils. It is these larger fibrils in the 'normal' tendon that are responsible for a large percentage of the tendon collagen CSA and for the very high tensile strength of these tendons; the tensile strength exhibited is probably due to the high density of intermolecular collagen cross-links. These observations suggest, at the least, that most of the original large-diameter fibrils in the ACL allografts are replaced by newly synthesized smaller diameter collagen fibrils (or undergo disaggregation, see below). The loss of the large-diameter fibrils from 6 months and older allografts and the predominance of the small-diameter fibrils seen in this study is the most likely explanation for the dramatic reduction in tensile strength of ACL allografts, and hence the observed increased AP laxity in a previous animal study by Shino *et al.* (1984).

These observations parallel those described above for ACL autografts, which also demonstrated within 6 months postimplantation the loss of large-diameter collagen fibrils of patellar tendon origin. It could be concluded, therefore, that the remodelling process has a similar timeframe in both ACL tendon allografts and patellar tendon ACL autografts. It further suggests that similar mechanisms of collagen degradation and neosynthesis of collagen may be occurring by the invading synovial stem cells which repopulate the ACL graft almost immediately after surgery.

A valid criticism of these studies could be that all the biopsies were obtained from the superficial region of the grafts and that this may not be representative of the bulk of the graft collagen. However, in the previous autograft study the biopsies were usually obtained from the middle of the autografts and the observations were no different from those in this allograft study. This suggests that the superficial region from which the biopsies were taken in this study is representative of the graft collagen.

Awaiting the appearance of large fibrils with close packing (perhaps under a Wolff's law tensile stimulus) as seen in normal ligament and tendon is probably futile. There is no current ultrastructural evidence available that large-diameter fibrils will eventually be formed and become a large proportion of the CSA of long-term ACL grafts or even that the packing of the small-diameter fibrils becomes closer within these grafts. If denser collagen fibril packing could be achieved, this might possibly enhance the collagen fibril CSA per unit area, which in turn might possibly increase the tensile strength of the graft by increased interfibril interactions as already discussed. The reason denser packing of fibrils is not seen in allo- or autografts may be due to an increased synthesis of small proteoglycans, particularly decorin and hyaluronan, preventing large collagen fibril formation (Scott 1990; see below).

It should be also mentioned that the conclusions drawn in this discussion are based on the assumption that large collagen fibrils of the allograft tendons do not undergo a process of disaggregation into smaller fibrils similar to that described by glycerol treatment of mature collagen fibrils, which is reversible (Leonardi *et al.* 1983). This is a possibility which must be seriously considered but is very difficult to verify experimentally without rigorous immuno-electron microscopy.

The remodelling of collagen in tendon auto-, allo- and xenografts has been elegantly quantified by the now classic work of Klein *et al.* (1972). They noticed at 3 months that xenografts lost 99%, allografts lost 63% and autografts 54% of their original collagen, demonstrating a clear antigenic influence on collagen turnover which was, however, still substantial—even in the autografts at 3 months. The remodelling of collagen during medial ligament repair in the rabbit has also been shown to be prolonged in that the collagen concentration takes many months to approach normal levels (Klein *et al.* 1972) and appears to be similar in larger animals (Woo *et al.* 1987a).

The observations and conclusions in this auto/allograft review throw into question the current timeframes for rehabilitation. It is generally concluded by most knee surgeons that the graft tissue will eventually mature, given enough time, and that graft tensile strength will also increase with time, especially if the athlete waits for up to 1 year for graft maturation. The observations in this study do not support this notion that graft tensile strength will gradually increase with time. However, collagen cross-link maturation could be very important in these grafts and this may be a mechanism for restoring some graft tensile strength even when the collagen fibrils remain of small diameter. Observations by Butler et al. (1987) that primate ACL autografts and ACL allografts using the patellar tendon were only about 30% the strength of normal ACL at 12 months postimplantation, strongly support the quantitative fibril observations outlined in this human auto/allograft study.

Comprehensive detailed clinical studies by Shelbourne (Shelbourne & Nitz 1990; Shelbourne & Davis 1999), and more recently by Barber-Westin et al. (1999), have demonstrated (contrary to expectations with the preceeding ACL graft small fibril data) that early accelerated ACL rehabilitation programmes have not led to increased AP laxity, which is a paradox when compared to the results of Beynon et al. (1997). It may be speculated that the early aggressive ACL rehabilitation advocated by Shelbourne may limit the collagen loss and may assist in early collagen fibril orientation and deposition, and hence may help to explain the lack of AP laxity with these programmes.

Excellent comprehensive reviews of all aspects of human ACL reconstruction are recommended further reading of this complex topic (Frank & Jackson 1997; Fu et al. 1999, 2000). ACL graft selection has been recently reviewed by Bartlett et al. (2001).

Goat ACL patellar tendon autograft collagen remodelling: quantitative collagen fibril analyses over 3 years

The aim of this study (Ng et al. 1995a, 1995b, 1996a, 1996b) was to quantify in detail the collagen fibril remodelling process in adult goat patellar tendon ACL autografts over a 3-year timeframe. Eleven mature female adult goats were used in this study. The middle one-third of the right patellar tendon was harvested and used as an ACL graft. The animals were sacrificed at the following time intervals: 6 weeks ($n = 3$), 12 weeks ($n = 2$), 24 weeks ($n = 2$), 52 weeks ($n = 3$) and 3 years ($n = 1$). The ACL grafts were then obtained and prepared for quantitative ultrastructural collagen fibril analyses.

The normal ACL ($t = 0, n = 5$) and ACL patellar tendon grafts ($n = 11$) were divided into thirds and 1 mm thick sections were cut from the femoral, middle and tibial thirds. This section was then cut into a strip and four sections obtained: two were deemed superficial and contained a synovial surface and two were deemed deep. The collagen fibril profiles were directly quantified from electron micrograph negatives using a specifically designed software program for automated computerized image analysis. The frequency of fibrils within 20 diameter size classes and the percentage area occupied for each diameter group of fibrils were automatically calculated as a mean (Fig. 4.31).

The results of the study were as follows:
1 Normal adult goat ACL, $t = 0$. The distribution was clearly bimodal with a large number of small fibrils < 100 nm in diameter and a group of larger fibrils > 100 nm in diameter (Fig. 4.32a). A small number of large fibrils of > 100 nm contributed about 45% of the total collagen fibril area; these large fibrils seen in the adult goat ACL are not seen in the normal adult human ACL.
2 Normal adult goat patellar tendon, $t = 0$. The collagen fibril distribution was quite different to the ACL with a more unimodal distribution. There were less small-diameter fibrils and more larger diameter fibrils > 100 nm than in the ACL, and these latter fibrils contributed 65% of the total collagen fibril area (Fig. 4.32b).
3 Patellar tendon ACL graft: tibial region versus femoral region (Figs 4.33 and 4.34). At 6 weeks postsurgery there was a large increase in the number of small-diameter collagen fibrils (< 100 nm) which was greatest at the tibial end. This number

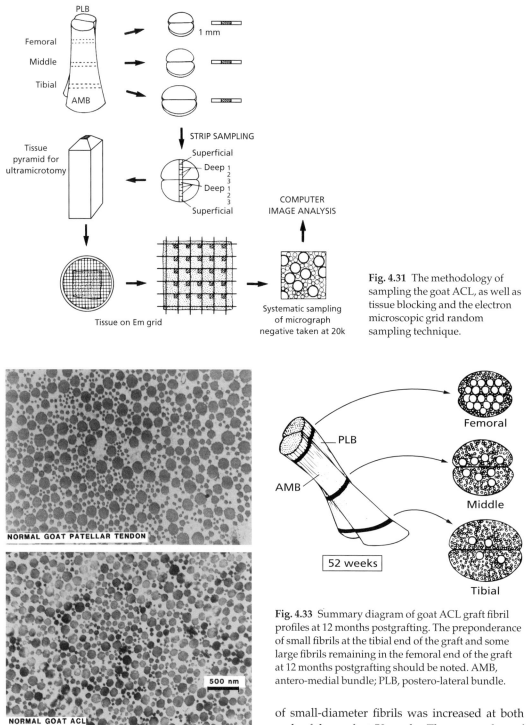

Fig. 4.31 The methodology of sampling the goat ACL, as well as tissue blocking and the electron microscopic grid random sampling technique.

(a)

NORMAL GOAT PATELLAR TENDON

(b)

NORMAL GOAT ACL

500 nm

Fig. 4.32 Electron micrographs of: (a) normal adult goat ACL, and (b) normal adult goat patellar tendon.

Fig. 4.33 Summary diagram of goat ACL graft fibril profiles at 12 months postgrafting. The preponderance of small fibrils at the tibial end of the graft and some large fibrils remaining in the femoral end of the graft at 12 months postgrafting should be noted. AMB, antero-medial bundle; PLB, postero-lateral bundle.

of small-diameter fibrils was increased at both ends of the graft at 52 weeks. There was a loss of the large-diameter fibrils (> 100 nm) which could be seen at 6 weeks, and at 52 weeks only a few

Fig. 4.34 Three-dimensional histograms of normal goat patellar tendon (PT) and anterior cruciate ligament (ACL) patellar tendon autografts at $t = 0, 3, 6, 12, 24$ and 48 weeks in relation to the femoral, middle and tibial regions of the ACL autografts. The vertical axis is the ratio of large fibrils (> 100 nm) to small fibrils (< 100 nm). Large fibrils are lost from the tibial end of the graft as early as 6 weeks postgrafting but some large fibrils still remain at the femoral end of the graft at 48 weeks (arrow 2). The predominance of large fibrils in the original PT used as the donor graft (arrow 1) should be noted.

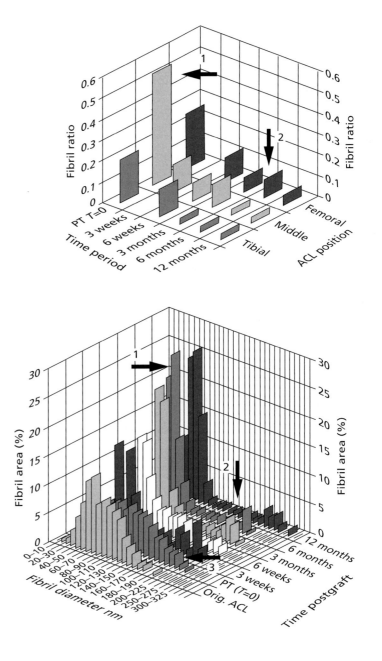

Fig. 4.35 Three-dimensional histograms of normal goat patellar tendon (PT), anterior cruciate ligament (ACL) and ACL autografts expressed as per cent area covered by the collagen fibrils versus age and fibril diameter. Again there is progressive loss of the large-diameter fibrils and the rapid replacement of these large fibrils (arrow 3) as early as 6 weeks after grafting, with a predominance of small fibrils at 12 months postgrafting (arrow 1). The lack of large fibrils at 12 months postgrafting (arrow 2) should be noted.

large fibrils remained at the femoral region. This is reflected if the ratio of large > 100 nm fibrils to small < 100 nm fibrils is plotted (Fig. 4.35).

4 Patellar tendon ACL graft superficial region versus deep region. The major observation was the complete loss of the large-diameter fibrils at 1 year from the superficial regions of the graft. There was also a concomitant increase in the num-ber of small-diameter fibrils in the deep region at 52 weeks not seen in the superficial regions. If one plots the ratio of large-diameter fibrils > 100 nm to small-diameter fibrils < 100 nm, the major fall in the ratio is seen in the superficial region reflecting the complete removal of the large-diameter fibrils in the superficial regions of the grafts at 52 weeks (Figs 4.32, 4.35 and 4.36).

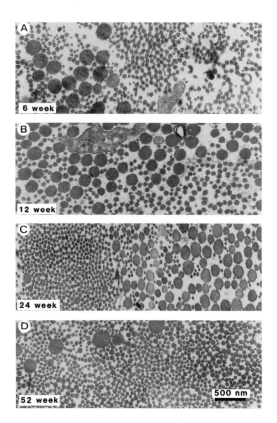

Fig. 4.36 Representative electron micrographs of ACL and patellar tendon autografts: (a) at 6 weeks, (b) at 12 weeks, (c) at 24 weeks, and (d) at 52 weeks postgrafting. The progressive loss of the large-diameter fibrils at $t = 0$ (see Fig. 4.32b) and the accumulation of small-diameter fibrils with increasing graft age should be noted.

The collagen fibril profile for each time group was compared to the control ACL and patellar tendon with Kolomogorov–Smirnov analyses. Differences were found between the patellar tendon collagen profile with the ACL grafts with the 12-, 24- and 52-week groups ($P = 0.005$, 0.07 and 0.1, respectively). All the grafts except the 6-week group contained mainly small fibrils (< 100 nm). The large fibrils were not repopulated in the 1-year grafts, but in the one graft studied at 3 years large fibrils > 100 nm were present. A positive correlation ($r = 0.6$, $P = 0.07$) was found between the percentage of fibrils of > 100 nm diameter with Young's modulus of the grafts, which was tested in a separate study.

This study has determined the anatomical regions of the ACL graft that undergo remodelling and that this process continues for up to 3 years postgrafting. This remodelling process changes the collagen fibril profile of the original patellar tendon to one containing a greater proportion of small-diameter fibrils. The remodelling process occurs from the most outer areas inwards, and is more vigorous in the tibial region of the graft. This would be consistent with synovial revascularization. The rapid depletion of the large fibrils in the grafts as early as 6 weeks is also consistent with the dramatic decrease in mechanical and material properties of such grafts (Fig. 4.35). This collagen fibril study in the goat also parallels that in the human ACL patellar tendon grafts and appears to be a useful model to follow collagen remodelling in the ACL graft.

A 3-year biomechanical and viscoelastic study of patellar tendon autografts for ACL reconstruction

In this study, 27 adult female goats were tested—four served as controls and the others received an autograft to the right knee with each left knee serving as an additional control (Ng *et al.* 1995a, 1995b). The animals with grafts were tested at 0 weeks ($n = 4$), 6 weeks ($n = 4$), 12 weeks ($n = 4$), 24 weeks ($n = 3$), 1 year ($n = 5$) and 3 years ($n = 3$) after surgery. The AP laxity of the knee joint, load–relaxation, and structural and mechanical properties of the graft were tested.

The AP laxity was significantly greater than that of the controls for all groups except at 3 years where the AP laxity almost approached normal. The mechanism of this return of AP laxity to near normal is not known but may be due to stiffening of the collateral ligament complexes or may be due to tibial and femoral condyle remodelling. Load–relaxation was greater than that of the control ACLs, but in the 1- and 3-year grafts load–relaxation was less than that of the patellar tendons with 5 min of sustained loading. Between 12 and 52 weeks, the stiffness and the modulus of the grafts were 44 and 49% those of the control

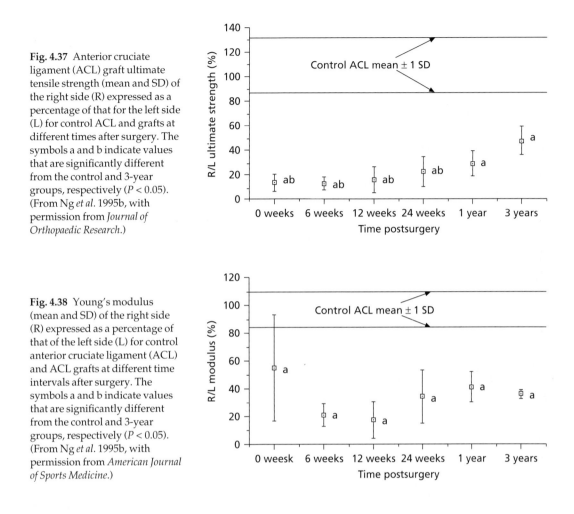

Fig. 4.37 Anterior cruciate ligament (ACL) graft ultimate tensile strength (mean and SD) of the right side (R) expressed as a percentage of that for the left side (L) for control ACL and grafts at different times after surgery. The symbols a and b indicate values that are significantly different from the control and 3-year groups, respectively ($P < 0.05$). (From Ng *et al.* 1995b, with permission from *Journal of Orthopaedic Research*.)

Fig. 4.38 Young's modulus (mean and SD) of the right side (R) expressed as a percentage of that of the left side (L) for control anterior cruciate ligament (ACL) and ACL grafts at different time intervals after surgery. The symbols a and b indicate values that are significantly different from the control and 3-year groups, respectively ($P < 0.05$). (From Ng *et al.* 1995b, with permission from *American Journal of Sports Medicine*.)

ligaments, respectively; the modulus was 37 and 46% that of the control ACLs and patellar tendons, respectively (Figs 4.37 and 4.38). The persistent inferior mechanical performance at 3 years suggests that ACL grafts in the goat may never attain normal ACL strength.

A 3-year study of collagen type and cross-links for ACL patellar tendon autografts in a goat model

The collagen matrix provides the tensile strength of ligaments. Previous animal studies have shown that ACL patellar tendon autografts contain mainly small-diameter collagen fibrils (< 100 nm) at 1 year postsurgery. The long-term collagen fibril profile and biochemical changes are not clear. This study examined goat ACL patellar tendon autografts up to 3 years postsurgery for collagen type and hydroxypyridinium (HP) cross-link density (Ng *et al.* 1995a, 1996a).

Twenty-two mature female goats received an ACL patellar tendon autograft to the right knee and were tested at 6 weeks ($n = 5$), 12 weeks ($n = 4$), 24 weeks ($n = 5$), 1 year ($n = 5$) and 3 years ($n = 3$). Two in each group were assigned for collagen typing and HP analyses. Two normal animals served as controls for collagen typing and HP analyses.

Type III collagen analyses with SDS gel electrophoresis showed an increase from 6 to 24 weeks and then decreased afterwards. At 3 years, the

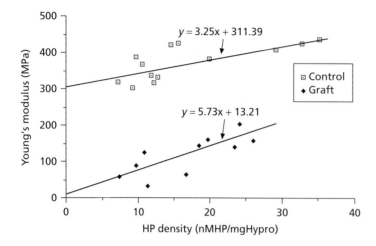

Fig. 4.39 The relationship between hydroxypyridinium (HP) cross-link density and Young's modulus of the ACL autografts ($r = 0.8$) and control ACL ($r = 0.7$). A significant positive correlation is shown for both tissues. The linear regression lines that predict the Young's moduli of ACL autografts and ACL controls from HP cross-link density are also shown. Hypro, hydroxproline. (From Ng *et al.* 1996a, with permission from *Journal of Orthopaedic Research*.)

grafts contained similar type III collagen amounts as the control ACL; the collagen was distributed generally throughout the grafts (not just in the perifascicular regions) as in the normal patellar tendon, as demonstrated by immunofluorescent labelling of the grafts with specific type III collagen antibodies.

The hydroxypyridinium cross-link density was low in the 6-, 12- and 24-week groups, but increased in the 1- and 3-year groups. The mean hydroxypyridinium cross-link density in the grafts was similar to the two control ACLs at less than 24 weeks, but at 1 and 3 years the hydroxypyridinium cross-link density was increased ($P < 0.09$). The hydroxypyridinium cross-link density of the left ACL of the unoperated goats was higher than the two controls, which could be due to the change in loading to the left knee in these animals (Fig. 4.39). A negative correlation was found between the percentage type III collagen and Young's modulus, but this was not significant.

A significant positive correlation ($P = 0.01$) was found between the hydroxypyridinium cross-link density and Young's modulus in both the ACL grafts ($r = 0.8$) and controls ($r = 0.7$). This is the first correlation to be made between a measurable biochemical parameter and a biomechanical parameter for ACL grafts and is very important in determining ACL graft tensile strength.

The grafts and control ACLs had comparable mean hydroxypyridinium cross-link densities but different Young's moduli, which implies hydroxypyridinium cross-link density is not the only determinant for material strength. Other factors such as collagen fibril size, density of packing and orientation may affect the Young's modulus. However, the good correlation on regression analysis suggests the hydroxypyridinium cross-link density may be an important indicator for ACL material strength. A previous study in MCL scars in rabbits has also demonstrated a positive relationship between hydroxypyridinium cross-link density and the failure stress of ligament scar (Frank *et al.* 1994, 1995). Chan *et al.* (1998) have also demonstrated a high correlation with pyridinoline content and failure loads with the healing patellar tendon in the rat.

These two similar observations in different species and different tissues indicates that hydroxypyridinium cross-link density is one of the important determinates for the tensile strength of ligament repair and during ACL graft remodelling. We currently do not understand the biological and mechanical factors that control collagen cross-linking and hence clinical therapies to improve and enhance collagen cross-link density are not yet available. There have been no studies on human ACL graft tissues and the hydroxypyridinium cross-link density to date.

Enhancement of ligament/tendon repair using tissue engineering technologies

Because of the long delay in achieving adequate tensile strength in ligament and tendon repairs to withstand the imposed tensile forces of daily living, researchers and clinicians have explored means to not only hasten the repair process in its three phases (as described above), but also to improve the quality of the repair scar tissue, which is known in the adult to be of poor mechanical quality. For example the normal rabbit MCL when cut surgically heals with the usual phases and a hypervascular disorganized scar tissue is left that is then remodelled over many weeks to years. Biomechanical testing of this scar tissue even at 1 year postinjury reveals it to be permanently weaker and less stiff than the normal MCL on both a structural and material basis. If the two ends of the ligament are opposed by sutures after severance and the gap minimized, the MCL can heal structurally to about 70–80% of the strength and structural stiffness of the normal MCL; but if a gap is left the healing is about 40–50% of the normal MCL. On a material basis (i.e. per CSA) in both the opposed and gap situations, the scar tissue only reaches a maximum of about 30% of normal MCL strength after years of healing (Frank *et al.* 1999).

The use of growth factors to attempt to enhance the healing phases of ligament and tendon has been pursued over the last decade since the isolation of growth factors such as transforming growth factor beta (TGF-β), insulin-like growth factor I (IGF-I) and IGF-II and also basic fibroblast growth factor (bFGF). These growth factors have been used both singly and in combinations using various delivery modes. The results have been rather disappointing in that more collagen can be deposited but it is not well organized and the collagen fibrils are usually of small diameter and hence does not lead to any long-term improvement of the quality of the repair tissue.

The use of mesenchyme stem cells is a useful strategy if the matrix synthetic capacity of these undifferentiated cells can be harnessed to enhance collagen deposition and its remodelling in the early phases of the healing response. The use of these cells is still in its early phases although results are encouraging (Young *et al.* 1998; Awad *et al.* 1999).

During the healing process in ligaments, Frank *et al.* (1999) noted several specific problems with the rabbit MCL scar tissue, which appeared to have mechanical implications (i.e. flaws, decreased collagen cross-links and persistence of small-diameter collagen fibrils). The latter has been identified in this chapter as the probable key explanation for the poor biomechanical performance of human and goat ACL auto- and allografts. The role of the small leucine-rich proteoglycans, such as decorin, fibromodulin and lumican, in controlling collagen fibrillogenesis *in vitro* has been well documented. Decorin stands out as an important molecule in controlling collagen fibril assembly (Vogel & Trotter 1987; Birk *et al.* 1995; Weber *et al.* 1996; Danielson *et al.* 1997).

Based on these and other observations, Frank and his co-workers hypothesized that inhibition of decorin expression during the early phases of ligament healing may enhance the size of newly synthesized collagen fibrils. They used an antisense method using binding of oligodeoxynucleotides to target decorin mRNA in collaboration with Nakamura *et al.* (1998). Remarkably, using this technology they were able to demonstrate that most antisense-treated scars contained bundles of aligned collagen with some restoration of the normal collagen crimp pattern. Even more remarkable was the appearance of large-diameter collagen fibrils in five of the six antisense-treated scars. Collagen fibril diameter analysis of average collagen fibril sizes for the antisense-treated scars, sense control scars, injection control scars and normal MCL were: 104.7 ± 51.1, 74.8 ± 11.00, 78.2 ± 11.9 and 189.1 ± 104.0 nm, respectively (Fig. 4.40). Correlated with these collagen fibril observations was an increase in the mechanical quality of the scar tissue. In other words, antisense scars were significantly (18–22%) less susceptible to elongation (creep) during low stress creep testing than both sense control and injection control scars. They failed at

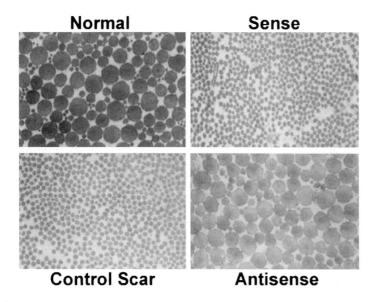

Fig. 4.40 A composite TEM of transverse sections of collagen fibrils in normal adult rabbit MCL (upper left) versus three 6-week healing scar groups: injected decorin 'sense' controls (upper right), injected control scar (bottom left) and antisense–decorin treated experimentals (bottom right). Note that five of the six antisense-treated 6-week MCL scars contained some patches of larger fibrils, as shown here, whilst none of the control scars contained any large fibrils. (From Frank *et al.* 1999, with permission from *Journal of Science and Medicine in Sport.*)

14.9 ± 6.62 MPa on average, which was significantly stronger (by 83–85%) when compared to both sense control (8.07 ± 3.45 MPa) and injection control scars (8.16 ± 3.86 MPa) (Fig. 4.41) (Frank *et al.* 1999).

This exciting work is the first to demonstrate that collagen fibril size can be manipulated during healing and can also improve the mechanical strength of the repair. This new knowledge may translate in the future to clinical therapies which may be able to more rapidly improve ligament and tendon tensile strength during the complex phases of healing.

Acknowledgements

The author is grateful to Dr Michael Benjamin, University of Cardiff for Fig. 4.1 and to Professor A.W. Parker for the use of Fig. 4.32 and also to Mrs Sue Simpson for preparation of the diagrams in the text. Thanks also go to orthopaedic colleagues Owen Deacon and Iain Mclean and other Australian orthopaedic surgeons for their continued interest in supplying human ACL graft biopsies and for their collaboration with the goat ACL autograft work.

References

Akeson, W.H., Amiel, D., Abel, M.F. *et al.* (1987) Effects of immobilization on joints. *Clinical Orthopaedics and Related Research* **219**, 28–37.

Amiel, D., Akeson, W.H., Harwood, F.L. & Frank, C.B. (1983) Stress deprivation effect on the metabolic turnover of the medial collateral ligament collagen: a comparison between nine and 12-week immobilization. *Clinical Orthopaedics and Related Research* **172**, 265–270.

Amiel, D., Frank, C., Harwood, F., Fronek, J. & Akeson, W. (1984) Tendons and ligaments: a morphological and biochemical comparison. *Journal of Orthopaedic Research* **1**, 257–265.

Amiel, D., Frey, C., Woo, S.L.-Y., Harwood, F. & Akeson, W. (1985) Value of hyaluronic acid in the prevention of contracture formation. *Clinical Orthopaedics and Related Research* **196**, 306–311.

Amiel, D., Frank, C.B., Harwood, F.L., Akeson, W.H. & Kleiner, J.B. (1987) Collagen alteration in medial collateral ligament healing in a rabbit model. *Connective Tissue Research* **16**, 357–366.

Amiel, D., Ishizue, K.K., Harwood, F.L., Kitayashi, L. & Akeson, W. (1989) Injury of the anterior cruciate ligament: the role of collagenase in ligament degeneration. *Journal of Orthopaedic Research* **7**, 486–493.

Aoki, M., Ogiwara, N., Ohta, T. & Nabeta, Y. (1998) Early active motion and weightbearing after cross-stitch Achilles tendon repair. *American Journal of Sports Medicine* **26**, 794–800.

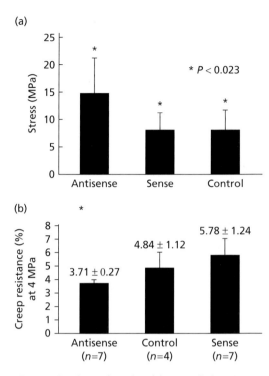

Fig. 4.41 Mechanical results of the 6-week decorin–antisense experiment. (a) Stress at the failure of antisense-treated scars was significantly greater than controls. (b) Creep testing at 4 MPa revealed that antisense-treated scars elongated significantly less than control scars and sense-injected scars after comparable stress histories *in vitro*. Note that all scars, including antisense-treated experimentals, remain inferior to normal ligaments in terms of both their strength and their creep resistance. Further improvement is required to approach normal ligament behaviour. (From Frank *et al*. 1999, with permission from *Journal of Science and Medicine in Sport*.)

Archambault, J.M., Wiley, J.P. & Bray, R.C. (1995) Exercise loading of tendons and the development of overuse injuries. A review of the current literature. *Sports Medicine* **20**, 77–79.

Arnoczky, S.P., Warren, R.F. & Ashlock, M.A. (1986) Replacement of the anterior cruciate ligament by an allograft. *Journal of Bone and Joint Surgery* **63A**, 376–385.

Awad, H.A., Butler, D.L., Bovin, G.P. *et al*. (1999) Autologous mesenchymal stem cell-mediated repair of tendon. *Tissue Engineering* **5**, 267–277.

Barber-Westin, S., Noyes, F.R. & Heckman, T.P. (1999) The effect of exercise and rehabilitation on anterior-posterior knee displacements after anterior cruciate ligament autograft reconstruction. *American Journal of Sports Medicine* **27**, 84–93.

Bartlett, R.J., Clatworthy, M.G. & Nguyen, T.N.V. (2001) Graft selection in reconstruction of the anterior cruciate ligament. Review article. *Journal of Bone and Joint Surgery* **83B**, 625–634.

Benjamin, M. & Evans, E.J. (1990) Fibrocartilage. A review. *Journal of Anatomy* **171**, 1–15.

Benjamin, M. & Ralphs, J.R. (1995) Development and functional anatomy of tendons and ligaments. In: *Repetitive Motion Disorders of the Upper Extremity* (Gordon, S.L., Blair, S.J. & Fine, L.J., eds). American Academy of Orthopaedic Surgeons, Rosemont, IL: 185–203.

Benjamin, M., Evans, E.J. & Copp, L. (1986) The histology of tendon attachments in man. *Journal of Anatomy* **149**, 89–100.

Benjamin, M., Qin, S. & Ralphs, J.R. (1995) Fibrocartilage associated with human tendons and their pulleys. *Journal of Anatomy* **187**, 625–633.

Beynon, B.D., Risberg, M., Tjomskand, O. *et al*. (1997) Evaluation of knee joint laxity and the structural properties of the anterior cruciate ligament graft in the human. A case report. *American Journal of Sports Medicine* **25**, 203–206.

Binkley, J.M. & Peat, M. (1986) The effects of immobilization on the ultrastructure and mechanical properties of the medial collateral ligament of rats. *Clinical Orthopaedics and Related Research* **203**, 301–308.

Birk, D.E., Nurminskaya, M.V. & Zycband, E.I. (1995) Collagen fibrillogenesis *in situ*: fibril segments undergo post-depositional modifications resulting in linear and lateral growth during matrix development. *Trends in Cell Biology* **8**, 404–410.

Butler, D.L., Grood, E.S, Noyes, F.R. *et al*. (1987) Mechanical properties of primate vascularized vs. nonvascularized patellar tendon grafts; changes over time. *Journal of Orthopaedic Research* **7**, 68–79.

Butler, D.L., Grood, E.S., Noyes, F.R. & Zernicke, R.F. (1979) Biomechanics of ligaments and tendons. In: *Exercise and Sports Sciences Reviews*, Vol. 6 (Hutton, R.S., ed.). Franklin Institute Press, Washington, DC: 125–181.

Butler, D.L., Kay, M.D. & Stouffer, D.C. (1985) Comparison of material properties in fascicle-bone units from human patellar tendon and knee ligaments. *Journal of Biomechanics* **18**, 1–8.

Cabaud, H.E., Feagin, J.F. & Rodkey, W.G. (1980) Acute anterior cruciate ligament injury and augmented repair: experimental studies. *American Journal of Sports Medicine* **8**, 79–86.

Caterson, B. & Lowther, D.A. (1978) Changes in the metabolism of the proteoglycan from sheep articular cartilage in response to mechanical stress. *Biochemica Biophysica Acta* **540**, 412–422.

Chan, B.P., Fu, S.C., Qin, L., Rolf, C. & Chan, K.M. (1998) Pyridinoline in relation to ultimate stress of the patellar tendon during healing: an animal study. *Journal of Orthopaedic Research* **16**, 597–603.

Chan, D. & Cole, W. (1984) *Analytical Biochemistry* **139**, 322–328.

Chaudhuri, S., Nguyen, H., Rangayyan, R.M., Walsh, S. & Frank, C.B. (1987) A Fourier domain directional filtering method for analysis of collagen alignment in ligaments. *IEEE Transactions of Biomedical Engineering* **34**, 509–518.

Chun, K.J., Butler, D.B., Bukovec, M.J. *et al.* (1989) Spatial variation in material properties in fascicle-bone units from human patellar tendon. *Transactions of Orthopaedic Research Society* **14**, 214.

Clancy, W.G., Narechania, R.G., Rosenberg, T.D., Gmeiner, J.G., Wisnefske, D.D. & Lange, T.A. (1981) Anterior and posterior cruciate reconstruction in Rhesus monkeys. An histological microangiographic and biochemical analysis. *Journal of Bone and Joint Surgery* **63A**, 1270–1284.

Clement, D.B., Taunton J.E. & Smart, G.W. (1984) Achilles tendinitis and peritendinitis: aetiology and treatment. *American Journal of Sports Medicine* **12**, 179–184.

Coleman, B.D., Khan, K., Kiss, Z.S., Bartlett, J., Young, D.A. & Wark, J.D. (2000) Open and arthroscopic patellar tenotomy for chronic patellar tendinopathy. *American Journal of Sports Medicine* **28**, 183–190.

Cooke, J.L., Khan, K.M., Harcourt, P.R. *et al.* (1997) A cross-sectional study of 100 athletes with jumper's knee managed conservatively and surgically. *British Journal of Sports Medicine* **31**, 332–336.

Danhers, L.E., Banes, A.J. & Burridge, K.W. (1986) The relationship of actin to ligament contraction. *Clinical Orthopaedics and Related Research* **210**, 246–251.

Daniel, D.M., Akeson, W.H. & O'Connor, J.J. (1990) *Knee Ligaments. Structure, Function, Injury and Repair.* Raven Press, New York.

Danielson, K.G., Baribault, H., Holmes, D.F., Graham, H., Kadler, K.E. & Iozzo, R.V. (1997) Target disruption of decorin leads to abnormal collagen fibril morphology and skin fragility. *Journal of Cell Biology* **136**, 729–743.

Deacon, O.W., McLean, I.D., Oakes, B.W., Cole, W.G., Chan, D. & Knight, M. (1991) Ultrastructural and collagen typing analyses of autogenous ACL grafts—an update. In: *Proceedings of the International Knee Society, May 1991*. Toronto.

Diamant, J., Keller, A., Baer, E., Litt, M. & Arridge, R.G.C. (1972) Collagen: ultrastructure and its relation to mechanical properties as a function of ageing. *Proceedings of the Royal Society of London, Series B* **180**, 293–315.

Engstrom, C.M., Hampson, B.A., Williams, J. & Parker, A.W. (1985) Muscle–tendon relations in runners. In: *Abstract Proceedings: Australian Sports Medicine Federation National Conference, Ballarat, 1985*: 56.

Enwemeka, C.S. (1989) The effects of therapeutic ultrasound on tendon healing. *American Journal of Physical Medicine and Rehabilitation* **68**, 283–287.

Enwemeka, C.S., Rodriguez, O., Gall, N.G. & Walsh, N.E. (1990) Morphometric analysis of collagen fibril populations in HeNe laser photostimulated tendons. *Journal of Clinical Laser Medicine and Surgery* **8**, 151–156.

Evans, E.J., Benjamin, M. & Pemberton, D.J. (1990) Fibrocartilage in the attachment zones of the quadriceps tendon and patellar ligament of man. *Journal of Anatomy* **171**, 155–162.

Fitton-Jackson, S. & Bassett, C.A.L. (1980) The response of skeletal tissues to pulsed magnetic fields. In: *Tissue Culture in Medical Research*, Vol. 2 (Richards, R.J. & Ranan, K.T., eds). Pergamon Press, Oxford: 21–29.

Frank, C. (1999) The pathophysiology of ligaments. In: *Orthopaedic Knowledge Update: Sports Medicine*, Vol. 2 (Arendt, E.A., ed.). American Academy of Orthopaedic Surgeons, Rosemont, IL: 29–36.

Frank, C. & Jackson, D.W. (1997) The science of reconstruction of the anterior cruciate ligament. Current concepts review. *Journal of Bone and Joint Surgery* **79A**, 1556–1576.

Frank, C., Schachar, N., Dittrich, D., Shrive, N., De Haas, W. & Edwards, G. (1983a) Electromagnetic stimulation of ligament healing in rabbits. *Clinical Orthopaedics and Related Research* **175**, 263–272.

Frank, C., Woo, S.L.-Y., Amiel, D., Gomez, M.A., Harwood, F.L. & Akeson, W.H. (1983b) Medial collateral ligament healing: a multidisciplinary assessment in rabbits. *American Journal of Sports Medicine* **11**, 379–389.

Frank, C.B., Eyre, D.R. & Shrive, N.G. (1994) Hydroxypyridinium cross-link deficiency in ligament scar. *Transactions of Orthopaedic Research Society* **19**, 13.

Frank, C., MacFarlane, B., Edwards, P., Rangayyan, R., Liu, Z.-Q., Walsh, S. & Bray, R. (1991) A quantitative analysis of matrix alignment in ligament scars: a comparison of movement versus immobilization in an immature rabbit model. *Journal of Orthopaedic Research* **9**, 219–227.

Frank, C., McDonald, D., Wilson, J., Eyre, D. & Shrive, N. (1995) Rabbit medial collateral ligament scar weakness is associated with decreased collagen pyridinoline crosslink density. *Journal of Orthopaedic Research* **13**, 15–165.

Frank, C., Shrive, N., Hiraoka, H., Nakamura, N., Kaneda, Y. & Hart, D. (1999) Optimization of the biology of soft tissue repair. *Journal of Science and Medicine in Sport* **2**, 190–210.

Friden, J., Sjostrom, M. & Ekblom, B. (1983) Myofibrillar damage following intense eccentric exercise in man. *International Journal of Sports Medicine* **4**, 170–176.

Frowen, P. & Benjamin, M. (1995) Variations in the quantity of uncalcified fibrocartilage at the insertions of the extrinsic calf muscles in the foot. *Journal of Anatomy* **186**, 417–421.

Fu, F.H., Bennett, C.H., Lattermann, C. & Ma, B. (1999) Current trends in anterior cruciate ligament reconstruction. Part 1. Biology and biomechanics of reconstruction. *American Journal of Sports Medicine* **27**, 821–830.

Fu, F.H., Bennett, C.H., Ma, B., Menetrey, J. & Lattermann, C. (2000) Current trends in anterior cruciate ligament reconstruction. Part 2. Operative procedures and clinical correlations. *American Journal of Sports Medicine* **28**, 124–130.

Garrett, W.E. (1996) Muscle strain injuries. *American Journal of Sports Medicine* **24**, S2–S8.

Grontvedt, T., Engbretsen, L., Benum, P., Fasting, O., Molster, A. & Strand, T. (1996) A prospective randomized study of three operations for acute rupture of the anterior cruciate ligament. *Journal of Bone and Joint Surgery* **78A**, 159–168.

Hart, D.P. & Danhers, L.E. (1987) Healing of the medial collateral ligament in rats. *Journal of Bone and Joint Surgery* **69A**, 1194–1199.

Hartig, D.E. & Henderson, J.M. (1999) Increasing hamstring flexibility decreases lower extremity overuse injuries in military basic trainees. *American Journal of Sports Medicine* **27**, 173–176.

Hasselman, C.T., Best, T.M., Hughes, C., Martinez, S. & Garrett, W.E. (1995) An explanation for the various rectus femoris strain injuries using previously undescribed muscle architecture. *American Journal of Sports Medicine* **23**, 493–499.

Heckman, J.D., Ryaby, J.P., McCabe, J., Frey, J.J. & Kilcoyne, R.F. (1994) Acceleration of tibial fracture healing by non-invasive, low intensity pulsed ultrasound. *Journal of Bone Joint Surgery* **76A**, 26–34.

Helbing, G. & Burri, C. (1977) Functional postoperative care after reconstruction of knee ligaments. In: *Injuries of the Ligaments and their Repair. Hand–Knee–Foot. Seventh International Symposium on Topical Problems in Orthopedic Surgery, Lucerne (Switzerland)* (Chachal, G., ed.). Thieme-Edition/PSG Publishing, Stuttgart: 161–165.

Jackson, D.W., Arnoczky, S.P., Frank, C.B., Woo, S.L.-Y. & Simon, T.M. (eds) (1993) *The Anterior Cruciate Ligament. Current and Future Concepts*. Raven Press, New York.

Jozsa, L. & Kannus, P. (1997) Healing and regeneration of tendons. In: *Human Tendons: Anatomy, Physiology and Pathology* (Jozsa, L. & Kannus, P., eds), Human Kinetics, Champaign, IL: 526–554.

Kannus, P., Jozsa, L., Renstrom, P. *et al.* (1992a) The effect of training, immobilization and remobilization on musculoskeletal tissue. Part 1: training and immobilization. *Scandinavian Journal of Medicine and Science in Sports* **2**, 100–118.

Kannus, P., Jozsa, L., Renstrom, P. *et al.* (1992b) The effect of training, immobilization and remobilization on musculoskeletal tissue. Part 2: remobilization and prevention of immobilization atrophy. *Scandinavian Journal of Medicine and Science in Sports* **2**, 164–176.

Kastelic, J. & Baer, E. (1980) Deformation in tendon collagen. In: *The Mechanical Properties of Biological Molecules* (Vincent, J. & Currey, J., eds), Symposium Society Experimental Biology, 397–435.

Kastelic, J., Galeski, A. & Baer, E. (1978) The multicomposite structure of tendon. *Connective Tissue Research* **6**, 11–23.

Katayose, M. & Magee, D.J. (2001) The cross-sectional area of supraspinatus as measured by diagnostic ultrasound. *Journal of Bone and Joint Surgery* **83B**, 565–571.

Ker, R.F., Dimery, N.J. & Alexander, R.McN. (1986) The role of tendon elasticity in hopping in a wallaby. *Journal of Zoology, London* **208A**, 417–428.

Kesava Reddy, G., Gum, S., Sthno-Bittel, L. & Enwemeka, C.S. (1998) Biochemistry and biomechanics of healing tendon: Part II. Effects of combined laser therapy and electrical stimulation. *Medicine and Science in Sports and Exercise* **30**, 794–800.

Khan, K.M., Tress, B.W., Hare, W.S.C. *et al.* (1998) Treat the patient, not the X-ray: advances in diagnostic imaging do not replace the need for clinical interpretation (Editorial). *Clinical Journal of Sports Medicine* **8**, 1–4.

Klein, L., Lunseth, P.A. & Aadalen, R. (1972) Comparison of functional and non-functional tendon grafts. Isotopic turnover and mass. *Journal of Bone Joint Surgery* **54A**, 1745–1753.

Knorzer, E., Folkhard, W., Geercken, W. *et al.* (1986) New aspects of the aetiology of tendon rupture. An analysis of time-resolved dynamic-mechanical measurements. *Archives of Orthopaedic and Traumatic Surgery* **105**, 113–120.

Komi, P.V. (1987) Neuromuscular factors related to physical performance. In: *Muscle and Nerve, Factors Affecting Performance. Proceedings of the 6th Biennial Conference, Cumberland College of Health Sciences, 1987* (Russo, P. & Balnave, R., eds), Sports Sciences & Research Centre, Cumberland College of Health Sciences, NSW, Australia: 114–132.

Komi, P.V., Salonen, M., Jarvinen, M. & Kokko, O. (1987) *In vivo* registration of achilles tendon forces in man. Methodological development. *International Journal of Sports Medicine* **8**, 3–8.

Kvist, M., Jozsa, L., Kannus, P. *et al.* (1991) Morphology and histochemistry of the myotendineal junction. *Acta Anatomica* **141** (199), 205.

Larsen, N. & Parker, A.W. (1982) Physical activity and its influence on the strength and elastic stiffness of knee ligaments. In: *Sports Medicine: Medical and Scientific Aspects of Elitism in Sport* (Howell, M.L. & Parker, A.W., eds), Proceedings of the Australian

Sports Medicine Federation, Gold Coast, Queensland, Australia. Vol. 8. 63–73.

Leonardi, L., Ruggeri, A., Roveri, N., Bigi, A. & Reale, E. (1983) Light microscopy, electron microscopy and X-ray diffraction analysis of glycerinated collagen fibrils. *Journal of Ultrastructure Research* **85**, 228–237.

MacFarlane, B.J., Edwards, P., Frank, C.B., Rangayyan, R.M. & Liu, Z.-Q. (1989) Quantification of collagen remodelling in healing nonimmobilized and immobilized ligaments. *Transactions of Orthopaedic Research Society* **14**, 300.

Mandelbaum, B.R., Myerson, M.S. & Forster, R. (1995) Achilles tendon ruptures. A new method of repair, early range of motion and functional rehabilitation. *American Journal of Sports Medicine* **23**, 392–395.

Matthew, C., Moore, M.J. & Campbell, L. (1987) A quantitative ultrastructural study of collagen fibril formation in the healing extensor digitorum longus tendon of the rat. *Journal of Hand Surgery* **12B**, 313–320.

McNeilly, C.M., Banes, A.J., Benjamin, M. & Ralphs, J.R. (1996) Tendon cells *in vivo* form a three dimensional network of cell processes linked by gap junctions. *Journal of Anatomy* **189**, 593–600.

Merrilles, M.J. & Flint, M.H. (1980) Ultrastructural study of the tension and pressure zones in a rabbit flexor tendon. *American Journal of Anatomy* **157**, 87–106.

Michna, M. (1984) Morphometric analysis of loading-induced changes in collagen-fibril populations in young tendons. *Cell and Tissue Research* **236**, 465–470.

Morgan, D.L., Proske, U. & Warren, D. (1978) Measurements of muscle stiffness and the mechanism of elastic storage of energy in hopping kangaroos. *Journal of Physiology, London* **282**, 253–261.

Nakamura, N., Timmermann, S.A., Hart, D.A. *et al.* (1998) A comparison of *in vivo* gene delivery methods for antisense therapy in ligament healing. *Gene Therapy* **5**, 1455–1461.

Ng, G.Y., Oakes, B.W., Deacon, O.D., McLean, I.D. & Eyre, D.R. (1995a) A three year correlation study of hydroxypyridinium cross-link density with Young's modulus of ACL-PT autograft in goats. In: *Transactions of Combined Orthopaedic Research Societies Meeting, USA, Canada and Japan, San Diego* (Oegema, T.R. & Nedza, P.S., eds). The Orthopaedic Research Society, Illinois: 98.

Ng, G.Y., Oakes, B.W., Deacon, O.D., McLean, I.D. & Lampard, D. (1995b) Biomechanics of patellar tendon autograft for reconstruction of anterior cruciate ligament in the goat. *Journal of Orthopaedic Research* **13**, 602–608.

Ng, G.Y., Oakes, B.W., Deacon, O.D., McLean, I.D. & Eyre, D.R. (1996a) Long-term study of the biochemistry and biomechanics of anterior cruciate ligament–patellar tendon autografts in goats. *Journal of Orthopaedic Research* **14**, 851–856.

Ng, G.Y., Oakes, B.W., McLean, I.D., Deacon, O.D. & Lampard, D. (1996b) The long-term biomechanical and viscoelastic performance of repairing anterior cruciate ligament after hemitransection injury in a goat model. *American Journal of Sports Medicine* **24**, 109–117.

Noonan, T.J. & Garrett, W.E. (1992) Injuries at the myotendinous junction. *Clinics in Sports Medicine* **11**, 783–806.

Noyes, F.R., Torvic, P.J., Hyde, W.B. & De Lucas, J.L. (1974) Biomechanics of ligament failure. 2. An analysis of immobilization, exercise and reconditioning effects in primates. *Journal of Bone and Joint Surgery* **56A**, 1406–1418.

Oakes, B.W. (1981) Acute soft tissue injuries—nature and management. *Australian Family Physician* **10** (Suppl.), 1–16.

Oakes, B.W. (1984) Hamstring injuries. *Australian Family Physician* **13**, 587–591.

Oakes, B.W. (1988) Ultrastructural studies on knee joint ligaments: quantitation of collagen fibre populations in exercised and control rat cruciate ligaments and in human anterior cruciate ligament grafts. In: *Injury and Repair of the Musculoskeletal Tissues* (Buckwalter, J. & Woo, S.L.-Y., eds). American Academy of Orthopaedic Surgeons, Rosemont, IL: 66–82.

Oakes, B.W. (1993) Collagen ultrastructure in the normal ACL and in ACL graft. In: *The Anterior Cruciate Ligament: Current and Future Concepts* (Jackson, D. *et al.*, eds). Raven Press, New York: 209–217.

Oakes, B.W., Parker, A.W. & Norman, J. (1981) Changes in collagen fibre populations in young rat cruciate ligaments in response to an intensive one month's exercise program. In: *Human Adaptation* (Russo, P. & Gass, G., eds). Department of Biological Sciences, Cumberland College of Health Sciences, Sydney, NSW, Australia: 223–230.

Oakes, B.W., Knight, M., McLean, I.D. & Deacon, O.W. (1991) Goat ACL autograft remodeling—quantitative collagen fibrils analyses over 1 year. Paper 65. In: *Transactions of Combined Meeting Orthopaedic Research Societies of USA, Japan and Canada, October 1991*: 60.

Oakes, B.W., Singleton, C. & Haut, R. (1998) Correlation of collagen fibril morphology and tensile modulus in the repairing and normal patella tendon. *Transactions of the Orthopaedic Research Society* **23**, 24.

Parker, A.W. & Larsen, N. (1981) Changes in the strength of bone and ligament in response to training. In: *Human Adaption* (Russo, P. & Gass, G., eds). Department of Biological Sciences, Cumberland College of Health Sciences, Sydney, NSW, Australia: 209–221.

Parry, D.A.D., Barnes G.R.G. & Craig, A.S. (1978) A comparison of the size distribution of collagen fibrils in connective tissues as a function of age and a possible relation between fibril size and distribution and mechanical properties. *Proceedings of Royal Society of London, Series B* **203**, 305–321.

Parry, D.A.D., Flint, M.H., Gillard, G.C. & Craig, A.S. (1982) A role for glycosaminoglycans in the development of collagen fibrils. *FEBS Letters* **149**, 1–7.

Piper, T.L. & Whiteside, L.A. (1980) Early mobilization after knee ligament repair in dogs: an experimental study. *Clinical Orthopaedics and Related Research* **50**, 277–282.

Proske, U. & Morgan, D. (1987) Tendon stiffness: methods of measurement and significance for the control of move-ment. A review. *Journal of Biomechanics* **20**, 75–82.

Rodeo, S. & Izawa, K. (1999) Pathophysiology of tendinous tissue. In: *Orthopaedic Knowledge Update: Sports Medicine* (Arendt, E.A. ed.), Vol. 2. American Academy of Orthopaedic Surgeons, Rosemont, IL: 29–36.

Rubin, C.T. & Lanyon, L.E. (1987) Osteoregulatory nature of mechanical stimuli: function as a determinant for adaptive remodelling in bone. *Journal of Orthopaedic Research* **5**, 300–310.

Rubin, C., Bolander, M., Ryaby, J.P. & Hadjiargyrou, M. (2001) The use of low intensity ultrasound to accelerate the healing of fractures. Current concepts review. *Journal of Bone and Joint Surgery* **83A**, 259–270.

Rufai, A., Ralphs, J.R. & Benjamin, M. (1995) Structure and histopathology of the insertional region of the human Achilles tendon. *Journal of Orthopaedic Research* **13**, 585–593.

Scott, J.E. (1990) Proteoglycan: collagen interactions and subfibrillar structure in collagen fibrils. Implications in the development and ageing of connective tissues. *Journal of Anatomy* **169**, 23–35.

Shadwick, R.E. (1986) The role of collagen crosslinks in the age related changes in mechanical properties of digital tendons. *Proceedings of North American Congress of Biomechanics* **1**, 137–138.

Shadwick, R.E. (1990) Elastic energy storage in tendons: mechanical differences related to function and age. *Journal of Applied Physiology* **68**, 1033–1040.

Shelbourne, K.D. & Davis, T.J. (1999) Evaluation of knee stability before and after participation in a functional sports agility program during rehabilitation after anterior cruciate ligament reconstruction. *American Journal of Sports Medicine* **27**, 156–172.

Shelbourne, K.D. & Nitz, P. (1990) Accelerated rehabilitation after anterior cruciate ligament reconstruction. *American Journal of Sports Medicine* **18**, 292–299.

Shino, K., Kawasaki, T., Hirose, H., Gotoh, I., Inoue, M. & Ono, K. (1984) Replacement of the anterior cruciate ligament by an allograft. *Journal of Bone and Joint Surgery* **66B**, 672–681.

Shino, K., Oakes, B.W., Inoue, M., Horibe, S., Nakata, K. & Ono, K. (1990) Human ACL allograft: collagen fibril populations studied as a function of age of the graft. *Transactions of the Annual Meeting of the Orthopaedic Research Society* **15**, 520.

Shino, K., Oakes, B.W., Inoue, M., Horibe, S. & Nakata, K. (1991) Human ACL allografts: an electron-microscopic analysis of collagen fibril populations. In: *Proceedings of the International Society of the Knee, May, Toronto, 1991.*

Shino, K., Oakes, B.W., Horibe, S., Nakata, K. & Nakamura, N. (1995) Human anterior cruciate ligament allografts. An electron microscopic analysis on collagen fibril populations. *American Journal of Sports Medicine* **23**, 203–209.

Speck, M. & Klaue, K. (1998) Early weight bearing and functional treatment after surgical repair of acute Achilles tendon rupture. *American Journal of Sports Medicine* **26**, 789–793.

Stanish, W., Rubinovich, R.M. & Curwin, S. (1986) Eccentric exercise in chronic Achilles tendinitis. *Clinical Orthopaedics and Related Research* **208**, 65–68.

Stehno-Bittel, L., Reddy, G.K., Gum, S. & Enwemeka, C.S. (1998) Biochemistry and biomechanics of healing tendon: Part 1. Effects of rigid plaster casts and functional casts. *Medicine and Science in Sports and Exercise* **30**, 788–793.

Tipton, C.M. & Vailas, A.C. (1989) Bone and connective tissue adaptations to physical activity. In: *Proceedings of the International Conference on Exercise, Fitness and Health, Toronto, 1988* (Bouchard, C. *et al.*, eds). Human Kinetics, Champaign, IL: 331–344.

Tipton, C.M., James, S.L., Mergner, W. & Tcheng, T.K. (1970) Influence of exercise on the strength of the medial collateral knee ligament of dogs. *American Journal of Physiology* **218**, 894–902.

Tipton, C.M., Matthes, R.D., Maynard, J.A. & Carey, R.A. (1975) The influence of physical activity on ligaments and tendons. *Medicine and Science in Sports* **7**, 165–175.

Tipton, C.M., Vailas, A.C. & Matthes, R.D. (1986) Experimental studies on the influences of physical activity on ligaments, tendons and joints: a brief review. *Acta Medica Scandinavica* **711** (Suppl.), 157–168.

Toole, B.P. & Lowther, D.A. (1968) The effect of chondroitin sulphate-protein on the formation of collagen fibrils *in vitro*. *Biochemical Journal* **109**, 857–866.

Vailas, A.C., Tipton, C.M., Matthes, R.D. & Gart, M. (1981) Physical activity and its influence on the repair process of medial collateral ligaments. *Connective Tissue Research* **9**, 25–31.

Viidik, A. (1973) Functional properties of connective tissues. *International Review of Connective Tissue Research* **6**, 127–215.

Viidik, A. (1980) Interdependence between structure and function. In: *Biology of Collagen* (Viidik, A., ed.). Academic Press, London: 257–280.

Viidik, A. (1996) Tendons and ligaments. In: *Extracellular Matrix*, Vol. 1 (Comper, W., ed.). Harwood Academic Publishers, Amsterdam: 303–327.

Viidik, A. & Ekholm, R. (1968) Light and electron microscopic studies of collagen fibres under strain. *Zeitschreift Antomie Entwicklungsgesch* **127**, 154–164.

Vogel, K.G. & Trotter, J.A. (1987) The effect of proteoglycans on the morphology of collagen fibrils formed *in vitro*. *Collagen Related Research* **7**, 105–114.

Walker, J. (1984) Deep transverse frictions in ligament healing. *Journal of Orthopaedic and Sports Physical Therapy* **6**, 89–94.

Weber, I.T., Harrison, R.W. & Iozzo, R.V. (1996) Model structure of decorin and implications for collagen fibrillogenesis. *Journal of Biological Chemistry* **271**, 31767–31770.

Weisman, G., Pope, M.H. & Johnson, R.J. (1980) Cyclical loading in knee ligament injuries. *American Journal of Sports Medicine* **8**, 24–30.

Williams, J.G.P. (1986) Achilles tendon lesions in sport. *Sports Medicine* **3**, 114–135.

Wilson, A.M. & Goodship, A.E. (1994) Exercise induced hyperthermia as a possible mechanism for tendon degeneration. *Journal of Biomechanics* **27**, 899–905.

Woo, S.L.-Y., Gomez, M.A., Sites, T.J., Newton, P.O., Orlando, C.A. & Akeson, W.H. (1987a) The biomechanical and morphological changes in the medial collateral ligament of the rabbit after immobilization and remobilization. *Journal of Bone and Joint Surgery* **69A**, 1200–1211.

Woo, S.L.-Y., Inoue, M., McGurk-Burleson, E. & Gomez, M.A. (1987b) Treatment of the medial collateral ligament injury. II: structure and function of canine knees in response to differing treatment regimes. *American Journal of Sports Medicine* **15**, 22–29.

Woo, S.L.-Y., An, K.-N., Frank, C.B. *et al.* (2000) Anatomy, biology and biomechanics of tendon and ligament. In: *Orthopaedic Basic Science Biology and Biomechanics of the Musculoskeletal System*, 2nd edn (Buckwalter, J.A., Einhorn, T.A. & Simon, S.R., eds). American Academy of Orthopaedic Surgeons, Rosemont, IL: 581–616.

Young, R.G., Butler, D.L., Weber, W., Caplan, A.I., Gordon, S.L. & Fink, D.J. (1998) Use of mesenchymal stem cells in a collagen matrix for Achilles tendon repair. *Journal of Orthopaedic Research* **16**, 406–413.

Chapter 5

Tissue Healing and Repair: Bone and Cartilage

K.-M. CHAN, HENRY C.L. HO AND CHRISTOPHER W.C. TONG

Healing and regeneration of bone

Structure of bone

Bone is a specialized form of connective tissue, which serves the following purposes.

1 It is a skeletal framework for the body.

2 It allows the different parts of the body, such as the appendages, to move in space through various degrees of freedom by means of joints controlled by the activity of their attached muscles and stabilized by ligaments.

3 It protects the vital organs such as the heart, lungs and abdominal viscera from external trauma.

4 It is a source of production for the elements of blood.

5 It plays a major part in mineral metabolism.

6 The bone marrow is an important part of the immune system.

The structure of bone, like that of other connective tissues, is composed of cellular elements and their surrounding matrix, which is unique in that it has an organic as well as an inorganic mineral component. The cells include bone-forming cells (osteoblasts), bone-resorbing cells (osteoclasts) and a stable population of maintenance cells (osteocytes). The relative activity of each of these cell types depends on the physiological or pathological state of this unique tissue. Under normal circumstances, in the absence of trauma, the osteocytes are lined up neatly in layers, like the skin of an onion, in the line of stress to form lamellar bone. In cortical bone of long bone diaphysis, these layers form whorls surrounding a central vascular channel contain-ing arterioles, venules, capillaries, nerves and lymphatics. These whorls are known as Haversian systems (Fig. 5.1). The osteocytes form connections with each other and are bathed in a limited and complex interconnecting fluid space called the canaliculi. In the metaphyseal portion of long bone, the lamellae are also stress orientated but form interlacing pillars called trabeculae, rather than Haversian systems, to support loads. Like many tissues in the body, bone is constantly undergoing remodelling in response to the loads that it is subjected to. There is a delicate balance between bone formation by osteoblasts and bone removal (resorption) by osteoclasts. The rate of

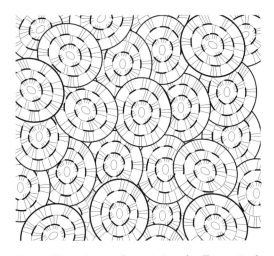

Fig. 5.1 Haversian canals consisting of well-organized layers of osteocytes interconnected by a system of canaliculi.

99

remodelling is more pronounced in trabecular bone and less in cortical bone.

The cells are derived from osteoprogenitor cells, which are themselves derived from immature mesenchymal cells of the inner cambium layer of the periosteum and endosteum lining the external and internal surfaces of bone, respectively. Under special circumstances, such as fractures, the rate of differentiation from osteoprogenitor cells to osteoblasts and osteoclasts is dramatically increased in an attempt to heal the fracture.

The strength of bone is derived from its matrix, which is produced and maintained by the osteoblasts and osteocytes. The matrix consists of an organic (40% of dry weight) and an inorganic (60%) component. The organic component is composed of mainly type 1 collagen fibres (90%), which are responsible for the tensile strength of bone, proteoglycans for its compressive strength, and other matrix proteins such as osteocalcin and osteonectin, which are important for the promotion of bone mineralization. Also present in trace amounts are growth factors and cytokines such as transforming growth factor (TGF-β), insulin-like growth factor (IGF) and interleukins 1 and 6 (IL-1 and IL-6), which aid the control of bone cell differentiation, activation, growth and turnover (Bostrom et al. 2000).

The inorganic component is the mineral portion consisting of calcium hydroxyapatite and osteocalcium phosphate (brushite), which are trapped in and between collagen molecules. These are responsible for the compressive strength of bone.

Fractures in sports

Fractures anywhere in the body have serious implications for the athlete since both the inhibition from pain and the disruption of skeletal framework significantly compromise the function of the affected part. Fractures sustained during sport are common. Templeton et al. (2000) found that sport accounted for 22.1% of all tibial diaphyseal fractures, of which 79.5% were sustained during soccer. In addition, the 10 activities that most commonly lead to injury for all ages are

cycling, Australian football, basketball, soccer, cricket, netball, rugby, roller skating/blading, skateboarding and trampolining (Finch et al. 1998). Furthermore, sports-related injuries cause significant morbidity. In a retrospective study by Shaw et al. (1997) on the epidemiology and outcome of 523 tibial diaphyseal fractures in footballers, only 73.9% of the patients had unimpaired sporting function after the injury and the average time to return to football was 7–8 months. Therefore, it is unlikely for a player to return to sport in the same season. The crux of the problem lies in the optimal time to return to full sporting activity without jeopardizing the structural integrity of the bone. Fractures may occur in any part of the bone, but specific areas such as those around the major joints will be discussed in greater detail since the interplay between early return of joint motion and perfect restoration and healing of the articular surface are of paramount importance if long-term osteoarthritis is to be avoided.

AIM AND PRINCIPLE OF FRACTURE TREATMENT

Fractures commonly encountered in athletic activities, usually arise from repeated stress and are commonly treated non-operatively. An example is the metatarsal fracture, also known as a march fracture. However, fractures arising from more major injuries can result in disruptions of larger structures such as the tibial plateau. The tibial plateau fracture is a good example of an injury that can have a major impact on an athlete's career and can indeed equate to permanent disability. The major concern here is to achieve accurate reduction of the fracture to restore a normal smooth articular surface followed by stable fracture fixation and to attain bone healing in as short a time as possible. As soon as bony integrity is achieved, weightbearing and mobilization can begin. Range of motion exercises of the joint should begin as soon as possible to prevent joint stiffness; they also have the role of promoting nutritional delivery and healing in the articular cartilage. Early safe mobilization also promotes the return of muscle function. While these are the basic principles behind the management of more complex periarticular fractures, the optimum rehabilitation strategy is yet to be defined.

The healing process of fractures after injury

The process of healing in bone is one of regeneration of bone, in contrast to healing in other tissues such as muscle where the defective tissue may be replaced to some degree by scar tissue. Fracture healing is a complex and well-orchestrated physiological process and much research has been invested in this field to achieve a better understanding of the natural pathways so that potential avenues of intervention to promote earlier fracture healing can be exploited. This has important therapeutic implications since the main concern for the athlete is how soon he or she can return to normal sport.

To understand fracture healing, it is important to appreciate the cellular events taking place at the fracture site (Fig. 5.2). Fracture healing can be broadly divided into primary and secondary healing. Primary healing, also known as primary cortical healing, involves a direct attempt by the cortex to re-establish mechanical continuity. In secondary fracture healing, the periosteum containing cells of osteogenic potential and the external soft tissues form a callus, which subsequently bridges the fracture gap and undergoes cartilaginous changes followed by replacement

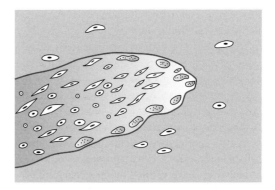

Fig. 5.3 Cutting cone: an important functional unit consisting of leading osteoclasts resorbing bone debris, thus creating a pathway for trailing osteoblasts and newly formed vessels to lay down immature bone.

with newly formed bone by the process of endochondral ossification. In the case of primary fracture healing, osteoclasts and osteoblasts function to remove bony debris and produce immature bone, respectively. This is followed by a vascular ingrowth to form the so-called 'cutting cone' (Fig. 5.3), which eventually leads to the re-establishment of Haversian systems. This process of primary fracture healing only takes place when there is a minimal fracture gap and rigid fracture fixation.

On the other hand, secondary fracture healing, which is the more common mode of healing found in fractures, involves an initial stage of fracture haematoma formation and the release of important signalling molecules including IL–1 and IL–6, TGF-β and platelet-derived growth factor (PDGF). The bone itself also releases PDGF, TGF-β, IGF-I, IGF-II and bone morphogenic protein (BMP). These function to orchestrate the various complex cellular changes taking place, which include the proliferation and differentiation of mesenchymal stem cells found in the periosteum into osteoblasts. During the first 10 days, these form new bone directly opposed to the cortex, a process known as intramembranous ossification. At the same time, the bridging callus, which is contributed by the periosteum and external soft tissues, undergoes cartilagenous transformation. At 2 weeks, calcification of the cartilage begins to

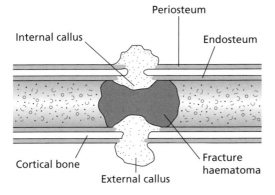

Periosteum

Internal callus

Endosteum

Cortical bone

Fracture haematoma

External callus

Fig. 5.2 Callus at the fracture site consisting of osteoblasts, osteoclasts, newly formed blood vessels and immature bone and cartilage.

take place. This tissue then becomes the target tissue for vascular ingrowth delivering osteoblasts to the area. The extent of this vascular invasion depends very much on the integrity of the surrounding blood supply to the periosteum, endosteum and soft tissue. Newly formed immature woven bone is laid down while the calcified cartilage matrix is digested away by chondroclasts. With time, under the influence of loading during rehabilitation, remodelling takes place and woven bone becomes substituted by mechanically competent and stress-orientated lamellar bone.

MECHANICAL FACTORS INFLUENCING THE HEALING PROCESS

With the above knowledge in mind, one has to have some evidence on which to devise a rehabilitation strategy. It is important to recognize those mechanical factors that can promote and retard the natural biology of fracture healing. Only then can the clinician devise a well thought-out rehabilitation plan that is based on scientific rather than anecdotal evidence.

Investigators (Cunningham *et al.* 1998) have studied the effects of strain rate and timing in the mechanical modulation of fracture healing. They studied the effects of applying cyclic interfragmentary micromovement at high and low strain rates at various stages of healing and discovered that a high strain rate, similar to that obtained during brisk walking, induces a greater amount of callus formation during the early phase of healing but significantly inhibits healing in the later period (6 weeks after fracture). They also predict that in the later (hard callus) phase, tissue damage may occur under abnormally high stresses and strains and recommend increasing the rigidity of fracture fixation until the fracture has healed. It has been suggested that as healing progresses, the rigidity of the fixation system should be increased in order to minimize such excessive strains (Kenwright & Gardener 1998). This can be achieved in clinical practice by the process of dynamization, whereby the fracture ends are jammed together further as the patient bears weight.

In addition, the amount of strain and hydrostatic pressure applied along the calcified surface of the fracture gap have also been found to affect the type of bone healing taking place. Using animal models, Claes *et al.* (1998) discovered that for strains of less than 5% and pressures of less than 0.15 MPa, predominantly intramembranous ossification was seen. Strains between 5 and 15% and hydrostatic pressures greater than 0.15 MPa stimulated endochondral ossification, and larger strains led to healing by fibrous connective tissue. The amount of strain also affected the production of TGF-β. Increased production was found for strains of up to 5% and a subsequent decrease for larger strains. The amount of strain taking place at the fracture site is clearly dependent on the type of fixation. A fracture fixed with a plate is much more likely to demonstrate less strain compared with one fixed with an Ilizarov ring fixator. Similarly, Augat *et al.* (1996) studied the effects of early weightbearing after fracture fixation using more flexible devices in the sheep long bone. Although there was an abundance of early soft callus formation, there was a significant delay in the healing of the osteotomy site. On the other hand, prevention of early full weightbearing and delayed full weightbearing resulted in a higher flexural rigidity of the fracture, an increased mechanical stiffness of the callus tissue, and an enhanced bone formation at the healing front (Augat *et al.* 1996).

The amount of stability that a fixation device imparts to a fracture will determine the optimum time to begin loading across the fractured bone. Sarmiento and Latta (1999) showed the beneficial effects of early weightbearing on fracture healing in their studies on rats and indeed confirmed Wolff's hypothesis that mechanical loading stimulates an osteogenic response in bone. The exact mechanism by which such mechanical influences act is still not defined but is certainly a fascinating area deserving further research. While recognizing the limitations of research models, one must remain critical about such data and question their validity when applied to clinical situations. For example, much of the research has been on animal experiments and the fracture pattern and behaviour may be quite different to that occurring in humans. The surgical method and technique of fracture fixation also influence the stability of the osteosynthesis and affects the surgeon's preferred method of rehabilitation. Therefore, the results of research experiments can only serve as a guide to the biological events taking place in a patient and cannot be strictly extrapolated.

The current practice of fracture fixation has now moved away from absolute rigid fixation using compression plates and rigid statically locked intramedullary nails to one of stable fixation allowing some micromovement to take place to stimulate early callus formation (Fig. 5.4). Indeed, some of the inherently more stable fractures such as the simple and minimally comminuted tibial shaft fractures may be treated primarily by a functional brace, allowing early weightbearing to stimulate micromotion. This method obviously spares the patient a surgical procedure, such as intramedullary nail fixation, and its surgical risks and allows a shorter rehabilitation time (Sarmiento & Latta 1999). Furthermore, the subsequent shortening and deformity found when bracing is used in the treatment of less stable tibial fractures might be functionally insignificant (Sarmiento & Latta 1999).

BIOLOGICAL FACTORS INFLUENCING THE HEALING PROCESS

In addition to using less rigid forms of fracture fixation, there is a growing trend towards using minimal fixation. Apart from the mechanical factors mentioned above, it is important to bear in mind that the chosen method of fixation must respect the local blood supply to the fracture because healing will not take place in the absence of an adequate blood supply due to a paucity of cellular elements and growth factors at the fracture site. The fixation device will ultimately fail if there is non-union of the fracture. Minimal fixation preserves the possibly already traumatized soft tissue envelope to the underlying bone and simultaneously allows more micromotion. The importance of a good blood supply is exemplified by the preponderance of fracture

non-union in the relatively less well vascularized distal tibial shaft fractures. The much better vascularized metaphysis, on the other hand, nearly always heals uneventfully.

Therefore, in a tibial plateau fracture, the fixation method usually now involves arthroscopically assisted reduction of the articular surface and percutaneous screw fixation supplemented by an external ring fixator. Few would advocate open reduction and plating of such injuries. Indeed, if plating is necessary, such as in long bone fractures of the forearm, minimally invasive techniques are being developed to slide the plate under the soft tissue after making a much smaller surgical wound. Plates such as the low-contact dynamic compression plate have also been designed with the aim of reducing the amount of pressure applied to the underlying periosteum and bone to minimize ischaemia.

Management of fracture

Although surgical stabilization and anatomical realignment remain the mainstay of treatment of most displaced fractures, it is still important to realize that the ultimate goal is to achieve solid bone union as early as possible. One must have the armamentarium to treat delayed or established non-unions and the assessment of such challenging problems is a test of one's understanding of the biological requirements of healing. Apart from surgical means of promoting union, such as bone grafting and bone marrow injection to reactivate the healing process, non-surgical methods, if found to be equally effective, would generally be the patient's choice.

Future research is directed at investigating such newer non-surgical methods. An example of an already widely used tool is ultrasound stimulation (US). This technique was first introduced by Duarte in 1983 and its effects have been confirmed in animal and clinical studies (Duarte 1983). However, the exact mechanism is still unknown, but a stimulation of the expression of numerous genes involved in the healing process including those encoding for aggrecan, IGF and TGF-β have been demonstrated (Hadjiargyrou *et al.*

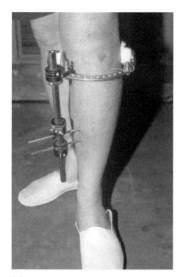

(a)

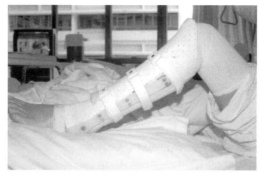

(c)

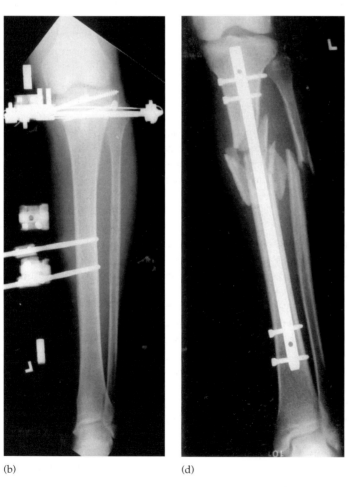

(b)   (d)

Fig. 5.4 (a) External fixator *in situ* to hold a comminuted tibial plateau fracture reduced. A minimally invasive technique of stable fracture fixation. (b) External fixator holding tibial plateau fracture reduced. (c) Sarmiento brace is useful for the treatment of tibial shaft fractures. (d) Intramedullary nail providing rigid internal fixation for tibial shaft fracture.

1998). An increase in the formation of soft callus formation and an earlier onset of endochondral ossification have been observed (Wang *et al.* 1994). In one animal study, US treatment resulted in a 1.5 times increase in the mean acceleration of fracture healing (Pilla *et al.* 1990). Heckman *et al.* (1994) reported a significant reduction in healing time in their multicentre, randomized, controlled clinical trial using low-intensity ultrasound for 20 min per day during the first week after a fracture. The use of ultrasound for the healing of fresh fractures has been approved by the American Food and Drug Administration.

Similarly, pulsed electromagnetic and electric fields have also been found to accelerate fresh fracture healing and augment healing in delayed union. It is believed that an exogenous electrical field applied at the fracture site can induce a mechanotransductive effect similar to that observed when bone is subjected to mechanical stress. Its use in clinical practice began in the 1970s. Deibert *et al.* (1994) demonstrated a 55–299% increase in strength of healed rabbit fibula that were subjected to daily ion resonance electromagnetic field stimulation. The exact cellular pathways responsible for this effect have not been well defined, but a stimulation of the secretion of numerous growth factors such as BMP-2, BMP-4, TGF-β and IGF-II *in vitro* have been demonstrated. Sedel *et al.* (1981) have extensively investigated the use of electromagnetic fields in the treatment of delayed union and non-union. Ryaby (1998) achieved an efficacy rate of 64–87% in the treatment of non-union of the tibia. However, large controlled, randomized, double-blind clinical trials are currently lacking.

In terms of pharmacological treatment, the potential clinical application of L-dopa, parathyroid hormone, bisphosphonates and zinc compounds, as well as the many different growth factors, in promoting fracture regeneration are under extensive investigation. To cite a few examples, a study by Holzer *et al.* (1999) showed that parentally administered parathyroid hormone to mid-diaphyseal fractures of rat femurs increased the callus area and strength and the bone density, thus calling for clinical trials in its use in healing fractures that are slow to heal.

Similarly, using a rat model, Sakai *et al.* (1999) applied a protein called activin, a member of the TGF-β family, topically to fibular fractures and demonstrated a dose-related increase in the callus volume and callus weight. An increase in the callus strength was also observed.

Research is currently taking place in order to discover the factors that have important signalling properties in these complex cellular events, as these may lead to new insights into the future development of new techniques for promoting fracture healing. One such example is BMP, which appears to be a subset of the TGF superfamily, and has an important role in early intramembranous ossification and in the differentiation of mesenchymal cells into chondrocytes by yet to be defined mechanisms. BMPs were discovered by Urist in 1965 (Urist 1965). They are present in many tissues, such as the kidney, peripheral and central nervous systems and the cardiorespiratory system. Johnson and colleagues demonstrated encouraging clinical results in 30 patients for the treatment of non-union and segmental bone defects using human BMP extracted from human bone incorporated into allografts to form a composite (Johnson & Urist 2000). However, large clinical trials are still lacking and the doses of BMP in these trials are far higher than that found in bone, leading to fears of inducing malignant change.

With so much still unknown to us, formulating the perfect rehabilitation programme for a particular fracture is very difficult. It is still very much subject to the orthopaedic surgeon's personal training and experience and the behaviour of the fracture as well as the patient's compliance. Understanding the complex cellular and biomechanical processes of fracture regeneration helps us institute rehabilitation based on concrete scientific evidence. However, there is no cookbook approach to any single fracture. The interpatient biology is bound to be different and, therefore, the healing ability is likely to be different as well. Thus, the progress of any fracture healing is still likely to be monitored by radiological means. However, the correlation between radiologica progress and actual mechanical strength of the bone may be difficult to establish. This, of course, poses further problems when one is designing clinical studies comparing different methods of rehabilitation. Furthermore, the forces acting through any part of the body at any one time cannot be measured easily. Such uncertainties are reflected by the numerous opinions available regarding the rehabilitation of a fracture. For example, for a given lower limb fracture, one surgeon may advise non-weightbearing mobilization whilst another may advise touch-down walking. To date, such advice cannot be supported by any sound scientific evidence and to conduct well-controlled prospective studies presents a major scientific challenge.

Healing and regeneration of articular cartilage

Structure of articular cartilage

Articular cartilage plays a vital role in the function of the musculoskeletal system by allowing almost frictionless motion to occur between the articular surfaces of a diarthrodial joint. Furthermore, articular cartilage distributes the loads of articulation over a larger contact area, thereby minimizing the contact stresses, and dissipating the energy associated with the load. These properties also allow the potential for articular cartilage to remain healthy and fully functional throughout the decades of life despite the very slow turnover rate of its collagen matrix.

The composition of articular cartilage consists of cells (chondrocytes), matrix proteins including collagen and proteoglycans, non-collagenous proteins, water and electrolytes.

CHONDROCYTES

The basic building blocks of the articular surface are the chondrocytes, which constitute around 5–10% of the wet weight of articular cartilage. Chondrocytes originate from undifferentiated mesenchymal marrow stem cells. These cells in turn progress through the calcified cartilage zone to become chondroblasts. The chondroblasts

become chondrocytes when they become isolated in lacunae, and the chondrocytes receive their nutritional support from the surrounding synovial fluid. Chondrocytes in skeletally mature articular cartilage do not divide but still remain alive via the glycolytic anaerobic metabolism pathway. As chondrocytes age, they exhibit a decrease in cellular activity, especially in the production of collagen and proteoglycan. The function of chondrocytes is to maintain the correct internal milieu of articular cartilage. They synthesize and maintain the various components of the matrix of articular cartilage. This includes the production of collagen, proteoglycans and non-collagenous proteins as well as enzymes (Mankin *et al.* 1994). They maintain the balance of synthesis and degradation of the protein macromolecular complex (Buckwalter & Mankin 1997).

COLLAGEN

Collagen contributes around 10% of the wet weight of articular cartilage. The predominant collagen type in articular cartilage, accounting for 90–95%, is type II collagen, while types VI, XI, X and XI are also found to lesser extents. Collagen is spread throughout the ground substance in the extracellular matrix and is formed by three polypeptide chains that are cross-linked covalently (Eyre 1980). Collagen fibres do not have a large resistance to compression due to their slenderness ratio. However, they are very strong in tension and are the primary component of cartilage, responsible for providing its tensile properties (Roth & Mow 1980) Articular cartilage is composed of distinct layers where the collagen fibres have different patterns of orientation (Fig. 5.5). These layers include the superficial zone, middle zone, deep zone, tidemark and calcified zone. In the superficial zone, collagen fibres are arranged in a parallel fashion relative to the joint surface. In the middle zone, collagen fibres are arranged in a criss-cross oblique fashion. In the deep zone collagen fibres are arranged perpendicular to the joint surface (Redler 1974). The tidemark is the boundary between the deep zone and the zone of calcified cartilage.

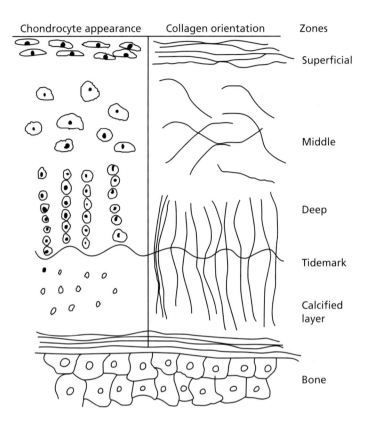

Fig. 5.5 Basic microstructural anatomy of articular cartilage.

PROTEOGLYCANS

Proteoglycans contribute around 10% of the wet weight of articular cartilage. Proteoglycans are composed of a protein core to which are attached many extended polysaccharide units called glycosaminoglycans (Muir 1983). The two main glycosaminoglycans found in articular cartilage are chondroitin sulphate and keratan sulphate. The vast majority of proteoglycans found in articular cartilage are known as aggregans, which bind with hyaluronan to form a large proteoglycan aggregate (Fig. 5.6). Chondrocytes produce aggrecan, link protein and hyaluronan, which are secreted into the extracellular matrix where they aggregate spontaneously (Muir 1983). The proteoglycan molecules contain repeating sulphate and carboxylate groups along their chains. These groups become negatively charged when placed in an aqueous solution. This negative charge attracts water molecules, which exerts a large swelling

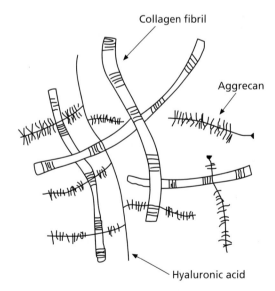

Fig. 5.6 This schematic diagram illustrates the interaction between the collagen molecules and the proteoglycan molecules in the articular cartilage extracellular matrix.

pressure and thus a tensile stress on the surrounding collagen network (Maroudas 1976).

The proteoglycan molecules are the main components in articular cartilage, providing resistance to compression forces within the articular cartilage. The balance of expanding total swelling pressure exerted by the proteoglycans and the constraining tensile force developed within the surrounding collagen network determines the degree of hydration in cartilage. A disruption of this balance, resulting from damage to the articular surface collagen network, has been shown to cause increased tissue hydration and significantly changes the ability of the articular cartilage to bear loads (Setton *et al.* 1993).

Mechanism of injury of articular cartilage

Direct blunt trauma, indirect impact loading or torsional loading of a joint can damage the articular cartilage and the calcified cartilage–subchondral bone region without disrupting the surrounding soft tissues. Examples of direct blunt trauma include falling from a height or striking a joint with a large hard object. Examples of indirect impact and torsional loading include a blow to a bone that forms the subchondral part of a joint or severe twisting of a joint that is loaded. Unfortunately, these injuries occur frequently in people taking part in sports and are hard to diagnose. The amount of cartilage damage from a given load depends on how rapidly this load is applied. Slowly applied loads and suddenly applied loads differ considerably in their effects.

As mentioned previously, the articular cartilage extracellular matrix consists of water and a macromolecular framework formed primarily of collagens and large aggregating proteoglycans. The collagens give the tissue its form and tensile strength, and the interaction of aggregating proteoglycans with water gives the articular cartilage its stiffness to compression, resilience and probably its durability. When the cartilage surface is loaded, fluid movement occurs within and out of the cartilage matrix. This movement of fluid serves to dampen and distribute loads within the cartilage and to the subchondral bone (Mow &

Rosenwasser 1988). When a load is applied slowly to the cartilage, the fluid movement within the cartilage allows the cartilage to deform and decreases the force applied to the matrix macromolecular framework. When a load is applied too rapidly, as occurs with a sudden impact or torsional joint loading of the joint surface, it may rupture the matrix macromolecular framework, damage cells and exceed the ability of articular cartilage to prevent subchondral bone damage by dampening and distributing loads.

Experimental studies have shown that blunt trauma can damage articular cartilage and the calcified cartilage–subchondral bone region, while leaving the articular surface intact (Donohue *et al.* 1983). Physiological levels of joint loading do not appear to cause joint injury, but impact loading above that associated with normal activities, but less than that required to produce cartilage disruption, can cause alterations of the cartilage matrix.

Types of chondral and osteochondral injury and their potential for healing

The response of articular cartilage to injury and the subsequent healing response incurred depends to a large extent on the type of cartilage injuries. Cartilage injuries can be divided into three main types: (i) chondral damage without visible tissue disruption; (ii) disruption of the articular cartilage alone with sparing of the underlying subchondral bone (an example of this would be the chondral flap injury); and (iii) articular cartilage injury involving the underlying subchondral bone (i.e. osteochondral fractures). The intensity and rate of muscle contraction affect the transmission of force to the articular cartilage. Age and genetic factors may influence the type of articular cartilage injury sustained by a particular individual (Buckwalter *et al.* 1996).

MATRIX AND CELL INJURIES

These are injuries where there is a damage to the chondral matrix and/or cells and/or subchondral bone without visible disruption of the articular surface. The proteoglycan content may decrease with a concomitant disruption of the collagen fibril network. If the basic matrix structure remains intact and enough viable cells remain, the cells can restore the normal tissue composition. However, if there is significant damage to the matrix or cell population, or if the tissue sustains further damage, then the lesion may progress to cartilage degeneration.

CHONDRAL FRACTURES AND CHONDRAL FLAPS

These are macroscopic disruptions to the articular cartilage tissue without involvement of the subchondral bone. No fibrin clot or inflammatory responses occur. The chondrocytes, however, will proliferate and synthesize new matrix macromolecules. New tissue does not fill the cartilage gap. Depending on the location and size of the lesion and the structural integrity, stability and alignment of the joint, the lesion may or may not progress to cartilage degeneration.

OSTEOCHONDRAL FRACTURES

Injuries which involve the articular cartilage and the underlying subchondral bone will elicit an inflammatory and bleeding response from the injured subchondral bone (Buckwalter et al. 1990). A clot will form in the subchondral bone defect and to various depths of the cartilage defect. This fibrin clot consists of mesenchymal stems cell that will differentiate into cartilage-forming cells. Platelets within the clot release vasoactive mediators and growth factors or cytokines, including TGF-β and PDGF (Buckwalter et al. 1996). Release of these growth factors appears to have an important role in the repair of osteochondral defects. In particular, they probably stimulate vascular invasion and migration of undifferentiated cells into the clot and influence the proliferative and synthetic activities of the cells. However, the repair tissue formed by these cells does not have the structural and biomechanical properties of articular hyaline cartilage but rather has properties resembling those of fibrocartilage.

Classification of articular cartilage injuries

The grading system devised by Outerbridge (1961) is a simple working tool for describing chondral lesions (Fig. 5.7). In grade I, the articular surface is swollen and soft and may be blistered. Grade II is characterized by the presence of fissures and clefts measuring less than 1 cm in diameter. Grade III is characterized by the presence of deep fissures extending to the subchondral bone and measuring more than 1 cm in diameter. Loose flaps and joint debris may also be noted. In grade IV, subchondral bone is exposed.

Treatment modalities of articular cartilage injuries

Various methods have been used to enhance the healing and repair of articular cartilage injuries. These include: (i) arthroscopic lavage and debridement; (ii) marrow stimulation techniques such as drilling, abrasion arthroplasty and microfracture; (iii) osteochondral autografting; and (iv) autologous chondrocyte implantation. The postoperative rehabilitation programme will vary depending on the method of treatment for the articular cartilage defect.

ARTHROSCOPIC LAVAGE AND DEBRIDEMENT

Arthroscopic lavage and debridement have been shown to produce measurable symptomatic improvement (Hubbard 1996, Levy et al. 1996). In a study by Levy et al. (1996), it was noted that debridement for acute small lesions (average size 42 mm^2) in 15 young soccer players allowed all players to return to soccer at 10.8 weeks after surgery, with six excellent and nine good results. However, the follow-up was short: only 1 year. Hubbard (1996) noted that grade IV femoral condyle lesions randomized to arthroscopic lavage versus debridement did better when debrided. The Lysholm scale score increased 28 points at 1 year and 21 points at 5 years in over 50% of patients. The defect size was not measured and

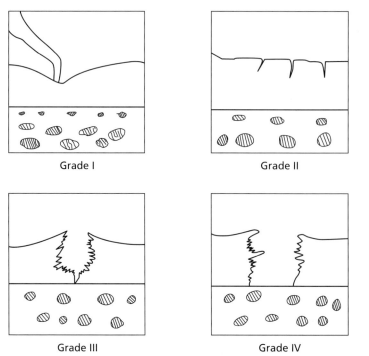

Grade I

Grade II

Grade III

Grade IV

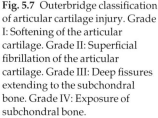

Fig. 5.7 Outerbridge classification of articular cartilage injury. Grade I: Softening of the articular cartilage. Grade II: Superficial fibrillation of the articular cartilage. Grade III: Deep fissures extending to the subchondral bone. Grade IV: Exposure of subchondral bone.

radiographic evidence of progression or follow-up arthroscopy was not performed in this study.

MARROW STIMULATION PROCEDURES: MICROFRACTURE AND DRILLING

The underlying principles of the various marrow stimulation techniques are similar. The concept is that the subchondral bone is breached (either with a drill or a microfracture pick) resulting in an inflammatory response; the resultant fibrin clot that forms will bring in mesenchymal stems cells, cytokines and growth factors, which will lead to a repair response in the articular cartilage defect. The repair material, however, is primarily fibrocartilage. Recently, the technique of micro-fracture has gained considerable popularity: the chondral defect is first debrided arthroscopically to a stable cartilage rim and any loose flaps of cartilage are removed. The calcified cartilage layer is removed by means of a curette paying attention not to violate the underlying subchondral bone. Arthroscopic surgical picks are then used to make multiple holes in the exposed subchondral bone. These holes are made 2–3 mm apart and

their function is to allow pluripotent cells from the underlying marrow to enter the defect and initiate a repair process. The advantages of the microfracture technique is that it is a simple procedure amenable to all surgeons who perform arthroscopic work. The cost is low as no sophisticated instruments or laboratory procedures are required. The use of a microfracture pick to breach the subchondral bone rather than using a drill should result in less thermal damage and cellular necrosis.

Steadman reported his 3–5 year results using the microfracture technique (Steadman *et al.* 1997). He noted pain relief in 75% of patients with 20% unchanged and 5% made worse. When it came to functionality and activities of daily living and work, 67% improved, 20% were unchanged and 13% were made worse. Sixty-five per cent were able to return to strenuous work and sports.

Recommendations for postoperative rehabilitation programmes after microfracture include protected weightbearing for 6–8 weeks and passive mobilization with a continuous passive mobilization (CPM) machine for 8 weeks. The benefits of CPM in the treatment of chondral defects using microfracture have been documented by Rodrigo and Steadman (1994) Postoperative weightbearing status depends on the location of the lesion. Patellar and trochlear grove lesions may be weightbearing and can tolerate a hinged knee brace with a 30° flexion stop. Patients come out of the brace when they are not weightbearing and go into a CPM machine from 10° to 90° for at least 8 h·day^{-1} (mostly at night). If the chondral defect is in the medial or lateral compartment, the patient is kept strictly to touch-down weightbearing, with a similar CPM protocol as used in patellofemoral lesions. The CPM machine is set at 1 cycle per minute with the largest range of motion that the patient finds comfortable. Following the 6–8-week period of protected weightbearing, patients are instructed to begin active range of motion exercises and progress to full weightbearing. No cutting, twisting or jumping sports are allowed until at least 4 months after surgery.

OSTEOCHONDRAL AUTOGRAFT TRANSPLANTATION

Osteochondral autograft transplantation involves the harvesting of small osteochondral plugs from the non-weightbearing portions of the knee and these plugs are transplanted into the cartilage defect in the weightbearing part of the knee. Most investigators agree that lesions < 2 cm^2 are most suitable so that donor site morbidity is avoided (Bobic 1996). The advantages of osteochondral grafting include a mature cartilage–bone unit transfer with rapid bone healing and a subsequent return to high-level function. The disadvantages include the technical difficulty in restoring the biconvex geometric congruity of the femoral condyle in the sagittal and coronal planes and the potential damage imparted to the cartilaginous cap of the individual plugs, dependent on the force required for insertion. Other questions regarding this technique remain unanswered. Concerns include the possible donor site morbidity relating to the harvest of the osteochondral plugs, and the fact that the tissue formed between the osteochondral plugs is fibrocartilage rather than articular cartilage.

Gambella and Glousman (1999) reported good to excellent results in a group of 150 patients treated with osteochondral grafting who had isolated medial and lateral femoral condyle and trochlear lesions. All physical examination parameters, including range of motion, effusion, tenderness and crepitation improved over time. Outcomes were adversely affected by poor mechanical alignment and patellofemoral chondromalacia. Second-look arthroscopies and histological biopsies were also performed and showed hyaline-like cartilage surfaces.

After osteochondral autograft transplantation, the patient is encouraged to move the knee in a hinged brace through an unrestricted range of motion but is strictly non-weightbearing for the first 6 weeks after surgery. After satisfactory assessment the patient can begin to gradually weightbear as tolerated. Graft healing is assessed both clinically and by 3-monthly serial cartilage-specific magnetic resonance imaging (MRI) scans. Patients are only allowed to return to full sporting activities after MRI evidence of full healing has been obtained.

AUTOLOGOUS CHONDROCYTE IMPLANTATION

In larger lesions, surgical resurfacing using autograft transfer can be a significant challenge. Restoration of articular surface in lesions > 2.5–3 cm^2 and up to 10–15 cm^2 can be accomplished by autologous chondrocyte implantation (ACI) (Brittberg et al. 1994, Minas & Peterson 1999). The technique of ACI involves a two-stage operation in the treatment of articular cartilage lesions. The first operation consists of arthroscopic surgery where the cartilage lesion is clearly defined and a sample of cartilage is harvested from the non-weightbearing area of the knee (usually over the lateral femoral ridge). This cartilage tissue is then sent to the laboratory where cartilage cells are grown and multiplied. The patient then undergoes a second operation, which is an open procedure around 6 weeks after the first operation. The harvested cells are then transplanted into the cartilage defect and the defect is covered with a piece of periosteum harvested from the proximal tibia. A hyaline cartilage repair tissue eventually fills the cartilage defect. The advantages of ACI include the potential to treat larger lesions, the use of autologous tissue and the reliability of obtaining hyaline-like tissues in the lesion. Disadvantages include the high cost of the procedure, the need for staged surgeries and an arthrotomy for reimplantation, as well as the possibility that the repair tissue is at best a rather unpredictable and inconsistent mosaic of bone, fibrous, fibrocartilaginous and hyaline tissue.

Since initiating the procedure of ACI in Sweden, Peterson and colleagues have performed over 1000 ACI procedures. Peterson *et al.* (2000) reported on the results of their first 101 patients who were treated with ACI. The results have been encouraging.

The postoperative rehabilitation protocol for ACI is based on an understanding of the natural history of the repair tissue generated with this technique (Gillogly *et al.* 1998, Minas & Peterson 1999). There are three phases of healing associated with ACI. The first phase (0–6 weeks) is the proliferative phase which occurs early after the cells are implanted. The second phase (7–12 weeks) involves a matrix production phase where the tissue becomes incorporated and integrated into the host. The final phase of healing is the maturation phase (13 weeks to 3 years), which can take an extended period of time as the repair fully matures with its stiffness closely resembling the surrounding articular cartilage. During the proliferative and matrix production phase, the principles of rehabilitation are early motion, which aids cellular orientation and the prevention of adhesions, protection of the graft from mechanical overload, and strengthening exercises that allow a functional gait. CPM and touch weightbearing are used during these early phases. Progression to full weightbearing is generally started between 4 and 6 weeks postoperatively. During the maturation phase, the knee is gradually loaded with increased strengthening exercises and various impact-loading activities. Following these principles during the repair maturation continuum will provide an optimum environment for the tissue to grow and mature.

References

Augat, P., Merk, J., Ignatius, A. *et al.* (1996) Early full weightbearing with flexible fixation delays fracture healing. *Clinical Orthopaedics and Related Research* **328**, 194–202.

Bobic, V. (1996) Arthroscopic osteochondral autograft transplantation in anterior cruciate ligament reconstruction: a preliminary clinical study. *Knee Surgery, Sports Traumatology, Arthroscopy* **3**, 262–264.

Bostrom, M.P.G., Boskey, A., Kaufman, J.K. & Einhorn, T.A. (2000) Form and function of bone. In: *Orthopaedic Basic Science*, 2nd edn (Busckwalter, J.A., ed.). American Academy of Orthopaedic Surgeons, Rosemont, IL: 320–333.

Brittberg, M., Lindahl, A., Nilsson, A. *et al.* (1994) Treatment of deep cartilage defects in the knee with autologous chondrocyte transplantation. *New England Journal of Medicine* **331**, 889–895.

Buckwalter, J.A. & Mankin, H.J. (1997) Articular cartilage. Part I: tissue design and chondrocyte-matrix interactions. *Journal of Bone and Joint Surgery* **79A**, 600–611.

Buckwalter, J.A., Rosenberg, L.C. & Hunziker, E.B. (1990) Articular cartilage: composition, structure, response to injury, and methods of facilitation of repair. In: *Articular Cartilage and Knee Joint Function: Basic Science and Arthroscopy* (Ewing, J.W., ed.). Raven Press, New York: 19–56.

Buckwalter, J.A., Einhorn, T.A., Bolander, M.E. & Cruess, R.L. (1996) Healing of musculoskeletal tissues. In: *Fractures* (Rockwood, C.A. & Green, D., eds). J.B. Lippincott, Philadelphia: 261–304.

Claes, L.E., Heigal, C.A., Neidlinger-Wilke, C. *et al.* (1998) Effects of mechanical factors on the fracture healing process. *Clinical Orthopaedics and Related Research* **355** (Suppl.), S132–S147.

Cunningham, A.E., Cunningham, J.L. & Kenwright, J. (1998) Strain rate and timing of stimulation in mechanical modulation of fracture healing. *Clinical Orthopaedics and Related Research* **355** (Suppl.), S105–115.

Deibert, M.C., McLeod, B.R., Smith, S.D. & Liboff, A.R. (1994) Ion resonance electromagnetic field stimulation of fracture healing in rabbits with fibular ostectomy. *Journal of Orthopaedic Research* **12** (6), 878–885.

Donohue, J.M., Buss, D., Oegema, T.R. & Thompson, R.C. (1983) The effects of indirect blunt trauma on adult canine articular cartilage. *Journal of Bone and Joint Surgery* **65A**, 948–956.

Duarte, L.R. (1983) The stimulation of bone growth by ultrasound. *Archives of Orthopaedic and Traumatic Surgery* **101**, 153–159.

Eyre, D.R. (1980) Collagen: molecular diversity in the body's protein scaffold. *Science* **207**, 1315–1322.

Finch, C., Vlauri, G. & Ozanne-Smith, J. (1998) Sport and active recreation injuries in Australia: evidence from emergency department presentations. *British Journal of Sports Medicine* **32** (3), 220–225.

Gambardella, R.A. & Glousman, R.E. (1999) Autogenous osteochondral grafting: a multicenter review of clinical results. *Proceedings of the 18th AANA Annual Meeting, 1999, Vancouver, BC, Canada*, p. 111.

Gillogly, S.D., Voight, M. & Blackburn, T. (1998) Treatment of articular cartilage defects of the knee with autologous chondrocyte implantation. *Journal of Orthopaedic and Sports Physical Therapy* **28**, 241–251.

Hadjiargyrou, M., Mcleod, K., Ryaby, J.P. & Rubin, C. (1998) Enhancement of fracture healing by low intensity ultrasound. *Clinical Orthopaedics and Related Research* **355** (Suppl.), S216–S219.

Heckman, J.D., Ryaby, J.P., McCabe, J., Frey, J.J. & Kilcoyne, R.F. (1994) Acceleration of tibial fracture-healing by non-invasive, low-intensity pulsed ultrasound. *Journal of Bone and Joint Surgery* **76A**, 26–34.

Holzer, G., Majeska, R.Y., Luny, M.W., Hartke, J.R. & Einhorn, T.A. (1999) Parathyroid hormone enhances fracture healing. A preliminary report. *Clinical Orthopaedics and Related Research* **366**, 258–263.

Hubbard, M.J.S. (1996) Articular debridement versus washout for degeneration of the medial femoral condyle. *Journal of Bone and Joint Surgery (British)* **78**, 217–219.

Johnson, E.E. & Urist, M.R. (2000) Human bone morphogenic protein allografting for reconstruction of femoral nonunion. *Clinical Orthopaedics* **371**, 61–74.

Kenwright, J. & Gardener, T. (1998) Mechanical influences on tibial fracture healing. *Clinical Orthopaedics and Related Research* **355** (Suppl.), S179–S190.

Levy, A.S., Lohnes, J., Sculley, S. *et al.* (1996) Chondral delamination of the knee in soccer players. *American Journal of Sports Medicine* **24**, 634–639.

Mankin, H.J., Mow, V.C., Buckwalter, J.A., Iannotti, J.P. & Ratcliffe, A. (1994) Form and function of articular cartilage. In: *Orthopaedic Basic Science* (Simon, S.R. ed.). American Academy of Orthopaedic Surgeons, Rosemont, IL: 1–44.

Maroudas, A. (1976) Balance between swelling pressure and collagen tension in normal and degenerative cartilage. *Nature* **260**, 808–809.

Minas, T. & Peterson, L. (1999) Advanced techniques in autologous chondrocyte transplantation. *Clinics in Sports Medicine* **18**, 13–44.

Mow, V.C. & Rosenwasser, M.P. (1988) Articular cartilage: biomechanics. In: *Injury and Repair of the Musculoskeletal Soft Tissues* (Woo, S.L. & Buckwalter, J.A. eds). American Academy of Orthopaedic Surgeons, Park Ridge, IL: 427–463.

Muir, H. (1983) Proteoglycans as organizers of the extracellular matrix. *Biochemical Society Transactions* **11**, 613–622.

Outerbridge, R.E. (1961) The etiology of chondromalacia patellae. *Journal of Bone and Joint Surgery* **43**, 752–757.

Peterson, L., Minas, T., Brittberg, M., Nilsson, A., Janssan, E. & Lindahl, A. (2000) Two to nine year outcomes after autologous chondrocyte transplantation of the knee. *Clinical Orthopaedics and Related Research* **374**, 212–234.

Pilla, A.A., Mont, M.A., Nasser, P.R. *et al.* (1990) Non-invasive low-intensity ultrasound accelerates bone healing in the rabbit. *Journal of Orthopaedic Trauma* **4**, 246–253.

Redler, I. (1974) A scanning electron microscopic study of human normal and osteoarthritic articular cartilage. *Clinical Orthopaedics and Related Research* **103**, 262–268.

Rodrigo, J. & Steadman, J.R. (1994) Improvement of full-thickness chondral defect healing in the human knee after debridement and microfracture using continuous passive motion. *American Journal of Knee Surgery* **7**, 109–116.

Roth, V. & Mow, V.C. (1980) The intrinsic tensile behaviour of the matrix of bovine articular cartilage and its variation with age. *Journal of Bone and Joint Surgery* **62A**, 1102–1117.

Ryaby, J.T. (1998) Clinical effects of electromagnetic and electric fields on fracture healing. *Clinical Orthopaedics and Related Research* **355** (Suppl.), S205–S215.

Sakai, R., Miwa, K. & Eto, Y. (1999) Local administration of activin promotes fracture healing in the rat fibula fracture model. *Bone* **25** (2), 191–196.

Sarmiento, A. & Latta, L. (1999) Functional fracture bracing. *Journal of the American Academy of Orthopaedic Surgeons* **7**, 66–75.

Sedel, L., Christel, P., Duriez, J. *et al.* (1981) Acceleration of repair of non-unions by electromagnetic fields. *Revue de Chirurgie Orthopedique et Reparatrice de l'Appareil Moteur* **67**, 11–13.

Setton, L.A., Zhu, W. & Mow, V.C. (1993) The biphasic poroviscoelastic behavior of articular cartilage role of the surface zone in governing the compression behavior. *Journal of Biochemistry* **26**, 581–592.

Shaw, A.D., Gustillo, T. & Court-Brown, C.M. (1997) Epidemiology and outcome of tibial diaphyseal fractures in footballers. *Injury* **28** (5–6), 365–367.

Steadman, J.R., Rodney, W.G., Singleton, S.B. & Briggs, K. (1997) Microfracture technique for full thickness chondral defects: technique and clinical results. *Operative Techniques in Orthopaedics* **7**, 200–205.

Templeton, P.A., Farrar, M.J., Williams, H.R., Bruguera, J. & Smith, R.M. (2000) Complications of tibial shaft soccer fractures. *Injury* **31** (6), 415–419.

Urist, M.R. (1965) Bone formation by autoinduction. *Science* **150**, 893–899.

Wang, S.J., Lewallen, D.G., Bolander, M.E. *et al.* (1994) Low intensity ultrasound treatment increases strength in a rat femoral fracture model. *Journal of Orthopaedic Research* **12**, 40–47.

PART 3

PRACTICAL ISSUES

Chapter 6

Physiological and Performance Consequences of Training Cessation in Athletes: Detraining

IÑIGO MUJIKA AND SABINO PADILLA

Introduction

Sports injuries are an unwanted but often inevitable component of competitive sports. Throughout their careers, most athletes will experience sport-related injuries that will keep them away from training and competition for variable periods of time. In addition to the injury-related functional impairment that the athlete will suffer, these periods of training cessation will also have a negative impact on his or her physiological status and performance level. Indeed, the principle of training reversibility or detraining implies that whereas regular exercise training brings about or preserves specific adaptations that enhance a subject's ability to tolerate the stress factors arising from training, and ultimately athletic performance (Gollnick *et al.* 1984; Houston 1986; Coyle 1988; Tidow 1995), training cessation results in a partial or complete reversal of these adaptations, which compromise athletic performance (Coyle 1988; Hawley & Burke 1998; Mujika & Padilla 2000a, 2001a). Recent reviews on detraining define this term as the partial or complete loss of training-induced anatomical, physiological and performance adaptations, as a consequence of training reduction or cessation (Mujika & Padilla 2000a, 2001a). This definition differentiates the process through which a trained individual loses some or all of his or her training-induced adaptations (e.g. reduced training, training cessation, bed rest confinement) and the lost adaptations themselves, which are the outcome of that process.

Athletes themelves, coaches, physicians and all professionals implicated in the process of getting an injured athlete back on the sports field should be aware of the physiological and performance consequences of training stoppage. Keeping these in mind during all three phases of the rehabilitation process contributes to limiting the negative functional impact of the inactivity associated with the sports injury, and therefore accelerates the recovery of preinjury fitness and performance level.

This chapter focuses on the detraining characteristics of highly trained athletes. However, when scientific data for highly trained athletes are lacking or insufficient, available results on moderately or recently trained subjects that might shed some light on different detraining-related issues will also be reported. In this respect, readers should bear in mind that detraining characteristics may not necessarily be identical in these two types of population (Lacour & Denis 1984; Hawley 1987; Moore *et al.* 1987; Coyle 1988; Neufer 1989; Coyle 1990; Fleck 1994; Wilber & Moffatt 1994; Mujika & Padilla 2000a, 2000b, 2001a, 2001b), and that observations made on laboratory-based training/detraining paradigms may not be directly extrapolated to athletes approaching their higher limits of adaptation.

Cardiorespiratory consequences of training cessation

Athletes in general, and endurance-trained athletes in particular, are characterized by quite impressive functional adaptations of their cardio-vascular and respiratory systems. However, it has often been reported that when the training stimulus is lacking or insufficient to maintain training-induced adaptations, such as during phases one and two of the rehabilitation process, there is a marked negative impact on these systems (Lacour & Denis 1984; Sjøgaard 1984; Hawley 1987; Coyle 1988, 1990; Fleck 1994; Wilber & Moffatt 1994; Mujika & Padilla 2000a, 2000b, 2001a).

Maximal oxygen uptake

Maximal oxygen uptake ($\dot{V}O_{2max}$) is a function of maximal delivery and utilization of oxygen. 'Central' oxygen delivery depends on maximal cardiac output and maximal arterial oxygen content, whereas 'peripheral' extraction of the delivered oxygen is expressed as the arterial–venous oxygen difference (Sutton 1992). All 'central' factors implicated in the oxygen transport system are likely to be affected by training cessation and suffer some degree of detraining.

According to data reported in the literature, training cessation induces a rapid reduction in maximal oxygen uptake ($\dot{V}O_{2max}$) in highly trained individuals with a large aerobic power (> 62 mL·kg^{-1}·min^{-1}) and an extensive training background (Moore et al. 1987), even when training stoppage lasts less than 4 weeks. Indeed, Houston et al. (1979) showed that 15 days of inactivity (7 days of leg casting followed by 8 days without training) led to 4% reductions in $\dot{V}O_{2max}$ in well-trained endurance runners. $\dot{V}O_{2max}$ also decreased by 4.7% in a group of endurance-trained runners who refrained from training for 14 days (Houmard et al. 1992, 1993). Coyle et al. (1986) studied eight endurance-trained subjects who stopped training for 2 or 4 weeks, and reported 6% $\dot{V}O_{2max}$ declines during upright exercise. Even more pronounced results were observed by Mankowitz et al. (1992), who reported a 12% decline in $\dot{V}O_{2max}$ during 14–22 days of training stoppage in a group of trained runners, and by Martin et al. (1986), who indicated

that 3–8 weeks of physical deconditioning in highly trained subjects brought about a 20% reduction of $\dot{V}O_{2max}$. Similar results have been repeatedly reported in team sport athletes. Male basketball players not training for 4 weeks once their competitive season was over showed a 13.8% $\dot{V}O_{2max}$ reduction (Ghosh et al. 1987), and 11 college soccer players decreased their $\dot{V}O_{2max}$ by 6.9% during 5 weeks of training cessation (Fardy 1969). Smorawinski et al. (2001) have recently shown a 16.5 and 10.4% $\dot{V}O_{2max}$ reduction in amateur cyclists and bodybuilders, respectively, as a result of 3 days of bed rest.

Conflicting results, however, are not lacking in the exercise science literature. Fifteen distance runners were shown to maintain $\dot{V}O_{2max}$ after 10 days of training cessation (Cullinane et al. 1986). The same was proven true for a group of trained cyclists and runners who also stopped training for 10 days (Heath et al. 1983), a group of female college swimmers not training for a similar period of time (Claude & Sharp 1991) and a group of soccer players after 3 weeks of training stoppage (Bangsbo & Mizuno 1988). These conflicting results could be partly explained by the different levels of physical activity performed by the athletes during the period of training stoppage.

Time and initial fitness level seem to determine the $\dot{V}O_{2max}$ loss during periods of training cessation. Indeed, seven endurance-trained subjects stopped training for 84 days, and their $\dot{V}O_{2max}$ declined by 7 and 16% in 21 and 56 days, respectively, it then stabilized at that level, which was still 17.3% higher than that of sedentary control subjects. A correlation of 0.93 was observed between $\dot{V}O_{2max}$ in the trained state and per cent $\dot{V}O_{2max}$ decline with inactivity (Coyle et al. 1984). Pavlik et al. (1986a, 1986b) reported on 40 observations referring to highly trained road cyclists and endurance runners who, for various reasons, stopped training for 60 days. They observed a linear decline in the athletes' $\dot{V}O_{2max}$ ($r = -0.55$) throughout the initial 45 days of training stoppage, with no further change thereafter. Sinacore et al. (1993) reported on five male and one female endurance-trained subjects who stopped training

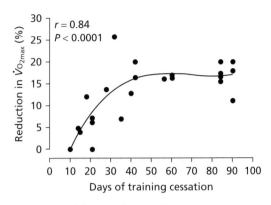

Fig. 6.1 Third degree polynomial regression between the number of days of training cessation and the percentage loss in maximal oxygen uptake ($\dot{V}O_{2max}$) in athletes, according to data reported in the literature.

for 12 weeks. $\dot{V}O_{2max}$ declined by 17.1%, and this decline was greatest in those subjects with the highest initial $\dot{V}O_{2max}$ values. Smorawinski et al. (2001) also observed a relationship between the initial $\dot{V}O_{2max}$ and the decrement in its value ($r = 0.73$) in amateur cyclists and bodybuilders confined to rest in bed for 3 days. Very long-term (2 years) training cessation has also been shown to be characterized by $\dot{V}O_{2max}$ declines of 6.3% in college badminton players (Miyamura & Ishida 1990).

These and other similar reported data (Drinkwater & Horvath 1972; Nemeth & Lowry 1984; Coyle et al. 1985; Martin et al. 1986; Allen 1989; Giada et al. 1995; Katzel et al. 1997; Nichols et al. 2000) indicate that the $\dot{V}O_{2max}$ of highly trained athletes decreases progressively and proportionally to the initial $\dot{V}O_{2max}$ during the initial 8 weeks of training cessation, this decline usually ranging between 4 and 20%. Most investigations, however, indicate that $\dot{V}O_{2max}$ ceases to decline thereafter (Fig. 6.1) and remains higher than that of untrained counterparts (Fardy 1969; Coyle et al. 1984, 1985), although one study reported that their subjects' $\dot{V}O_{2max}$ fell down to sedentary values (Drinkwater & Horvath 1972). This partial retention of $\dot{V}O_{2max}$ by highly trained athletes may be due to the accumulated effect of long-term training, but it might also be due to the inherent, genetically determined physiological capabilities of these athletes (Wilber & Moffatt 1994).

Blood volume

The observed reduction in cardiovascular function during short periods of training cessation (see Fig. 6.2) can to a large extent be attributed to a decline in blood volume, which may be apparent within the first 2 days of inactivity (Thompson et al. 1984; Cullinane et al. 1986). Houmard et al. (1992) considered that part of the reduction in $\dot{V}O_{2max}$ observed in a group of distance runners after 14 days of training withdrawal was due to a 5.1% reduction in estimated resting plasma volume. Identical 5% decreases in plasma volume have been observed by other authors in distance runners who ceased training for 10 days (Thompson et al. 1984; Cullinane et al. 1986). Moreover, eight endurance athletes who refrained from training for 2 or 4 weeks were reported to suffer 9 and 12% declines in blood and plasma volumes during upright exercise, respectively (Coyle et al. 1986).

The mechanisms responsible for these declines have not been clearly established. However, marked reductions in plasma protein content are likely to play an important part. In a study with previously untrained individuals as subjects, 16 young males underwent 4 weeks of endurance training and heat acclimatization followed by 4 weeks of training stoppage. The latter resulted in reduced $\dot{V}O_{2max}$ (3.6%) and blood volume (4.7%). Red cell volume decreased by 98 mL, plasma volume by 248 mL, total plasma protein by 16 g and plasma albumin by 12 g. Moreover, plasma volume changes were directly related to plasma protein dynamics, as loss of protein appeared to be responsible for 97% of the reduction in plasma volume (Pivarnik & Senay 1986). In addition, 6 days of training cessation have been shown to fully reverse the effects of short-term training (6 days) on resting plasma volume and concentrations of aldosterone and adrenaline (epinephrine) during submaximal intensity exercise, but not those of arginine vasopressin. According to the authors of the study, these observations implicate plasma volume as a significant variable in modifying the exercise response of fluid and electrolyte hormones (Shoemaker *et al.* 1998). In contrast, Raven *et al.* (1998) reported that a reduction of daily aerobic activity (active deconditioning) for 8 weeks resulted in a significant 7% $\dot{V}o_{2max}$ decrease in eight untrained women and 11 untrained men. None the less, total blood volume (4.0%) and plasma volume (3.1%) did not decrease significantly, and the baseline haemodynamic variables analysed by the investigators were unaltered by the deconditioning period. These data suggest that some of the changes in $\dot{V}o_{2max}$ accompanying physical deconditioning may be independent of changes in total blood volume and plasma volume (Raven *et al.* 1998).

Heart rate

RESTING HEART RATE

Whereas resting heart rate has been shown to increase significantly after only 3 days of bed rest in endurance athletes (Smorawinski *et al.* 2001), it has been reported not to change in athletes following short-term (10 days) training cessation (Cullinane *et al.* 1986). Resting heart rate did not change in five Olympic rowers and one canoeist during 6–34 weeks of training stoppage following the 1988 Seoul Olympic Games (Maron *et al.* 1993), but it increased by 6.4% in 2–12 weeks of injury-induced training cessation in physical education students (Bánhegyi *et al.* 1999).

SUBMAXIMAL HEART RATE

As a consequence of the above-mentioned reduction in blood volume, the heart rate at submaximal exercise intensities increases by approximately 5–10%. Coyle *et al.* (1986), observed an 11% higher heart rate during submaximal exercise after a group of endurance athletes spent 2–4 weeks away from training. Heart rate while performing submaximal exercise (75 and 90% of $\dot{V}o_{2max}$) increased by 11 beats·min^{-1} in a group of endurance runners after 14 days without training (Houmard *et al.* 1992). Madsen *et al.* (1993) also observed heart rates of 6–7 beats·min^{-1} higher at submaximal exercise intensities after 4 weeks of insufficient training stimulus in nine endurance athletes.

Changes in athletes' submaximal exercise heart rates have also been reported after longer periods of training cessation. Seven endurance-trained subjects exercised at the same absolute submaximal intensity in a trained state and during 84 days of no training. Their heart rates increased from 84 to 93% of maximal values during the initial 56 days of inactivity, but stabilized thereafter. Exercise of the same relative submaximal intensity, on the other hand, elicited almost identical percentages of maximal heart rate (Coyle *et al.* 1985). Eleven college soccer players showed increased heart rate at submaximal exercise intensities during 5 weeks without training (Fardy 1969). This result, along with a shortened length of the cardiac isovolumetric contraction phase at rest, led the author of the study to suggest that inactivity brought about an increase in the sympathoadrenergic tone of the players. Increased submaximal heart rates were also observed in adolescent (15–18 years) female athletes as a result of 12 (Drinkwater & Horvath 1972) and 23 (Michael *et al.* 1972) weeks of training cessation following the track season. In addition, the latter investigators also observed a progressive 16% increase in postexercise recovery heart rate, but stated that both submaximal and recovery heart rate increases seemed to level off after the initial 7 weeks of training stoppage. In line with the above results, six college football players showed an increased heart rate during submaximal exercise after 9 weeks of training cessation following their competitive season. Their values, nevertheless, remained lower than those of sedentary counterparts (Penny & Wells 1975). Giada *et al.* (1998) observed that heart rates at a power output of 100 W increased from 108 to 114 beats·min^{-1} in young cyclists, and from 100 to 106 beats·min^{-1} in older cyclists after 2 months of training cessation.

The training stoppage also influences heart rate during maximal intensity exercise, increasing it by about 5–10%. Cullinane *et al.* (1986) measured a 5% increase in maximal heart rate in 15 runners after 10 days of training cessation. Fourteen days of training cessation also resulted in 9 beats·min^{-1} higher maximal heart rate in a group of endurance runners (Houmard *et al.* 1992). Madsen *et al.* (1993), on the other hand, reported unchanged maximal heart rates after 4 weeks of insufficient training stimulus in nine endurance athletes. In contrast, in an 84-day training cessation follow-up study on seven endurance-trained subjects, maximal heart rate increased by 4–5% after the initial 12–21 days without training, but it did not change thereafter (Coyle *et al.* 1984).

Stroke volume

The reduced maximal aerobic capacity observed in highly trained subjects after short periods of training cessation seems to be a consequence of the decline in stroke volume arising from the reduced blood volume that characterizes detraining (Coyle *et al.* 1984). Coyle *et al.* (1986) observed that stroke volume fell by 12% during upright exercise in a group of endurance athletes who stopped training for 2–4 weeks. This effect was reversed after plasma volume expansion, but this intervention did not restore $\dot{V}o_{2max}$, which remained 3% lower than in the trained state. This observation suggests that the reduction in blood volume associated with detraining limits ventricular filling during upright exercise and is largely responsible for the inactivity-induced decline in cardiovascular function. Stroke volume declined by 10% after the initial 12 of 84 days without training in seven endurance-trained subjects, and averaged 10–14% below trained levels during 12–84 days of training stoppage. These values did not differ from the controls. The authors indicated that the decline in $\dot{V}o_{2max}$ during the initial 21 days of training cessation was associated with a decreased stroke volume

(Coyle *et al.* 1984). The same group reported that 3–8 weeks of physical deconditioning in highly trained subjects, which brought about a 20% reduction of $\dot{V}o_{2max}$, resulted in a significant 17.2% reduction in stroke volume during upright exercise (Martin *et al.* 1986). On the other hand, Pavlik *et al.* (1986a, 1986b) indicated that the resting stroke volume index (mL·beat^{-1}·m^{-2}) and ejection fraction rose in a group of highly trained road cyclists and endurance runners during 60 days of training cessation. These changes were paralleled by a linear decrease in $\dot{V}o_{2max}$ until the 45th day of training withdrawal. In contrast, Smorawinski *et al.* (2001) recently reported on a significant decrease in resting stroke volume in a group of endurance athletes after 3 days of bed rest, but not in bodybuilders. The authors did not elucidate whether these differences depended on the subjects' habitual physical training mode and endurance activity level or the genetic factors associated with aerobic capacity.

Cardiac output

Cardiac output decreases during exercise in highly trained athletes during periods of training cessation. This decrease takes place because the above-mentioned increase in exercise heart rate is not enough to counterbalance the decline in stroke volume. Coyle *et al.* (1984) reported that estimated maximal cardiac output stabilized at 8% below trained values after 21 days of training cessation in endurance athletes, not falling beyond that level between the 21st and 84th days without training. These authors also observed a progressive shift from 84 to 94% of maximal cardiac output between the trained and detrained (84 days without training) states when subjects exercised at the same absolute submaximal intensity, whereas exercise of the same relative submaximal intensity elicited almost identical percentages of cardiac output (Coyle *et al.* 1985). Slightly but significantly higher cardiac ouputs were also elicited during submaximal supine exercise following 8 weeks of training cessation in highly trained subjects (Martin *et al.* 1986).

Detrained cyclists' and runners' cardiac index ($L \cdot m^{-2} \cdot min^{-1}$) increased at rest as a result of the increased stroke volume index (Pavlik *et al.* 1986a, 1986b). Also, resting cardiac output of 55 physical education students not training for 2–12 weeks due to injury increased by 10.1% (Bánhegyi *et al.* 1999). On the other hand, submaximal and maximal cardiac output was unchanged in endurance athletes and bodybuilders as a result of 3 days of bed rest (Smorawinski *et al.* 2001).

Cardiac dimensions and circulation

Short-term training cessation has also been shown to result in altered cardiac dimensions in highly trained athletes (Fig. 6.2). Martin *et al.* (1986), for instance, reported significant reductions in left ventricular end-diastolic dimension (11.8%), left ventricular wall thickness (25.0%) and increased mean blood pressure during upright exercise in athletes who did not take part in physical training for 3 weeks. These investigators attributed these changes to a reduction in left ventricular

mass (19.5%). The increased mean blood pressure during upright exercise measured by these and other authors (Coyle *et al.* 1986) could indeed be due to a reduced left ventricular mass, coupled with a higher total peripheral resistance, which increased by 8% after 2–4 weeks of training cessation (Coyle *et al.* 1986). Cullinane *et al.* (1986), on the other hand, did not observe any change in the cardiac dimensions and the blood pressure of 15 distance runners following 10 days of training stoppage. During longer periods of training cessation (8 weeks), the left ventricular end-diastolic dimension of highly trained athletes declined in parallel with stroke volume when performing upright exercise (Martin *et al.* 1986). Meanwhile, left ventricular posterior wall thickness decreased progressively by 25%, but left ventricular mass was unaltered after the decline observed following the first 3 weeks of deconditioning.

Six Olympic-level athletes (five rowers and one canoeist) were shown to decrease their maximal left ventricular wall thickness by 23% (range 15–33%) and their left ventricular mass by 22%

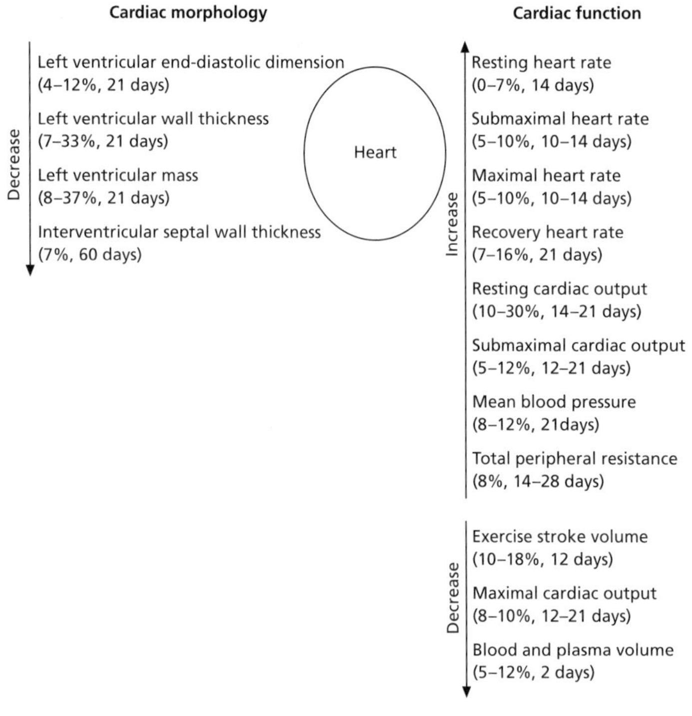

Cardiac morphology

Decrease

Left ventricular end-diastolic dimension
(4–12%, 21 days)

Left ventricular wall thickness
(7–33%, 21 days)

Left ventricular mass
(8–37%, 21 days)

Interventricular septal wall thickness
(7%, 60 days)

Heart

Cardiac function

Increase

Resting heart rate
(0–7%, 14 days)

Submaximal heart rate
(5–10%, 10–14 days)

Maximal heart rate
(5–10%, 10–14 days)

Recovery heart rate
(7–16%, 21 days)

Resting cardiac output
(10–30%, 14–21 days)

Submaximal cardiac output
(5–12%, 12–21 days)

Mean blood pressure
(8–12%, 21days)

Total peripheral resistance
(8%, 14–28 days)

Decrease

Exercise stroke volume
(10–18%, 12 days)

Maximal cardiac output
(8–10%, 12–21 days)

Blood and plasma volume
(5–12%, 2 days)

Fig. 6.2 Morphological and physiological changes most likely to occur at the cardiac level, and minimum reported time of training cessation necessary for these changes to take place in athletes.

(range 8–37%) during 6–34 weeks of training stoppage following the 1988 Seoul Olympic Games. No changes in blood pressure or resting heart rate were observed. It was concluded that deconditioning may be associated with a considerable reduction in ventricular septal thickness in elite athletes, suggesting that this population had a physiological form of left ventricular hypertrophy induced by training (Maron *et al.* 1993). Studying a group of young (24 ± 6 years) and a group of older (55 ± 5 years) amateur cyclists during 2 months of training stoppage, Giada *et al.* (1998) reported a reduced posterior wall thickness index (6.6%) and interventricular septal wall thickness index (6.5%) in the young athletes. In the older athletes, detraining was characterized by a reduced left ventricular end-diastolic diameter index (3.4%), left ventricular end-diastolic volume index (9.9%) and left ventricular mass index (15.7%). The authors concluded that in the young athletes, thickness was greatly reduced whereas ventricular cavities remained unchanged, the final result being a slight and non-significant reduction in left ventricular mass. Conversely, in the older athletes, the significant reduction in left ventricular mass was the result of reduced cardiac cavities, whereas thickness of the free wall and septum remained unchanged. It was suggested that in the elderly subjects cardiac adaptation to aerobic training takes place mainly through a higher degree of diastolic filling of the left ventricle with a greater utilization of Starling's mechanism, which makes up for the reduced chronotropic capacity.

Giannattasio *et al.* (1992) reported that former professional sprint runners and hammer throwers had left ventricular end-diastolic diameter and mass indexes similar to those of sedentary subjects after 4–5 years of training cessation. They also indicated that the impairment of the cardiopulmonary reflex that they observed in athletes is to a great extent reversible with training cessation-induced regression of cardiac hypertrophy. Pavlik *et al.* (1986a, 1986b) observed that diastolic relative muscular wall thickness, interventricular septum thickness and left ventricular posterior wall thickness remained unchanged

and above control values in road cyclists and endurance runners during 60 days of inactivity. The same was true for end-diastolic and end-systolic volumes. Small and opposite non-significant changes were observed in relative left ventricular end-diastolic volume (which tended to increase) and relative left ventricular end-systolic volume (which tended to decrease), resulting in a linearly increased ejection fraction until the 30th day of no training ($r = 0.40$), which reached control level. The stroke volume index also increased until the 40th day ($r = 0.40$). Since the resting heart rate remained low throughout the follow-up period, the resting cardiac index grew linearly until day 40 ($r = 0.47$), reaching the control level by the third week, then exceeding it. No further change was observed between the 45th and 60th days. Left ventricular mean circumferential shortening velocity followed a similar increasing trend until day 30 ($r = 0.44$). Mean arterial blood pressure remained practically stable throughout the study, but relative total peripheral resistance declined continuously ($r = -0.45$). Based on their observations, these authors concluded that the cardiovascular regulation undergoes a peculiar shift during training cessation in that a persisting cardiac enlargement and bradycardia is associated with a temporarily unstable autonomic control due to relatively high levels of both sympathetic and parasympathetic activity. This imbalance often leads to a hyperkinesis-like syndrome when an athlete stops endurance training abruptly. These conclusions coincide with a clinical entity known as 'detraining syndrome' (also referred to as 'relaxation syndrome'), which arises when athletes with a long endurance-training history suddenly abandon their regular physical activity (Mujika & Padilla 2000a). It is characterized by a tendency to dizziness and fainting, non-systematic precordial disturbances, sensations of cardiac arrhythmia, extrasystolia and palpitation, headaches, loss of appetite, gastric disturbances, profuse sweating, insomnia, anxiety and depression (Israel 1972; S'Jongers 1976).

Bánhegyi *et al.* (1999), on the other hand, studying a group of 22 female and 23 male physical education students who were forced to stop exercising due to injury, reported slight reductions in relative left ventricular wall thickness and relative left ventricular muscle mass (2.6 and 2.7%, respectively). They also observed increased resting heart rate (6.4%) and cardiac output (10.1%). When comparing these results with their own previous observations on highly trained cyclists (Pavlik et al. 1986a, 1986b), they concluded that the earliest modifications in echocardiographic parameters are likely to appear in the autonomous regulation of the heart, first in sympathetic activity, then in parasympathetic tone. The change in morphological parameters, if any, would appear much later. This time course would be the result of the fast response of the nervous regulatory component, and it would depend on the previous conditioning level of the athlete, as athletes of excellent condition not training for several weeks were only shown to increase resting sympathetic autonomous activity, whereas less well-trained athletes' changes in the components of cardiac function occur sooner and in a faster sequence (an elevation of resting sympathetic activity becomes manifest in an increased resting cardiac output, a drop in resting parasympathetic tone in a faster heart rate, and also some of the morphological parameters may show modifications).

Interestingly, three out of 10 highly trained masters athletes (59 ± 8 years) developed new asymptomatic ischaemic-appearing, exercise-induced ST segment depression on their exercise electrocardiogram (ECG) during 3 months of training stoppage (Katzel et al. 1997). After 5–8 years of follow-up, two of the three athletes with silent ischaemia experienced major cardiac events (sudden death, cardiac bypass surgery), whereas the other seven athletes did not have any cardiovascular events. These observations led the authors to suggest that silent ischaemia after a 3-month period of training stoppage in highly trained older athletes may be a predictor of future cardiac events (Begum & Katzel 2000).

Mean and systolic blood pressures have been shown to increase along with total peripheral resistance during 9–12 weeks without training in six endurance cyclists and runners (Martin et al. 1986) and in six college football players (Penny & Wells 1975). The values of the latter, however, remained lower than those of sedentary counterparts. It should also be noted that there have been reports of unchanged blood pressure in seven young female track athletes (aged 14–17 years) following 12 weeks of training cessation at the end of their competitive season (Drinkwater & Horvath 1972), and in Olympic rowers and canoeists not training for 6–34 weeks (Maron et al. 1993).

Ventilatory function

According to several reports in the literature, ventilatory function suffers a rapid deterioration when highly trained athletes stop exercising. Maximal exercise ventilation decreased in parallel with $\dot{V}o_{2max}$ (2–7%) in six runners after 15 days without training (Houston et al. 1979). Also, male basketball players not training for 4 weeks after their competitive season showed a deterioration of cardiorespiratory efficiency, as indicated by reduced maximal ventilation (9.3%), O_2 pulse (12.7%) and increased ventilatory equivalent (3.9%) (Ghosh et al. 1987). In the above-mentioned investigations, maximal ventilatory volume decreased in parallel with $\dot{V}o_{2max}$. A much higher decline in maximal ventilation (21.3%) has been observed in endurance athletes after just 3 days of bed rest (Smorawinski et al. 2001). Cullinane et al. (1986) did not observe a decreased maximal ventilatory volume in male long-distance runners after 10 days of inactivity, but they did observe a significantly lower maximal O_2 pulse.

Reports on the negative effects of longer periods of training cessation on ventilatory volume during maximal exercise have also been published. Indeed, maximal ventilation decreased by 10, 10.3 and 14.5% in 11 college soccer players in 5 weeks (Fardy 1969), young female track athletes in 12 weeks (Drinkwater & Horvath 1972) and five badminton players in 2 years (Miyamura & Ishida 1990), respectively. In addition, the latter athletes' hypercapnic ventilatory responsiveness was shown to increase significantly. Also, ventilatory volume shifted from 53 to 71% of the maximal after 56 days without training in endurance athletes (Coyle *et al.* 1985). Drink-water and Horvath (1972) and Michael *et al.* (1972) also observed markedly increased sub-maximal ventilatory volume and ventilatory equivalent in female athletes during long-term training cessation.

Metabolic consequences of training cessation

When an athlete reduces his or her habitual level of physical training to a level which is insufficient to maintain previously acquired adaptations, metabolic detraining occurs. This is primarily characterized by marked changes in the pattern of substrate availability and utilization during exercise, which most often result in altered lactate kinetics that are detrimental to sports performance (Hawley 1987; Neufer 1989; Wilber & Moffatt 1994; Mujika & Padilla 2000a&b, 2001a).

Substrate availability and utilization

RESPIRATORY EXCHANGE RATIO

One of the metabolic consequences of a short period of insufficient training stimulus in athletes is an increased respiratory exchange ratio (RER)

at submaximal and maximal exercise intensities (Table 6.1). Moore *et al.* (1987) observed in an athletic population that 3 weeks of training stop-page brought about a shift in RER from 0.89 to 0.95 at an exercise intensity of 60% of $\dot{V}o_{2max}$. In another investigation, seven endurance-trained athletes exercised at the same absolute sub-maximal intensity when they trained and during 84 days of training cessation; the RER increased from 0.93 to 1.00. Exercise of the same relative submaximal intensity elicited almost identical percentages of maximal heart rate, ventilation and cardiac output, but RER increased from 0.93 to 0.96 (Coyle *et al.* 1985). Also, the RERs of nine highly trained endurance athletes shifted from 0.89 to 0.91 when cycling at 75% of $\dot{V}o_{2max}$ after 4 weeks of insufficient training (Madsen *et al.* 1993). Maximal RER also increased from 1.03 to 1.06 after 14 days without training in a group of endurance-trained runners (Houmard *et al.* 1992). Finally, Drinkwater and Horvath (1972) reported higher RER values during submaximal and maximal exercise in female athletes 12 weeks after the end of the track season, and Smorawinski *et al.* (2001) observed higher RER values both at rest and at submaximal exercise intensities in endurance athletes confined to bed for 3 days. Taken as a whole, these results clearly indicate a shift towards an increased reliance on carbohy-drate as an energy substrate for exercising mus-cles, concomitantly with a decreased contibution from lipid metabolism.

Table 6.1 Studies reporting changes in the exercise respiratory exchange ratio (RER) as a result of training cessation in athletes.

Days of training cessation	Exercise intensity	Trained vs detrained RER	Reference
12	74% $\dot{V}o_{2max}$	0.93 vs 0.97	Coyle *et al.* 1985
14	100% $\dot{V}o_{2max}$	1.03 vs 1.06	Houmard *et al.* 1992
21	74% $\dot{V}o_{2max}$	0.93 vs 0.98	Coyle *et al.* 1985
21	60% $\dot{V}o_{2max}$	0.89 vs 0.95	Moore *et al.* 1987
28	75% $\dot{V}o_{2max}$	0.89 vs 0.91	Madsen *et al.* 1993
56	74% $\dot{V}o_{2max}$	0.93 vs 0.99	Coyle *et al.* 1985
84	74% $\dot{V}o_{2max}$	0.93 vs 1.00	Coyle *et al.* 1985
84	100% $\dot{V}o_{2max}$	0.97 vs 1.10	Drinkwater & Horvath 1972

GLUCOSE AND LIPID METABOLISM

There have been several reports of a rapid decline in sensitivity for insulin-mediated whole-body glucose uptake during short-term inactivity. Burstein *et al.* (1985) studied insulin-stimulated glucose disposal and erythrocyte insulin receptor binding in seven endurance-trained athletes (six runners and one swimmer) after 12 h, 60 h and 7 days of training stoppage. Plasma glucose did not change throughout the study period, but plasma insulin increased significantly between the second and seventh days without training. The metabolic clearance rate of glucose, measured by the euglycaemic clamp technique, decreased from 15.6 ± 1.8 mL·kg^{-1}·min^{-1} at the 12 h time point after the last training bout, to 10.1 ± 1.0 mL·kg^{-1}·min^{-1} at 60 h, and to 8.5 ± 0.5 mL·kg^{-1}·min^{-1} after 7 days. The last two values were not different from those of the sedentary controls (7.8 ± 1.2 mL·kg^{-1}·min^{-1}). There was also a $21.4 \pm 1.8\%$ decrease in insulin receptor binding to isolated young erythrocytes between 12 and 60 h postexercise, apparently due to a reduced receptor number, rather than the affinity. These authors concluded that the increase in peripheral insulin action seen in trained athletes is rapidly reversed, and that modulation of *in vivo* insulin response by training stoppage may be at least partially mediated by changes in insulin receptor number. Five days of training stoppage were enough in endurance athletes to decrease insulin sensitivity to levels found in untrained counterparts (Mikines *et al.* 1989a). These authors, using the sequential hyperglycaemic clamp technique, reported that glucose-induced β-cell secretion increased slightly towards untrained levels during the same period, indicating that β-cells are subjected to an adaptation during training (Mikines *et al.* 1989b). Hardman *et al.* (1998) measured a 15.8% higher postprandial serum insulin response in endurance athletes after 6.5 days without exercise.

In a similar short-term inactivity study (6 days) in endurance runners, it was shown that glucose disposal rates after insulin infusion fell by 14.2–29.5%, despite 10.0–21.9% higher plasma insulin. Insulin clearance and muscle GLUT-4 glucose

transporter protein were also reduced by 8–29 and 17.5%, respectively. These results indicated that short-term inactivity decreases insulin action in endurance runners, suggesting that a reduction in muscle GLUT-4 transporter level may play a role in the decrease in glucose disposal rates (Vukovich *et al.* 1996). McCoy *et al.* (1994) reported that 10 days of training stoppage in trained triathletes resulted in a 43.3% increase in the area under the insulin response curve during an oral glucose tolerance test, but still remained 24.3% below values of untrained control subjects. No change was observed following training cessation in the glucose response to the test, but GLUT-4 protein levels decreased by 33.2%, in parallel with a 28.6% reduction in citrate synthase activity, suggesting that glucose transport and oxidation are regulated by the muscle activity level. In keeping with the previous findings, the area under the glucose and insulin curves increased, respectively, by 65 and 73% during 7–10 days of training cessation in endurance-trained athletes. Resting metabolic rate fell by 4%, and the RER during the oral glucose tolerance test increased by the same amount. However, no change was observed in the calf and forearm blood flow. These data indicated a deterioration in glucose tolerance and energy metabolism, but these changes did not seem to be mediated by limb blood flow (Arciero *et al.* 1998).

Heath *et al.* (1983) also studied the effects of 10 days of training cessation on glucose tolerance and insulin sensitivity in a group of trained cyclists and runners. Glucose tolerance was significantly reduced, as shown by a 10–25% increase in blood glucose concentration and a 55–120% increase in plasma insulin concentration in response to an oral glucose tolerance test. A single bout of exercise, however, returned post-glucose tolerance test glucose and insulin levels to almost initial trained values, giving support to the authors' hypothesis that residual effects of the last bouts of exercise play an important role in the trained individuals' improved glucose tolerance and blunted insulin response to a glucose load. Following 14 days of training cessation, an increased area under the glucose curve

(14.8%) was observed in 12 endurance runners. The insulin curve also increased in endurance (30.3%) and strength (23.3%) in athletes during an oral glucose tolerance test. The insulin sensitivity index decreased by 23.7% in the former, and 16.0% in the latter. The authors, however, observed no change in GLUT-4 content, either in endurance runners or in weightlifters. This lack of change was evident despite a 25.3% decrease in citrate synthase activity in the endurance runners. It was concluded that the decrement in insulin sensitivity with training cessation was not associated with a decrease in GLUT-4 protein content, and that muscle oxidative capacity does not necessarily change in tandem with GLUT-4 protein content (Houmard et al. 1993).

On the other hand, 2 weeks of training cessation from endurance running has been shown to yield a condition that favours the storage of adipose tissue, as shown by a marked increase (86%) in adipose tissue lipoprotein lipase activity, coupled with a marked decrease (45–74%) in muscle lipoprotein lipase activity (Simsolo et al. 1993). Moreover, endurance-trained subjects in the fasted state have been reported to increase their concentrations of triacylglycerol (47%), very low-density lipoprotein cholesterol (28.2%) and the ratio of total cholesterol : high-density lipoprotein cholesterol (7.5%) during 6.5 days without exercise. Concentrations of non-esterified fatty acids, on the other hand, decreased during the same period by 43.5%. Due to a higher rate of triacylglycerol removal, probably related to their high lipoprotein lipase activity because of their well-vascularized skeletal muscle mass, endurance-trained subjects usually exhibit low levels of postprandial lipaemia. However, 6.5 days without training increased postprandial lipaemia by 42.2%, as shown by the increased area under the plasma triacylglycerol versus time curve, indicating that frequent exercise is necessary to maintain a low level of postprandial lipaemia in endurance-trained subjects (Hardman et al. 1998). Ten days of training cessation also resulted in a 15% reduction in high-density lipoprotein cholesterol and a 10% increase in low-density lipoprotein cholesterol in endurance-trained ath-

letes (Thompson et al. 1984). Also, marathon runners have been shown to increase their plasma levels of lipoprotein(a) and apolipoprotein A1 by 24.2 and 16.0%, respectively, during 1 month of suspended physical activity of all types. Moreover, high-density lipoprotein cholesterol decreased by 14.6% as compared with post-marathon race values (Bonetti et al. 1995). Giada et al. (1995) studied the effects of 2 months of training stoppage in a group of young (24 ± 6 years) and a group of older (55 ± 5 years) amateur cyclists. Compared with the values recorded at the peak of their seasonal preparation, body fat increased by 4 and 2% in young and older athletes, respectively. Triglycerides (14.5 and 22.2%) and the low-density lipoprotein cholesterol : high-density lipoprotein cholesterol ratio (21.4 and 26.3%) increased significantly in both groups, whereas apolipoprotein A1 (8.4 and 8.6%), high-density lipoprotein cholesterol (10.2 and 8.7%), high-density lipoprotein$_2$ cholesterol (10.5 and 12%) and high-density lipoprotein$_3$ cholesterol (7.7 and 4.5%) decreased significantly. In addition, fibrinogen and very low-density lipoprotein cholesterol also increased in the group of young cyclists (5.2 and 34.0%, respectively). The authors of this study concluded that a 2-month interruption in aerobic training changed antiatherogenic lipoprotein profile and body composition unfavourably in both groups, and, therefore, that age did not seem to have a significant influence on the plasma lipid response to training stoppage.

Mankowitz et al. (1992) observed, in a group of trained runners, that 14–22 days of training stoppage resulted in a 7.7% reduction in fasting high-density lipoprotein cholesterol concentration, and a 21% reduction in postheparin lipoprotein lipase activity. No significant changes were observed in body fat, estimated plasma volume, lipoprotein(a), total cholesterol, triglycerides and low-density lipoprotein cholesterol. On the other hand, the mean areas under the concentration versus time curves for chylomicron-retinyl esters increased by 41% and for chylomicron remnant-retinyl esters increased by 37% after training cessation. It was concluded that detraining was characterized by reduced fasting concentrations of high-density lipoprotein cholesterol and a decreased metabolism of chylomicrons—changes that are associated with an increased incidence of atherosclerosis.

During 2 months of training stoppage, six highly trained female swimmers were shown to have increased their body mass by 4.8 kg, of which 4.3 kg was fat mass. This represented an increase in body fat of about 4%. Interestingly, no change was observed in lipid and energy intake during this period, and the energy equivalent of the fat gain (170 MJ) closely matched the habitual energy cost of daily training, suggesting that the fat gain was related to a failure to reduce energy and fat intake to a level commensurate with the new energy and lipid expenditure, perhaps in order to promote the restoration of lipid balance (Alméras et al. 1997).

RESTING METABOLIC RATE

The influence of training cessation on the resting metabolic rate of athletes has not been clearly established. In one report, resting metabolic rate was shown to fall by 4% in a group of endurance-trained athletes during 7–10 days without training, indicating a reduced energy metabolism (Arciero et al. 1998). However, other authors reported that the resting metabolic rate was not affected by 3 weeks of training stoppage in trained males, which led the authors to suggest that exercise training does not potentiate resting metabolic rate (LaForgia et al. 1999).

Blood lactate kinetics

It has been clearly established that highly trained athletes respond to submaximal exercise of the same absolute intensity with higher blood lactate concentrations after only a few days of training cessation. In a recent investigation, the blood lactate threshold of endurance athletes was negatively affected after only 3 days of bed rest, falling from 71 to 60% of $\dot{V}o_{2max}$ (Smorawinski et al. 2001). Competitive swimmers' skeletal muscle metabolic characteristics have been reported

to suffer dramatic changes affecting blood lactate kinetics in as little as 1–4 weeks of training cessation. Indeed, muscle respiratory capacity decreased by 50% after 1 week of inactivity in a group of eight swimmers. When subjects performed a standardized 183 m submaximal swim, postswim blood lactate was 2.3 times higher, pH significantly lower (7.183 vs 7.259), bicarbonate concentration 22.7% lower, and base deficit twice as high (Costill et al. 1985). A group of 24 college swimmers not training for 4 weeks after 5 months of competitive training showed a 5.5 mmol·L^{-1} increase in blood lactate concentration following a standardized 183 m submaximal swim, which was also indicative of a reduction in the muscle oxidative capacity, and/or a change in the swimmers' mechanical efficiency (Neufer et al. 1987). Similar results were observed by Claude and Sharp (1991) in seven female swimmers who refrained from training for 10 days.

Endurance runners and cyclists performing an exercise task of the same relative submaximal intensity before and after 84 days of training stoppage showed a shift in blood lactate concentration from 1.9 to 3.2 mmol·L^{-1}, along with a marked decline in the muscle respiratory capacity (Coyle et al. 1985). An increased blood lactate concentration at submaximal exercise intensity has also been reported in six college American football players after 9 weeks of postseason break (Penny & Wells 1975). Moreover, the lactate threshold has been shown to decline with 84 days of inactivity from 79.3 to 74.7% of $\dot{V}o_{2max}$, but to remain above sedentary control values of 62.2% (Coyle et al. 1985). Pavlik et al. (1986b) reported on 40 observations on highly trained road cyclists and endurance runners who, for various reasons, stopped training for 60 days. They observed a linear decline in the athletes' lactate threshold ($r = -0.58$) throughout the initial 45 days of training stoppage, with no further change thereafter. Nichols et al. (2000) reported on a female masters athlete (49.5 years) who due to injury was forced to refrain from training for a period of 32 days. Compared to values assessed 2 days preinjury, when the subject was at the peak of her competitive season, power output

Table 6.2 Main metabolic changes most likely to occur, and minimum reported time of training cessation necessary for these changes to take place in athletes.

Metabolic change	Percentage change	Minimum time (days)
↑ Maximal respiratory exchange ratio	3–13	14
↑ Submaximal respiratory exchange ratio	2–8	12
↓ Resting metabolic rate	0–4	7–10
↓ Insulin-mediated glucose uptake	14–46	2.5
↑ Postprandial insulin response	10–22	6.5
↓ Insulin clearance	8–29	6
↓ Muscle GLUT-4 protein content	0–33	6
↓ Muscle lipoprotein lipase activity	21–75	14
↑ Adipose tissue lipoprotein lipase activity	86	14
↑ Body fat	0–4 percentage points	60
↑ Postprandial lipaemia	42	6.5
↑ Triacylglycerol	0–47	6.5
↓ Non-esterified fatty acids	44	6.5
↓ High-density lipoprotein cholesterol	8–15	10
↑ Low-density lipoprotein cholesterol	0–10	10
↑ Very low-density lipoprotein cholesterol	28–34	6.5
↑ Lipoprotein(a)	0–24	30
↓ Chylomicron metabolism	37–41	14–22
↑ Submaximal blood lactate	150–231	7
↓ Lactate threshold	4–17	21
↓ Blood bicarbonate	8–24	7
↓ Muscle glycogen	20–39	7

at the lactate threshold decreased by 16.7%, and power output at a blood lactate concentration of 4 mmol·L^{-1} by 18.9%. The athlete needed approximately 11 weeks to return to her pre-injury level of fitness. A meta-analysis study by Londeree (1997) has confirmed that there is a decline in the lactate threshold with training cessation.

Muscle glycogen

Muscle glycogen concentration declines rapidly with training cessation in highly trained athletes. This decline is associated with a rapid reduction in glucose to glycogen conversion and glycogen synthase activity. In eight competitive swimmers, the deltoid muscle glycogen concentration declined by 20% in the first week of training cessation after the competitive season, and by 8–10% per week without training thereafter (Costill et al. 1985). Pre-exercise muscle glycogen has also been shown to be reduced by 20% in a group of triathletes,

cyclists and runners undergoing 4 weeks of insufficient training (Madsen et al. 1993). Moreover, short-term (5 days) training stoppage has been shown to be enough in seven endurance-trained athletes to decrease glucose to glycogen conversion and glycogen synthase activity towards sedentary values (Mikines et al. 1989a).

A summary of the main metabolic consequences of training cessation in athletes can be found in Table 6.2.

Muscular consequences of training cessation

One of the most important characteristics of skeletal muscle is its dynamic nature. Skeletal muscle tissue has an extraordinary plasticity that enables it to adapt to variable states of functional demands, neuromuscular activity and hormonal signals, by reversibly changing its functional characteristics and structural composition (Saltin & Gollnick 1983; Hoppeler 1986; Kannus et al.

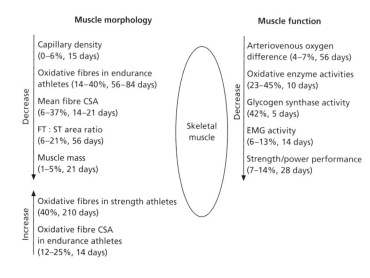

Fig. 6.3 Morphological and physiological changes most likely to occur at the skeletal muscle level, and minimum reported time of training cessation necessary for these changes to take place in athletes.

1992b; Gordon & Pattullo 1993). Training-induced skeletal muscle adaptations are such that the trained muscle increases its tolerance to exercise (Houston 1986). On the other hand, as shown in Fig. 6.3, skeletal muscle tissue also readjusts to the reduced physiological stressors during periods of injury, when there is reduced training or complete training cessation (Sjøgaard 1984; Houston 1986; Hawley 1987; Costill 1988; Coyle 1988, 1990; Fleck 1994; Wilber & Moffatt 1994; Tidow 1995; Mujika & Padilla 2001b).

Muscle structure

MUSCLE CAPILLARIZATION

Given the contradictory results that have been reported in the literature, it is fair to state that the effects of training stoppage on capillary density in athletes have not been clearly established. Houston et al. (1979) reported a 6.3% reduction in capillary density after only 15 days of training cessation in well-trained endurance runners. Similarly, in semiprofessional soccer players, the number of capillaries around ST fibres decreased significantly from 6.0 to 5.8 after 3 weeks of training cessation (Bangsbo & Mizuno 1988). In contrast with these results, Coyle et al. (1984) reported that seven endurance-trained subjects' trained-state muscle capillarization was unchanged after

as long as 84 days without training, and that capillarization in this population was about 50% higher than in sedentary controls. These authors discussed that the retention of the increased capillary density contributed to the observed partial maintenance of the ability to attain a high percentage of $\dot{V}O_{2max}$ without large increases in blood lactate concentration.

MUSCLE FIBRE DISTRIBUTION

The consequences of training cessation on muscle fibre distribution seem to depend on the duration of the inactive period. Six highly trained distance runners wore a walking plaster cast for 7 days, then refrained from training for 8 additional days, but this was not enough to induce any change in their muscle fibre distribution (Houston et al. 1979). The same was true in the case of four soccer players not training for 3 weeks (Bangsbo & Mizuno 1988), and 12 strength-trained athletes not training for 14 days (Hortobágyi et al. 1993). Longer periods of training cessation, on the other hand, have been reported to induce significant changes in the fibre distribution of athletes participating in various sports. Coyle et al. (1985) observed a large progressive shift from FTa to FTb fibres in endurance runners and cyclists, the latter increasing from 5% in the trained state to 19%

after 56 days of training cessation. Sinacore *et al.* (1993) studied muscle fibre distribution in five male and one female endurance-trained subjects who stopped training for 12 weeks. They observed a 26% increase in the proportion of FTb fibres, and a concomitant 40% decrease in the proportion of FTa fibres. Larsson and Ansved (1985) reported that the proportion of ST fibres in four elite oarsmen decreased by 14–16% during the 4-year period following their retirement from competition. An opposite tendency towards a higher oxidative fibre population has been observed in strength athletes. Indeed, a case study on one elite power lifter indicated that the oxidative muscle fibre population was 1.4 times greater after 7 months without training (Staron *et al.* 1981), and Häkkinen and Alén (1986) reported a reduction in percentage FT muscle fibres (from 66 to 60%) in an elite bodybuilder who underwent training cessation for 13.5 months. Nevertheless, 14–15-year-old soccer players showed unchanged muscle fibre distribution after 4–8 weeks of training cessation (Amigó *et al.* 1998), and female dancers have also been shown not to change their fibre type distribution after long-term (32 weeks) training cessation, suggesting, beyond the possible limitations inherent to the mucle biopsy technique, that their high percentage of ST fibres may have been the result of natural selection rather than a training-induced adaptation (Dahlström *et al.* 1987).

MUSCLE FIBRE SIZE

Mean fibre cross-sectional area (CSA) has been shown to change during short-term training stoppage. Bangsbo and Mizuno (1988) studied samples of the gastrocnemius muscle of male soccer players undergoing 3 weeks of training cessation and reported a 7% decline in the mean fibre CSA. This change was primarily due to a 12.4% decline in FTa fibre area, from 6022 to 5278 μm^2. Similar results have been observed in 12 weightlifters, whose FT fibre CSA declined by 6.4% in 14 days of training stoppage. It is worth mentioning that plasma concentrations of growth hormone (58.3%), testosterone (19.2%) and the

testosterone : cortisol ratio (67.6%) increased during the study period, whereas cortisol and creatine kinase enzyme levels decreased, respectively, by 21.5 and 82.3%. The investigators concluded, on the one hand, that short-term training stoppage in strength athletes specifically affected FT fibre size, and on the other hand, that changes in the hormonal milieu accompanying inactivity were propitious for an enhanced anabolic process, but the absence of the overload training stimulus prevented the materialization of such changes at the tissue level (Hortobágyi *et al.* 1993; Houmard *et al.* 1993). In contrast, 14 days of training stoppage did not result in a changed muscle fibre CSA in a group of endurance runners (Houmard *et al.* 1992); it even increased slightly (from 4.05 to $4.52 \cdot 10^3 \mu m^2$ in ST fibres, and from 4.20 to $5.22 \cdot 10^3 \mu m^2$ in FTa fibres) in a similar group of runners (Houston *et al.* 1979). This change can be considered a reversal of the training-induced reduction in oxidative fibre size which facilitates diffusion by reducing its distance.

Longer periods of training stoppage also brought about declines in FT and ST fibre CSA, the FT : ST area ratio and muscle mass in athletes. It has been shown that rugby league players' CSA of FT fibres decreased to a greater extent than ST fibres, the former being 23% larger at the end of the season, but only 9% larger after 6 weeks without training. Further, an atrophy of the muscle bulk was suggested by the author in view of the fact that body mass decreased from 79.8 to 76.0 kg, but body fat content remained relatively constant during the inactive period (Allen 1989). A 49.5-year-old female masters athlete's fat-free mass decreased by 1.8 kg and body fat increased by 2.1% during 32 days of training stoppage due to injury (Nichols *et al.* 2000). In line with these reports, LaForgia *et al.* (1999) observed a small (0.7 kg) decrease in fat-free mass during a 3-week period without training in trained males. After 7 months of training cessation, an average atrophy of 37.1% was observed in all fibre types of a power lifter, along with a large fat–weight loss (Staron *et al.* 1981). Also, an elite bodybuilder's fat-free mass, thigh and arm girth, and average fibre area decreased by 9.3, 0.5, 11.7 and 8.3%, respectively, after 13.5 months without training. In addition, the FT : ST fibre area ratio decreased from 1.32 to 1.04 (Häkkinen & Alén 1986). Häkkinen *et al.* (1981) also observed a reduction in the FT : ST muscle fibre area ratio from 1.11 to 1.04, and a reduced muscle mass following 8 weeks of training stoppage in strength-trained athletes, as well as decreased FT and ST fibre areas after 12 weeks without training (Häkkinen *et al.* 1985). Larsson and Ansved (1985) observed a 10% decrease in the relative area of ST fibres in oarsmen after long-term cessation of their athletic activity, and Amigó *et al.* (1998) reported a reduction in the diameter of ST and FT muscle fibres in adolescent soccer players 4–8 weeks after the competitive season. Dahlström *et al.* (1987), on the other hand, measured a large increase in fibre areas after 32 weeks of training cessation in female dancers, suggesting again that smaller fibres were an endurance training-induced adaptation to decrease the oxygen diffusion distance.

Muscle function

ARTERIOVENOUS OXYGEN DIFFERENCE

As stated above, in addition to the 'central' factors already discussed, $\dot{V}o_{2max}$ is also a function of the maximal 'peripheral' extraction of the delivered oxygen, which is traditionally expressed as the arteriovenous oxygen difference (Sutton 1992). The authors are aware of only one study reporting data on the arteriovenous oxygen difference during training cessation in highly trained individuals (Coyle *et al.* 1984). According to that study, 21 days without training did not bring about any change in the maximal arteriovenous oxygen difference of seven endurance-trained athletes (15.1, 15.1 and 15.4 mL·100 mL^{-1} at days 0, 12 and 21 of training cessation, respectively). After 56 and 84 days without training, on the other hand, values fell to 14.5 (4% reduction) and 14.1 mL·100 mL^{-1} (7% reduction), respectively. Based on these results, the authors suggested that whereas the initial $\dot{V}o_{2max}$ loss observed in

athletes during training cessation is due to a decreased stroke volume, the decreased arterial–mixed venous oxygen difference would be responsible for the reduction in $\dot{V}o_{2max}$ observed between the third and 12th weeks of training cessation (Coyle *et al.* 1984).

MYOGLOBIN CONCENTRATION

In a 12-week training cessation study, Coyle *et al.* (1984) reported that myoglobin concentration in the gastrocnemius muscle of seven endurance-trained runners and cyclists (43.3 mg·g protein^{-1}) did not change significantly after 3 (41.0 mg·g protein^{-1}) and 12 weeks (40.7 mg·g protein^{-1}) of training cessation. In addition, these muscle myoglobin concentrations were not different from those of eight sedentary controls (38.5 mg·g protein^{-1}). In a case study, Nemeth and Lowry (1984) reported on the myoglobin content in ST and FT fibres of the vastus lateralis muscle of a 47-year-old cyclist, at peak training and after 6 and 84 days of training cessation. The myoglobin levels remained unchanged despite a 16.7% decline in $\dot{V}o_{2max}$ and a 15–35% decrease in the activities of oxidative enzymes during the period of training restriction. It was concluded that a change in training condition that leads to changes in the oxidative enzymes of human muscle fibres does not affect myoglobin levels of the same cells.

ENZYMATIC ACTIVITIES

Skeletal muscle oxidative capacity decreases markedly as a consequence of training cessation, as reflected by large reductions in mitochondrial enzyme activities. Indeed, Coyle *et al.* (1984, 1985) observed that seven endurance-trained subjects' citrate synthase activity declined from 10.0 to 7.7 mol·kg protein^{-1}·h^{-1} during the initial 3 weeks of training cessation, then continued declining to 6.0 mol·kg protein^{-1}·h^{-1} by the 56th day, and stabilized thereafter. Succinate dehydrogenase, β-hydroxyacyl-coenzyme A (CoA) dehydrogenase and malate dehydrogenase declined roughly in parallel with citrate synthase (i.e. by about

20% in 3 weeks and 40% in 56 days of training stoppage), also stabilizing thereafter at that level, which was still 50% higher than that of sedentary counterparts. Very similar observations were made by Chi *et al.* (1983) after 42–84 days of training stoppage in endurance athletes—where citrate synthase, succinate dehydrogenase, β-hydroxyacyl-CoA dehydrogenase, malate dehydrogenase and β-hydroxybutyrate dehydrogenase declined by an average of 36% during that period. As in the previous study, detrained-state oxidative enzyme values were also 40% higher than controls. Interestingly, these authors also showed that mitochondrial enzyme levels decreased almost to untrained levels in ST fibres, but remained 50–80% higher in FT fibres. During 7 weeks of training followed by 3 weeks of training cessation, Moore *et al.* (1987) observed a 45% decline in citrate synthase activity in previously trained athletes, even though pretraining citrate synthase activity did not change in response to the initial 7 weeks of training. Also, Houmard *et al.* (1992, 1993) reported a 25.3% decline in citrate synthase activity in a group of 12 distance runners who stopped training for 14 days. Similar results (27% decline in citrate synthase and β-hydroxyacyl-CoA dehydrogenase) have been reported in soccer players not training for 3 weeks (Bangsbo & Mizuno 1988), triathletes (28.6% decline in citrate synthase activity) not training for 10 days (McCoy *et al.* 1994) and adolescent soccer players (37.5% decline in citrate synthase activity) not training for 4–8 weeks (Amigó *et al.* 1998). Madsen *et al.* (1993) reported a 12% lower β-hydroxyacyl-CoA dehydrogenase activity after 4 weeks of insufficient training in nine endurance athletes, and Houston *et al.* (1979) measured a 24% lower succinate dehydrogenase in six distance runners who did not train for 15 days. A similar 25% lower succinate dehydrogenase has been observed in six rugby league players' lateral head of the gastrocnemius muscle 6 weeks after the end of their competitive season (Allen 1989). Nemeth and Lowry (1984) reported that the activities of β-hydroxyacyl-CoA dehydrogenase, citrate synthase and malate dehydrogenase fell by approximately 15–35% during 84

days of training cessation in the vastus lateralis muscle of a masters cyclist. Moreover, 16 male and female runners' skeletal muscle lipoprotein lipase activity was reduced by 45–75% during 2 weeks of training cessation, whereas this enzyme's activity increased by 86% at the adipose tissue level. The adipose tissue lipoprotein lipase : muscle lipoprotein lipase ratio increased from 0.51 to 4.45, which was indicative of a tendency for the storage of circulating lipids in the adipose tissue (Simsolo *et al.* 1993). Houston (1986) suggested that the observed declines in mitochondrial enzymatic activities are primarily regulated by altered protein synthesis rates. Moreover, these declines appear to be associated with the concomitant long-term reductions in $\dot{V}o_{2max}$ and arteriovenous oxygen difference (Coyle *et al.* 1984; Allen 1989).

Small non-systematic changes in glycolytic enzyme activities have also been reported during periods of training cessation in highly trained athletic populations. For instance, hexokinase decreased significantly by about 17%, phosphorylase did not change, phosphofructokinase increased non-significantly (about 16%) and lactate dehydrogenase increased significantly by about 20% in endurance athletes not training for 84 days (Coyle *et al.* 1985). Chi *et al.* (1983) also observed an identical 17% decline in hexokinase, whereas phosphorylase, phosphofructokinase and lactate dehydrogenase increased by 3.6–21.1% in 42–84 days without training. Houston *et al.* (1979), on the other hand, reported a 13% lower mean lactate dehydrogenase activity after 15 days of training cessation. Competitive swimmers not training for 4 weeks showed non-significant declines in phosphorylase and phosphofructokinase activities in their posterior deltoid muscle (Costill *et al.* 1985). Phosphofructokinase has also been shown to decline by 16% in rugby players not training for 6 weeks (Allen 1989), and by 54.5% in adolescent soccer players 4–8 weeks after their competitive season (Amigó *et al.* 1998). In addition, Mikines *et al.* (1989a) reported that glycogen synthase activity dropped by 42% after only 5 days without training in seven endurance-trained subjects.

MITOCHONDRIAL ATP PRODUCTION

No studies reporting on the consequences of training cessation on highly trained athletes' mitochondrial ATP production rates seem to be available in the exercise science literature. However, using recently trained individuals as subjects, Wibom *et al.* (1992) reported a 12–28% decrease in mitochondrial ATP production rate during 3 weeks of training cessation consecutive to 6 weeks of endurance training. This decrease was attributed to a 4–17% reduction in individual mitochondrial enzyme activities. Because highly trained athletes' mitochondrial enzyme activities are markedly affected by training stoppage (see above), it can be inferred that a marked reduction in mitochondrial ATP production would also take place in athletes undergoing a training cessation period. It is worth noticing, however, that the mitochondrial ATP production rate remained 37–70% above pretraining levels in the above-mentioned study on previously sedentary subjects (Wibom *et al.* 1992).

Training cessation and endurance performance

It has been repeatedly shown that the endurance performance of highly trained athletes suffers a rapid deterioration when the training stimulus disappears or is insufficient to maintain training-induced adaptations (Table 6.3). Smorawinski *et al.* (2001) have recently reported that peak power output during a graded, incremental cycle test to exhaustion declined by 14.3% in a group of endurance athletes after only 3 days of bed rest, and by 10% in strength-trained athletes. Female competitive swimmers were 2.6% slower in a 366 m swim after only 10 days without training (Claude & Sharp 1991). Exercise time to exhaustion has also been reported to be reduced during training cessation—by 9.2% (Houmard *et al.* 1992, 1993) and 25% (Houston *et al.* 1979) in 2 weeks, and by 7.6% (Coyle *et al.* 1986) and 21% (Madsen *et al.* 1993) in 4 weeks. The latter investigators suggested that altered substrate utilization and/or altered Mg^{2+} transport from the extracellular to the intracellular area, which could inhibit Ca^{2+} release from the sarcoplasmic reticulum, could have contributed to the reduced endurance performance after training stoppage. Interestingly, Houmard *et al.* (1992) suggested that the short-term training cessation-induced performance impairment observed in their 12 distance runners was primarily due to the loss in cardiorespiratory fitness they had suffered, rather than to altered mechanical efficiency, because they did not observe a decline in running economy at submaximal exercise intensities (75 and 90% of $\dot{V}o_{2max}$).

Swimming performance (100 and 200 m) has also been shown to drop by 3–13% in national and international level swimmers during the inactive period in between two training seasons (Mujika *et al.* 1995). Also, exercise time to exhaustion has been reported to decline by 23.8% in 5 weeks

Table 6.3 Studies reporting changes in endurance performance measures as a result of training cessation in athletes.

Days of training cessation	Performance measure	Percentage decrease	Reference
10	366 m swim	2.6	Claude & Sharp 1991
14	Exercise time to exhaustion	9.2	Houmard *et al.* 1992, 1993
14	Exercise time to exhaustion	25	Houston *et al.* 1979
28	Exercise time to exhaustion	7.6	Coyle *et al.* 1986
28	Exercise time to exhaustion	21	Madsen *et al.* 1993
≈30	100, 200 m swim	3–13	Mujika *et al.* 1995
32	Peak power output	18.2	Nichols *et al.* 2000
35	Exercise time to exhaustion	23.8	Fardy 1969
60	Peak power output	3.5–8.8	Giada *et al.* 1998

of training cessation in 11 college soccer players (Fardy 1969), and endurance-trained female runners' oxygen uptake during a standardized submaximal exercise task increased significantly by about 3–8% after 12 weeks of training cessation (Drinkwater & Horvath 1972). In line with these results, Coyle *et al.* (1985) observed that a submaximal exercise bout requiring a $\dot{V}o_2$ of 3.11 ± 0.23 L·min^{-1} ($74 \pm 2\%$ of $\dot{V}o_{2max}$) when their athletes were trained, elicited a $\dot{V}o_2$ of 3.20 ± 0.25 L·min^{-1} ($90 \pm 3\%$ of $\dot{V}o_{2max}$) after 84 days without training. Compared with values obtained at the peak of their training season, amateur cyclists aged 24 ± 6 and 55 ± 5 years have been shown to decrease their peak power output by, respectively, 3.5 and 8.8% during 2 months without training (Giada *et al.* 1998). Finally, an injured female masters athlete who could not train for 32 days, decreased her peak power output by 18.2% and her muscular resistance to fatigue measured by a timed ride to exhaustion at 110% of peak power output by 16.6%, as compared with values assessed when she was at the peak of her competitive season, 2 days before getting injured (Nichols *et al.* 2000).

Training cessation and strength performance

According to the available body of data, athletes can maintain or suffer a limited decay in their muscular strength during short periods of training stoppage. Fourteen days of training cessation did not significantly change 12 weightlifters' one repetition maximum bench press (–1.7%) and squat (–0.9%) performance, isometric (–7%) and isokinetic (–2.3%) concentric knee extension force, and vertical jump (1.2%) values. On the other hand, isokinetic eccentric knee extension force and surface electromyograph (EMG) activity of the vastus lateralis decreased by 12 and 8.4–12.7%, respectively. These results lead to the conclusion that eccentric strength was specifically affected in strength athletes inactive for a short period of time, but that other aspects of neuromuscular performance were unaltered (Hortobágyi *et al.* 1993). College swimmers have

been shown to maintain their muscular strength measured on a swim bench during 4 weeks of training cessation. However, their swim power, indicative of their ability to apply force during swimming, declined by 13.6% (Neufer *et al.* 1987). Longer periods of training cessation result in more pronounced declines in the strength performance of strength-trained athletes, but this loss is still limited to 7–12% during periods of inactivity ranging from 8 to 12 weeks. Häkkinen *et al.* (1981) reported 11.6 and 12.0% decreases in squat–lift and leg extension forces, respectively, following 8 weeks of training stoppage. In addition, maximal bilateral and unilateral isometric force decreased by 7.4 and 7.6%, respectively. This was coupled with decreased averaged maximal bilateral (5.6%) and unilateral (12.1%) integrated EMG. The latter change took place within the first 4 weeks of training cessation (Häkkinen & Komi 1983). Results from the same group of investigators have shown that both muscle atrophy and a diminished neural activation are responsible for the decline in maximal force that takes place during 12 weeks of training cessation, because FT and ST fibre areas, muscle mass and maximal integrated electrical activity were shown to diminish with inactivity (Häkkinen *et al.* 1981, 1985; Häkkinen & Komi 1983). Studying six endurance-trained subjects during 12 weeks of training cessation, Sinacore *et al.* (1993) observed a significant reduction in the percentage of initial torque after 30 s of recovery following a 1 min bout of fatiguing exercise of the quadriceps femoris. Changes in FTa and FTb fibre distributions paralleled changes in the rate of torque recovery following the 12-week period of training stoppage. The rate of torque recovery after a standard bout of fatiguing exercise was related to $\dot{V}o_{2max}$ and may have reflected local muscle endurance exercise adaptations.

Retention of training-induced adaptations

Overuse or any other type of injury can keep athletes from performing their habitual exercises and/or from maintaining their usual training intensity level. In view of the negative effects on physiological characteristics and performance criteria induced by an insufficient training stimulus, any strategy aiming to avoid or reduce detraining would seem worthwhile for the injured or the less active athlete. These strategies, which generally include performing either a reduced training programme or an alternative form of training (i.e. to cross-train), are briefly summarized below.

Reduced training

Reduced training has recently been defined as a non-progressive, standardized reduction in the quantity of training, which may maintain or even improve many of the positive physiological and performance adaptations gained with training (Mujika & Padilla 2000a). From a cardiorespiratory viewpoint, this strategy has been shown to be a valuable procedure to retain many of the training-induced adaptations for at least 4 weeks in highly trained athletes (Neufer *et al.* 1987; Houmard *et al.* 1989, 1990a, 1990b; McConell *et al.* 1993; Martin *et al.* 1994; Ciuti *et al.* 1996), and even longer in moderately trained individuals (Hickson & Rosenkoetter 1981; Hickson *et al.* 1982, 1985; Houmard *et al.* 1996). As a matter of fact, during periods of reduced training not forced by injury, highly trained athletes have been shown to not change their: $\dot{V}o_{2max}$ (Neufer *et al.* 1987; Houmard *et al.* 1989, 1990a, 1990b; Madsen *et al.* 1993; Martin *et al.* 1994); resting (McConell *et al.* 1993), submaximal (Houmard *et al.* 1989, 1990b; McConell *et al.* 1993) and maximal (Houmard *et al.* 1989; Madsen *et al.* 1993) heart rates; submaximal (Houmard *et al.* 1989; McConell *et al.* 1993) and maximal (Madsen *et al.* 1993; McConell *et al.* 1993) exercise ventilatory volumes; and exercise time to exhaustion (Houmard *et al.* 1989, 1990b; McConell *et al.* 1993; Martin *et al.* 1994). Specific athletic performance, on the other hand, can decline rapidly in highly trained athletes despite the use of reduced training strategies (Neufer *et al.* 1987; Madsen *et al.* 1993; McConell *et al.* 1993).

From a metabolic perspective, it has been shown that submaximal exercise (65, 85 and 95% $\dot{V}o_{2max}$) RER can increase slightly during periods of reduced training (Houmard *et al.* 1990b; McConell *et al.* 1993). Exercise blood lactate concentration has been reported not to change (Houmard *et al.* 1989, 1990b) or to increase (Neufer *et al.* 1987; McConell *et al.* 1993). Unchanged insulin action and GLUT-4 concentrations have also been reported as a result of reduced training in recently trained individuals (Houmard *et al.* 1996).

At the muscle level, research indicates that athletes can readily maintain their lean body mass (Houmard *et al.* 1989, 1990a, 1990b; McConell *et al.* 1993), oxidative enzyme activities (Houmard *et al.* 1990b) and muscular strength (Neufer *et al.* 1987; Houmard *et al.* 1990b; Tucci *et al.* 1992; Martin *et al.* 1994) by means of reduced training programmes. The retention of these characteristics may be related to a stable hormonal milieu, as suggested by the unchanged testosterone, cortisol and testosterone : cortisol ratio that have been observed in trained distance runners during 3 weeks of reduced training (Houmard *et al.* 1990a).

A growing body of data in the exercise and sports science literature indicate that maintaining training intensity during periods of reduced training and tapering is of paramount importance for athletes in order to retain training-induced physiological and performance adaptations (Van Handel *et al.* 1988; Neufer 1989; Houmard 1991; Shepley *et al.* 1992; McConell *et al.* 1993; Houmard & Johns 1994; Mujika 1998; Mujika *et al.* 2000, 2002). Training volume, on the other hand, can be reduced to a great extent without risking detraining effects. Indeed, it has been indicated that this reduction can reach 60–90% of the previous weekly volume, depending on the duration of the reduced training period (Costill *et al.* 1985, 1991; Cavanaugh & Musch 1989; Neufer 1989; Houmard *et al.* 1990a, 1990b, 1994; Houmard 1991; D'Acquisto *et al.* 1992; Johns *et al.* 1992; Shepley *et al.* 1992; McConell *et al.* 1993; Gibala *et al.* 1994; Houmard & Johns 1994; Martin *et al.* 1994; Mujika *et al.* 1995, 1996, 2000, 2002; Mujika 1998). Reports from the literature also indicate that if training-induced physiological and performance adaptations are to be maintained by highly trained athletes during periods of reduced training frequencies, these reductions should be moderate, not exceeding 20–30% (Neufer *et al.* 1987; Houmard *et al.* 1989; Neufer 1989; Houmard 1991; Houmard & Johns 1994; Mujika 1998; Mujika *et al.*, 2002).

For additional information on the physiological and performance consequences of periods of reduced training stimulus, readers can consult the reviews by Houmard (1991), Houmard and Johns (1994), Mujika (1998) and Neufer (1989).

Cross-training

It has been suggested that cross-training, defined here as the participation in an alternative training mode exclusive to the one normally used (Loy *et al.* 1995), could be a useful means to avoid or limit detraining during recovery from a sport-specific injury. The limited body of data available in the literature on the effects of cross-training as opposed to training cessation suggest that whereas moderately trained individuals may maintain fitness and delay deconditioning by performing dissimilar training modes (Moroz & Houston 1987; Claude & Sharp 1991), similar-mode cross-training would be necessary in more highly trained individuals (Loy *et al.* 1995).

Thorough information on the possible benefits and practical use of cross-training in sports can be found in a review by Loy *et al.* (1995).

Cross-transfer effect

During prolonged periods of inactivity, neural (increased motor unit synchronization and activation) and muscular (hypertrophy, increased content of creatine phosphate and glycogen) adaptations induced by strength training (Häkkinen *et al.* 1985) may be in jeopardy. Interestingly, however, a cross-transfer effect (also referred to as cross-education and cross-training) of training-induced strength gains between ipsilateral (i.e. trained limb) and contralateral (i.e. untrained limb) limbs has been repeatedly described in the literature (Hellenbrandt *et al.* 1947; Coleman 1969; Shaver 1975; Krotkiewski

et al. 1979; Moritani & deVries 1979; Houston *et al.* 1983; Narici *et al.* 1989; Kannus *et al.* 1992a; Housh & Housh 1993; Weir *et al.* 1994; Housh *et al.* 1996). This phenomenon has obvious implications in limiting muscular detraining during periods of unilateral casting, rehabilitation from injuries or following joint surgery.

Conclusions

Sports injuries imply periods of training cessation or a marked reduction in the habitual physical activity level of athletes, and an insufficient training stimulus brings about a partial or complete loss of previously acquired physiological and performance adaptations, i.e. detraining. Cardiorespiratory consequences of training cessation in athletes include a rapid $\dot{V}O_{2max}$ decline, though it usually remains above values of sedentary controls. The $\dot{V}O_{2max}$ loss results from an almost immediate reduction in total blood and plasma volumes, the latter being caused by a reduced plasma protein content. Exercise heart rate increases during maximal and submaximal intensities, but not sufficiently to counterbalance the reduced stroke volume. Therefore, maximal and submaximal cardiac output drops, whereas it may increase at rest. Cardiac dimensions, including ventricular volumes and wall thickness, often decrease. Blood pressure and total peripheral resistance, on the other hand, increase, and ventilatory efficiency is most usually impaired after short periods of training cessation.

A shift towards a higher reliance on carbohydrate as a fuel for exercising muscles is a primary consequence of training cessation from a metabolic standpoint. Even short-term insufficient training results in an increased respiratory exchange ratio at maximal and submaximal exercise intensities. Glucose tolerance and whole-body glucose uptake are rapidly and markedly reduced, due to a decline in insulin sensitivity coupled with a reduced muscle GLUT-4 transporter protein content. Muscle lipoprotein lipase activity decreases while it increases at the adipose tissue level, thus favouring the storage of adipose tissue. In addition, the training-induced antiatherogenic lipoprotein profile is reversed. Blood lactate concentration increases at submaximal exercise intensities, and the lactate threshold is apparent at a lower percentage of $\dot{V}_{O_{2max}}$. These changes, coupled with a base deficit, result in a higher postexercise acidosis. Trained muscle's glycogen concentration suffers a rapid decline, reverting to sedentary values within a few weeks of training cessation.

Skeletal muscle tissue is characterized by its dynamic nature and extraordinary plasticity, which allows it to adapt to variable levels of functional demands. When these demands are insufficient to retain training-induced adaptations, muscular detraining occurs. This implies alterations in both muscle structure and muscle function. Muscle capillary density could decrease in athletes within 2–3 weeks of training cessation, but this possibility has not been clearly established. Muscle fibre distribution remains unchanged during the initial weeks of training cessation, but there may be a decreased proportion of ST fibres and a large shift from FTa to FTb fibres in endurance athletes, and an increased oxidative fibre population in strength-trained athletes within 8 weeks of training stoppage. A general decline in muscle fibre CSA is rapidly measurable during training cessation in strength and sprint-orientated athletes, whereas fibre area may increase slightly in endurance athletes. The arteriovenous oxygen difference, unchanged following 3 weeks without training, declines after 8 weeks of continued inactivity. Myoglobin concentration, on the other hand, does not seem to be affected by training cessation. Rapid and progressive reductions in oxidative enzyme activities result in a reduced mitochondrial ATP production. These, along with the reduced arteriovenous oxygen difference, are directly related to the decline in $\dot{V}_{O_{2max}}$ observed in athletes undergoing long-term training cessation. These muscular characteristics remain, nevertheless, above sedentary values in the detrained athlete. Glycolytic enzyme activities show non-systematic changes during periods of training cessation.

The general loss in cardiorespiratory fitness, metabolic efficiency and muscle respiratory capacity results in a rapid decline in the trained athletes' endurance performance. This has been shown by impaired performance measures in all-out swims, peak power output and time to exhaustion tests. In contrast, force production declines slowly and in relation to decreased EMG activity. Strength performance in general is thus readily retained for up to 4 weeks of training cessation, but highly trained athletes' eccentric force and sport-specific power may suffer significant declines within this timeframe.

Reduced training strategies have been shown to delay the onset of detraining at the cardiorespiratory, metabolic and muscular levels in highly trained athletes. A maintenance of training intensity appears to be the key factor for an athlete to retain training-induced physiological and performance adaptations during periods of reduced training, whereas training volume can be reduced by as much as 60–90%. Training frequency reductions, on the other hand, should be more moderate, not exceeding 20–30%.

Performing alternative training modes exclusive to the one normally used by an athlete (i.e. cross-training) may delay detraining, as long as similar-mode exercises are performed. However, even dissimilar-mode cross-training may be beneficial to the moderately trained subject.

Finally, given that a cross-transfer effect between ipsilateral and contralateral limbs is often observed during periods of unilateral strength training, exercising the healthy limb should be recommended during periods of unilateral casting, rehabilitation from injuries or following joint surgery.

References

Allen, G.D. (1989) Physiological and metabolic changes with six weeks detraining. *Australian Journal of Science and Medicine in Sport* **21**, 4–9.

Alméras, N., Lemieux, S., Bouchard, C. & Tremblay, A. (1997) Fat gain in female swimmers. *Physiology and Behavior* **61**, 811–817.

Amigó, N., Cadefau, J.A., Ferrer, I., Terrados, N. & Cussó, R. (1998) Effect of summer intermission on skeletal muscle of adolescent soccer players. *Journal of Sports Medicine and Physical Fitness* **38**, 298–304.

Arciero, P.J., Smith, D.L. & Calles-Escandon, J. (1998) Effects of short-term inactivity on glucose tolerance, energy expenditure, and blood flow in trained subjects. *Journal of Applied Physiology* **84**, 1365–1373.

Bangsbo, J. & Mizuno, M. (1988) Morphological and metabolic alterations in soccer players with detraining and retraining and their relation to performance. In: *Science and Football: Proceedings of the First World Congress of Science and Football* (Reilly, B. *et al.*, eds). E. & F.N. Spon, London: 114–124.

Bánhegyi, A., Pavlik, G. & Olexó, Z. (1999) The effect of detraining on echocardiographic parameters due to injury. *Acta Physiologica Hungarica* **86**, 223–227.

Begum, S. & Katzel, L.I. (2000) Silent ischemia during voluntary detraining and future cardiac events in master athletes. *Journal of the American Geriatrics Society* **48**, 647–650.

Bonetti, A., Tirelli, F., Arsenio, L., Cioni, F., Strata, A. & Zuliani, U. (1995) Lipoprotein(a) and exercise. *Journal of Sports Medicine and Physical Fitness* **35**, 131–135.

Burstein, R., Polychronakos, C., Toews, C.J., MacDougall, J.D., Guyda, H.J. & Posner, B.I. (1985) Acute reversal of the enhanced insulin action in trained athletes. *Diabetes* **34**, 756–760.

Cavanaugh, D.J. & Musch, K.I. (1989) Arm and leg power of elite swimmers increase after taper as measured by biokinetic variable resistance machines. *Journal of Swimming Research* **5**, 7–10.

Chi, M.M.-Y., Hintz, C.S., Coyle, E.F. *et al.* (1983) Effects of detraining on enzymes of energy metabolism in individual human muscle fibers. *American Journal of Physiology* **244**, C276–C287.

Ciuti, C., Marcello, C., Macis, A. *et al.* (1996) Improved aerobic power by detraining in basketball players mainly trained for strength. *Sports Medicine, Training and Rehabilitation* **6**, 325–335.

Claude, A.B. & Sharp, R.L. (1991) The effectiveness of cycle ergometer training in maintaining aerobic fitness during detraining from competitive swimming. *Journal of Swimming Research* **7**, 17–20.

Coleman, A.E. (1969) Effect of unilateral isometric and isotonic contractions on the strength of the contralateral limb. *Research Quarterly for Exercise and Sport* **40**, 490–495.

Costill, D.L. (1988) Detraining: loss of muscular strength and power. *Sports Medicine Digest* **10**, 4.

Costill, D.L., Fink, W.J., Hargreaves, M., King, D.S., Thomas, R. & Fielding, R. (1985) Metabolic characteristics of skeletal muscle during detraining from competitive simming. *Medicine and Science in Sports and Exercise* **17**, 339–343.

Costill, D.L., Thomas, R., Robergs, R.A. *et al.* (1991) Adaptations to swimming training: influence of training volume. *Medicine and Science in Sports and Exercise* **23**, 371–377.

Coyle, E.F. (1988) Detraining and retention of training-induced adaptations. In: *Resource Manual for Guidelines for Exercise Testing and Prescription* (Blair, S.N., *et al.*, eds). Lea & Febiger, Philadelphia: 83–89.

Coyle, E.F. (1990) Detraining and retention of training-induced adaptations. *Sports Science Exchange* **2**, 1–5.

Coyle, E.F., Martin III, W.H., Sinacore, D.R., Joyner, M.J., Hagberg, J.M. & Holloszy, J.O. (1984) Time course of loss of adaptations after stopping prolonged intense endurance training. *Journal of Applied Physiology* **57**, 1857–1864.

Coyle, E.F., Martin III, W.H., Bloomfield, S.A., Lowry, O.H. & Holloszy, J.O. (1985) Effects of detraining on responses to submaximal exercise. *Journal of Applied Physiology* **59**, 853–859.

Coyle, E.F., Hemmert, M.K. & Coggan, A.R. (1986) Effects of detraining on cardiovascular responses to exercise: role of blood volume. *Journal of Applied Physiology* **60**, 95–99.

Cullinane, E.M., Sady, S.P., Vadeboncoeur, L., Burke, M. & Thompson, P.D. (1986) Cardiac size and $\dot{V}o_{2max}$ do not decrease after short-term exercise cessation. *Medicine and Science in Sports and Exercise* **18**, 420–424.

D'Acquisto, L.J., Bone, M., Takahashi, S., Langhans, G., Barzdukas, A.P. & Troup, J.P. (1992) Changes in aerobic power and swimming economy as a result of reduced training volume. In: *Swimming Science VI* (MacLaren, D., Reilly, T. & Lees, A., eds). E. &. F.N. Spon, London: 201–205.

Dahlström, M., Esbjörnsson, M., Jansson, E. & Kaijser, L. (1987) Muscle fiber characteristics in female dancers during an active and an inactive period. *International Journal of Sports Medicine* **8**, 84–87.

Drinkwater, B.L. & Horvath, S.M. (1972) Detraining effects on young women. *Medicine and Science in Sports* **4**, 91–95.

Fardy, P.S. (1969) Effects of soccer training and detraining upon selected cardiac and metabolic measures. *Research Quarterly* **40**, 502–508.

Fleck, S.J. (1994) Detraining: its effects on endurance and strength. *Strength and Conditioning* **16**, 22–28.

Ghosh, A.K., Paliwal, R., Sam, M.J. & Ahuja, A. (1987) Effect of 4 weeks detraining on aerobic and anaerobic capacity of basketball players and their restoration. *Indian Journal of Medical Research* **86**, 522–527.

Giada, F., Vigna, G.B., Vitale, E. *et al.* (1995) Effects of age on the response of blood lipids, body composition, and aerobic power to physical conditioning and deconditioning. *Metabolism* **44**, 161–165.

Giada, F., Bertaglia, E., De Picoli, B. *et al.* (1998) Cardiovascular adaptations to endurance training and detraining in young and older athletes. *International Journal of Cardiology* **65**, 149–155.

Giannattasio, C., Seravalle, G., Cattaneo, B.M. *et al.* (1992) Effect of detraining on the cardiopulmonary reflex in professional runners and hammer throwers. *American Journal of Cardiology* **69**, 677–680.

Gibala, M.J., MacDougall, J.D. & Sale, D.G. (1994) The effects of tapering on strength performance in trained athletes. *International Journal of Sports Medicine* **15**, 492–497.

Gollnick, P.D., Moore, R.L., Riedy, M. & Quintinskie Jr, J.J. (1984) Significance of skeletal muscle oxidative enzyme changes with endurance training and detraining. *Medicine and Sport Science* **17**, 215–229.

Gordon, T. & Pattullo, M.C. (1993) Plasticity of muscle fiber and motor unit types. *Exercise and Sport Sciences Reviews* **21**, 331–362.

Häkkinen, K. & Alen, M. (1986) Physiological performance, serum hormones, enzymes and lipids of an elite power athlete during training with and without androgens and during prolonged detraining. A case study. *Journal of Sports Medicine* **26**, 92–100.

Häkkinen, K. & Komi, P.V. (1983) Electromyographic changes during strength training and detraining. *Medicine and Science in Sports and Exercise* **15**, 455–460.

Häkkinen, K., Komi, P.V. & Tesch, P.A. (1981) Effect of combined concentric and eccentric strength training and detraining on force-time, muscle fiber and metabolic characteristics of leg extensor muscles. *Scandinavian Journal of Sports Science* **3**, 50–58.

Häkkinen, K., Alén, M. & Komi, P.V. (1985) Changes in isometric force- and relaxation-time, electromyographic and muscle fibre characteristics of human skeletal muscle during strength training and detraining. *Acta Physiologica Scandinavica* **125**, 573–585.

Hardman, A.E., Lawrence, J.E.M. & Herd, S.L. (1998) Postprandial lipemia in endurance-trained people during a short interruption to training. *Journal of Applied Physiology* **84**, 1895–1901.

Hawley, J.A. (1987) Physiological responses to detraining in endurance-trained subjects. *Australian Journal of Science and Medicine in Sport* **19**, 17–20.

Hawley, J. & Burke, L. (1998) *Peak Performance Training and Nutritional Strategies for Sport*. Allen & Unwin, St Leonards, NSW, Australia.

Heath, G.W., Gavin III, J.R., Hinderliter, J.M., Hagberg, J.M., Bloomfield, S.A. & Holloszy, J.O. (1983) Effects of exercise and lack of exercise on glucose tolerance and insulin sensitivity. *Journal of Applied Physiology* **55**, 512–517.

Hellenbrandt, F.A., Parrish, A.M. & Houtz, S.J. (1947) Cross education: the influence of unilateral exercise on the contralateral limb. *Archives of Physical Medicine* **28**, 76–85.

Hickson, R.C. & Rosenkoetter, M.A. (1981) Reduced training frequencies and maintenance of increased aerobic power. *Medicine and Science in Sports and Exercise* **13**, 13–16.

Hickson, R.C., Kanakis Jr, C., Davis, J.R., Moore, A.M. & Rich, S. (1982) Reduced training duration effects on aerobic power, endurance, and cardiac growth. *Journal of Applied Physiology* **53**, 225–229.

Hickson, R.C., Foster, C., Pollock, M.L., Galassi, T.M. & Rich, S. (1985) Reduced training intensities and loss of aerobic power, endurance, and cardiac growth. *Journal of Applied Physiology* **58**, 492–499.

Hoppeler, H. (1986) Exercise-induced ultrastructural changes in skeletal muscle. *International Journal of Sports Medicine* **7**, 187–204.

Hortobágyi, T., Houmard, J.A., Stevenson, J.R., Fraser, D.D., Johns, R.A. & Israel, R.G. (1993) The effects of detraining on power athletes. *Medicine and Science in Sports and Exercise* **25**, 929–935.

Houmard, J.A. (1991) Impact of reduced training on performance in endurance athletes. *Sports Medicine* **12**, 380–393.

Houmard, J.A. & Johns, R.A. (1994) Effects of taper on swim performance. Practical implications. *Sports Medicine* **17**, 224–232.

Houmard, J.A., Kirwan, J.P., Flynn, M.G. & Mitchell, J.B. (1989) Effects of reduced training on submaximal and maximal running responses. *International Journal of Sports Medicine* **10**, 30–33.

Houmard, J.A., Costill, D.L., Mitchell, J.B., Park, S.H., Fink, W.J. & Burns, J.M. (1990a) Testosterone, cortisol, and creatine kinase levels in male distance runners during reduced training. *International Journal of Sports Medicine* **11**, 41–45.

Houmard, J.A., Costill, D.L., Mitchell, J.B., Park, S.H., Hickner, R.C. & Roemmich, J.N. (1990b) Reduced training maintains performance in distance runners. *International Journal of Sports Medicine* **11**, 46–52.

Houmard, J.A., Hortobágyi, T., Johns, R.A. *et al.* (1992) Effect of short-term training cessation on performance measures in distance runners. *International Journal of Sports Medicine* **13**, 572–576.

Houmard, J.A., Hortobágyi, T., Neufer, P.D. *et al.* (1993) Training cessation does not alter GLUT-4 protein levels in human skeletal muscle. *Journal of Applied Physiology* **74**, 776–781.

Houmard, J.A., Scott, B.K., Justice, C.L. & Chenier, T.C. (1994) The effects of taper on performance in distance runners. *Medicine and Science in Sports and Exercise* **26**, 624–631.

Houmard, J.A., Tyndall, G.L., Midyette, J.B. *et al.* (1996) Effect of reduced training and training cessation on insulin action and muscle GLUT-4. *Journal of Applied Physiology* **81**, 1162–1168.

Housh, D.J. & Housh, T.J. (1993) The effect of unilateral velocity-specific concentric strength training. *Journal of Orthopaedic and Sports Physical Therapy* **17**, 252–256.

Housh, T.J., Housh, D.J., Weir, J.P. & Weir, L.L. (1996) Effects of eccentric-only resistance training and detraining. *International Journal of Sports Medicine* **17**, 145–148.

Houston, M.E. (1986) Adaptations in skeletal muscle to training and detraining. The role of protein synthesis and degradation. In: *Biochemistry of Exercise VI* (Saltin, B., ed.). Human Kinetics, Champaign, IL: 63–74.

Houston, M.E., Bentzen, H. & Larsen, H. (1979) Inter-relationships between skeletal muscle adaptations and performance as studied by detraining and retraining. *Acta Physiologica Scandinavica* **105**, 163–170.

Houston, M.E., Froese, E.A., Valeriote, S.P., Green, H.J. & Ranney, D.A. (1983) Muscle performance, morphology and metabolic capacity during strength training and detraining: a one leg model. *European Journal of Applied Physiology* **51**, 25–35.

Israel, S. (1972) Le syndrome aigu de relâche ou de désentraînement: problème lié au sport de compétition. *Bulletin du Comité National Olympique de la République Démocratique Allemande* **14**, 17.

Johns, R.A., Houmard, J.A., Kobe, R.W. *et al.* (1992) Effects of taper on swim power, stroke distance and performance. *Medicine and Science in Sports and Exercise* **24**, 1141–1146.

Kannus, P., Alosa, D., Cook, L. *et al.* (1992a) Effect of one-legged exercise on the strength, power and endurance of the contralateral leg. *European Journal of Applied Physiology* **64**, 117–126.

Kannus, P., Josza, L., Renström, P. *et al.* (1992b) The effects of training, immobilization and remobilization on musculoskeletal tissue. 1. Training and immobilization. *Scandinavian Journal of Medicine and Science in Sports* **2**, 100–118.

Katzel, L.I., Busby-Whitehead, M.J., Hagberg, J.M. & Fleg, J.L. (1997) Abnormal exercise electrocardiograms in master athletes after three months of deconditioning. *Journal of the American Geriatrics Society* **45**, 744–746.

Krotkiewski, M., Aniansson, A., Grimby, G., Björntorp, P. & Sjöström, L. (1979) The effect of unilateral isokinetic strength training on local adipose and muscle tissue morphology, thickness, and enzymes. *European Journal of Applied Physiology* **42**, 271–281.

Lacour, J.R. & Denis, C. (1984) Detraining effects on aerobic capacity. *Medicine and Sport Science* **17**, 230–237.

LaForgia, J., Withers, R.T., Williams, A.D. *et al.* (1999) Effect of 3 weeks of detraining on the resting metabolic rate and body composition of trained males. *European Journal of Clinical Nutrition* **53**, 126–133.

Larsson, L. & Ansved, T. (1985) Effects of long-term physical training and detraining on enzyme histochemical and functional skeletal muscle characteristics in man. *Muscle and Nerve* **8**, 714–722.

Londeree, B.R. (1997) Effect of training on lactate/ventilatory thresholds: a meta-analysis. *Medicine and Science in Sports and Exercise* **29**, 837–843.

Loy, S.F., Hoffmann, J.J. & Holland, G.J. (1995) Benefits and practical use of cross-training in sports. *Sports Medicine* **19**, 1–8.

Madsen, K., Pedersen, P.K., Djurhuus, M.S. & Klitgaard, N.A. (1993) Effects of detraining on endurance capacity and metabolic changes during prolonged exhaustive exercise. *Journal of Applied Physiology* **75**, 1444–1451.

Mankowitz, K., Seip, R., Semenkovich, C.F., Daugherty, A. & Schonfeld, G. (1992) Short-term interruption of training affects both fasting and post-prandial lipoproteins. *Atherosclerosis* **95**, 181–189.

Maron, B.J., Pelliccia, A., Spataro, A. & Granata, M. (1993) Reduction in left ventricular wall thickness after deconditioning in highly trained Olympic athletes. *British Heart Journal* **69**, 125–128.

Martin, D.T., Scifres, J.C., Zimmerman, S.D. & Wilkinson, J.G. (1994) Effects of interval training and a taper on cycling performance and isokinetic leg strength. *International Journal of Sports Medicine* **15**, 485–491.

Martin III, W.H., Coyle, E.F., Bloomfield, S.A. & Ehsani, A.A. (1986) Effects of physical deconditioning after intense endurance training on left ventricular dimensions and stroke volume. *Journal of the American College of Cardiology* **7**, 982–989.

McConell, G.K., Costill, D.L., Widrick, J.J., Hickney, M.S., Tanaka, H. & Gastin, P.B. (1993) Reduced training volume and intensity maintain aerobic capacity but not performance in distance runners. *International Journal of Sports Medicine* **14**, 33–37.

McCoy, M., Proietto, J. & Hargreaves, M. (1994) Effect of detraining on GLUT-4 protein in human skeletal muscle. *Journal of Applied Physiology* **77**, 1532–1536.

Michael, E., Evert, J. & Jeffers, K. (1972) Physiological changes of teenage girls during five months of detraining. *Medicine and Science in Sports* **4**, 214–218.

Mikines, K.J., Sonne, B., Tronier, B. & Galbo, H. (1989a) Effects of acute exercise and detraining on insulin action in trained men. *Journal of Applied Physiology* **66**, 704–711.

Mikines, K.J., Sonne, B., Tronier, B. & Galbo, H. (1989b) Effects of training and detraining on dose–response relationship between glucose and insulin secretion. *American Journal of Physiology* **256**, E588–E596.

Miyamura, M. & Ishida, K. (1990) Adaptive changes in hypercapnic ventilatory response during training and detraining. *European Journal of Applied Physiology* **60**, 353–359.

Moore, R.L., Thacker, E.M., Kelley, G.A. *et al.* (1987) Effect of training/detraining on submaximal exercise responses in humans. *Journal of Applied Physiology* **63**, 1719–1724.

Moritani, T. & deVries, H.A. (1979) Neural factors versus hypertrophy in the time course of muscle strength gain. *American Journal of Physical Medicine* **58**, 115–130.

Moroz, D.E. & Houston, M.E. (1987) The effects of replacing endurance running training with cycling in female runners. *Canadian Journal of Sport Science* **12**, 131–135.

Mujika, I. (1998) The influence of training characteristics and tapering on the adaptation in highly trained individuals: a review. *International Journal of Sports Medicine* **19**, 439–446.

Mujika, I. & Padilla, S. (2000a) Detraining: loss of training-induced physiological and performance adaptations. Part I. Short-term insufficient training stimulus. *Sports Medicine* **30**, 79–87.

Mujika, I. & Padilla, S. (2000b) Detraining: loss of training-induced physiological and performance adaptations. Part II. Long-term insufficient training stimulus. *Sports Medicine* **30**, 145–154.

Mujika, I. & Padilla, S. (2001a) Cardiorespiratory and metabolic characteristics of detraining in humans. *Medicine and Science in Sports and Exercise* **33**, 413–421.

Mujika, I. & Padilla, S. (2001b) Muscular characteristics of detraining in humans. *Medicine and Science in Sports and Exercise* **33**, 1297–1303.

Mujika, I., Chatard, J.-C., Busso, T., Geyssant, A., Barale, F. & Lacoste, L. (1995) Effects of training on performance in competitive swimming. *Canadian Journal of Applied Physiology* **20**, 395–406.

Mujika, I., Busso, T., Lacoste, L., Barale, F., Geyssant, A. & Chatard, J.-C. (1996) Modeled responses to training and taper in competitive swimmers. *Medicine and Science in Sports and Exercise* **28**, 251–258.

Mujika, I., Goya, A., Padilla, S., Grijalba, A., Gorostiaga, E. & Ibáñez, J. (2000) Physiological responses to a 6-day taper in middle-distance runners: influence of training intensity and volume. *Medicine and Science in Sports and Exercise* **32**, 511–517.

Mujika, I., Goya, A., Ruiz, E., Grijalba, A., Santisteban, J. & Padilla, S. (2002) Physiological and performance responses to a 6-day taper in middle-distance runners: influence of training frequency. *International Journal of Sports Medicine* **23**, 367–373.

Narici, M.V., Roi, G.S., Landoni, L., Minetti, A.E. & Cerretelli, P. (1989) Changes in force, cross-sectional area and neural activation during strength training and detraining of the human quadriceps. *European Journal of Applied Physiology* **59**, 310–319.

Nemeth, P.M. & Lowry, O.H. (1984) Myoglobin levels in individual human skeletal muscle fibers of different types. *Journal of Histochemistry and Cytochemistry* **32**, 1211–1216.

Neufer, P.D. (1989) The effect of detraining and reduced training on the physiological adaptations to aerobic exercise training. *Sports Medicine* **8**, 302–321.

Neufer, P.D., Costill, D.L., Fielding, R.A., Flynn, M.G. & Kirwan, J.P. (1987) Effect of reduced training on muscular strength and endurance in competitive swimmers. *Medicine and Science in Sports and Exercise* **19**, 486–490.

Nichols, J.F., Robinson, D., Douglass, D. & Anthony, J. (2000) Retraining of a competitive master athlete following traumatic injury: a case study. *Medicine and Science in Sports and Exercise* **32**, 1037–1042.

Pavlik, G., Bachl, N., Wollein, W., Lángfy, G. & Prokop, L. (1986a) Effect of training and detraining on the resting echocardiographic parameters in runners and cyclists. *Journal of Sports Cardiology* **3**, 35–45.

Pavlik, G., Bachl, N., Wollein, W., Lángfy, G. & Prokop, L. (1986b) Resting echocardiographic parameters after cessation of regular endurance training. *International Journal of Sports Medicine* **7**, 226–231.

Penny, G.D. & Wells, M.R. (1975) Heart rate, blood pressure, serum lactate, and serum cholesterol changes after the cessation of training. *Journal of Sports Medicine* **15**, 223–228.

Pivarnik, J.M. & Senay Jr, L.C. (1986) Effects of exercise detraining and deacclimation to the heat on plasma volume dynamics. *European Journal of Applied Physiology* **55**, 222–228.

Raven, P.B., Welch-O'Connor, R.M. & Shi, X. (1998) Cardiovascular function following reduced aerobic activity. *Medicine and Science in Sports and Exercise* **30**, 1041–1052.

Saltin, B. & Gollnick, P.D. (1983) Skeletal muscle adaptability: significance for metabolism and performance. In: *Handbook of Physiology: Skeletal Muscle* (Peachey, L.D., Adrian, R.H., Geiger, S.R., eds). American Physiological Society, Bethesda. Williams & Wilkins, Baltimore: 555–631.

Shaver, L.G. (1975) Cross-transfer effects of conditioning and deconditioning on muscular strength. *Ergonomics* **18**, 9–16.

Shepley, B., MacDougall, J.D., Cipriano, N., Sutton, J.R., Tarnopolsky, M.A. & Coates, G. (1992) Physiological effects of tapering in highly trained athletes. *Journal of Applied Physiology* **72**, 706–711.

Shoemaker, J.K., Green, H.J., Ball-Burnett, M. & Grant, S. (1998) Relationships between fluid and electrolyte hormones and plasma volume during exercise with training and detraining. *Medicine and Science in Sports and Exercise* **30**, 497–505.

Simsolo, R.B., Ong, J.M. & Kern, P.A. (1993) The regulation of adipose tissue and muscle lipoprotein lipase in runners by detraining. *Journal of Clinical Investigation* **92**, 2124–2130.

Sinacore, D.R., Coyle, E.F., Hagberg, J.M. & Holloszy, J.O. (1993) Histochemical and physiological correlates of training- and detraining-induced changes in the recovery from a fatigue test. *Physical Therapy* **73**, 661–667.

Sjøgaard, G. (1984) Changes in skeletal muscles capillarity and enzyme activity with training and detraining. *Medicine and Sport Science* **17**, 202–214.

S'Jongers, J.J. (1976) Le syndrome de désentraînement. *Bruxelles-Médical* **7**, 297–300.

Smorawinski, J., Nazar, K., Kaciuba-Uscilko, H. *et al.* (2001) Effects of 3-day bed rest on physiological responses to graded exercise in athletes and sedentary men. *Journal of Applied Physiology* **91**, 249–257.

Staron, R.S., Hagerman, F.C. & Hikida, R.S. (1981) The effects of detraining on an elite power lifter. A case study. *Journal of the Neurological Sciences* **51**, 247–257.

Sutton, J.R. (1992) Limitations to maximal oxygen uptake. *Sports Medicine* **13**, 127–133.

Thompson, P.D., Cullinane, E.M., Eshleman, R., Sady, S.P. & Herbert, P.N. (1984) The effects of caloric restriction or exercise cessation on the serum lipid and lipoprotein concentrations of endurance athletes. *Metabolism* **33**, 943–950.

Tidow, G. (1995) Muscular adaptations induced by training and de-training. A review of biopsy studies. *New Studies in Athletics* **10**, 47–56.

Tucci, J.T., Carpenter, D.M., Pollock, M.L., Graves, J.E. & Leggett, S.H. (1992) Effect of reduced frequency of training and detraining on lumbar extension strength. *Spine* **17**, 1497–1501.

Van Handel, P.J., Katz, A., Troup, J.P., Daniels, J.T. & Bradley, P.W. (1988) Oxygen consumption and blood lactic acid response to training and taper. In: *Swimming Science V* (Ungerechts, B.E., Wilke, K. & Reischle, K., eds). Human Kinetics, Champaign, IL: 269–275.

Vukovich, M.D., Arciero, P.J., Kohrt, W.M., Racette, S.B., Hansen, P.A. & Holloszy, J.O. (1996) Changes in insulin action and GLUT-4 with 6 days of inactivity in endurance runners. *Journal of Applied Physiology* **80**, 240–244.

Weir, J.P., Housh, T.J. & Weir, L.L. (1994) Electromyographic evaluation of joint angle specificity and cross-training after isometric training. *Journal of Applied Physiology* **77**, 197–201.

Wibom, R., Hultman, E., Johansson, M., Matherei, K., Constantin-Teodosiu, D. & Schantz, P.G. (1992) Adaptation of mitochondrial ATP production in human skeletal muscle to endurance training and detraining. *Journal of Applied Physiology* **73**, 2004–2010.

Wilber, R.L. & Moffatt, R.J. (1994) Physiological and biochemical consequences of detraining in aerobically trained individuals. *Journal of Strength and Conditioning Research* **8**, 110–124.

Chapter 7

Physiological and Functional Implications of Injury

CHRISTOPHER J. STANDAERT AND STANLEY A. HERRING

Introduction

As even the casual reader of this text can discern, musculoskeletal injury in the athlete can involve a wide range of anatomical structures and physiological variables. Understanding the ways in which injury and treatment affect the athlete's physical performance is central to developing both an acute treatment strategy and a long-term management plan for the athlete. Injury clearly can involve significant tissue damage, resulting in pain and reduced physical performance. However, injury needs to be viewed in the setting of the entire athlete, not just the local area of acute tissue damage. Prior injuries, strength or flexibility imbalance, skill, technique, or any of a number of other factors affecting the full functional kinetic chain can have a strong bearing on how to approach rehabilitation in a given individual.

As described by Kibler (1998), the term 'kinetic chain' refers to the sequencing of individual body segments or joints that must be moved in a specific order and manner to allow for the efficient accomplishment of a given task. The task of pitching a baseball is an example of one such task (Fig. 7.1). This skill, along with most of those in the throwing or hitting sports, actually involves two separate chains of motion: one extends from the ground and planting leg through the hip and trunk to the landing leg; the other extends from the ground and planting leg through the pelvis and trunk to the shoulder, elbow, wrist and, ultimately, the hand (Kibler 1998). Injuries or deficits anywhere along these chains can decrease the efficiency of the task and cause overload on other areas with resultant dysfunction or tissue failure. In considering the local and systemic effects of injury and inactivity, it becomes apparent that any element of the kinetic chain can either be a possible causative factor in injury or be at risk for the deleterious effects of injury. In the case of a baseball pitcher with a sore shoulder, for example, the local tissue injury in the shoulder may be partly related to relative muscular imbalance in the shoulder or inflexibility in the lumbar spine. Resting the pitcher with the intent of allowing the

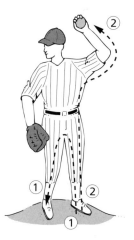

Fig. 7.1 Illustration of the kinetic chains involved in pitching a baseball. The first chain extends from the ground and planting leg to the hip, trunk and down the landing leg. The second chain runs from the ground and planting leg to the hip and trunk then to the shoulder, elbow, wrist and hand of the throwing arm. (Adapted from Kibler 1998.)

acute inflammation in the shoulder to resolve may result in numerous less desirable consequences. These might include reductions in endurance, strength, mobility or neuromuscular control, all of which are necessary for the production of appropriate arm speed, positioning and release necessary to achieve optimal ball speed and movement. Awareness of the potential for these deficits is crucial in the rehabilitation of the athlete. This chapter will present a format for understanding injury in this context and include a discussion of the physiological and functional implications of injury as they relate to rehabilitation.

Rehabilitation

Sports injuries are an extremely common event for athletes (see Chapter 1). Reports of injury rates and severity vary widely by sport and also by methods of measurement (Henry *et al.* 1982; Keller *et al.* 1987; Saal 1991; Bennell & Crossley 1996; Murtaugh 2001). None the less, reported injury rates can be extremely high, including a 12.7% incidence of injury in adolescent wrestlers during participation in a single tournament (Lorish *et al.* 1992), a greater than 50% injury rate for high school football players for a single season (DeLee & Farney 1992), a 69% injury rate for a professional basketball team over 7 years (Henry *et al.* 1982) and a lifetime incidence of > 70% for interfering shoulder pain in elite swimmers (McMaster & Troup 1993). The natural history of soft tissue injuries is not necessarily benign, either—a recent study on ankle sprains in the general population (the vast majority of which were not treated with extensive rehabilitation) reported that 72.6% of subjects had persisting symptoms 6–18 months after injury (Braun 1999). An initial injury may also have a significant impact on the risk of further injury. A review on injuries in soccer players noted that prior injury was one of the factors most strongly associated with new injury and that 20% of 'minor' injuries were followed by a more severe injury within 2 months (Keller *et al.* 1987). Macera (1992) also noted that there is a strong effect of previous injury on the risk of further injury in runners. The precise reasons

for the increased risk of reinjury are not entirely clear, but several possibilities exist, including incomplete recovery from the initial injury, incomplete rehabilitation, uncorrected biomechanical problems, or physiological, anthropomorphical or technique issues related to an individual athlete (Keller *et al.* 1987; Rutherford *et al.* 1990; Macera 1992; Taylor *et al.* 1993; Jonhagen *et al.* 1994). Clearly, athletic injuries have a significant impact on a large number of athletes, teams and sporting events. Interventions that may lessen the ultimate impact of an injury upon an athlete's performance, including comprehensive rehabilitation, may have a dramatic effect not just for the individual athlete, but for sports competition as a whole.

The rehabilitation plan for an individual athlete is based upon an assessment of the athlete's specific injury and more global functional properties, along with an understanding of the functional consequences of the injury and treatment. First, the actual tissue injury must be diagnosed accurately. The presentation of the injury, or the clinical symptom complex (Herring 1990), needs to be identified, as do the type of injury and the physiological and biomechanical factors associated with its occurrence. Finally, the acute method of treatment needs to be established with a thorough knowledge of the local or systemic effects of the chosen modality (e.g. immobilization, surgery, etc.). From this base, an appropriate rehabilitation strategy can be developed that addresses the full functional capacity of the athlete (Herring & Kibler 1998).

Although injury is often associated with focal tissue damage, the goal of treatment for an injured athlete extends far beyond achieving tissue homeostasis. The athlete's goal is to return to sport at the highest level of performance possible. This means that medical professionals have to deal with all aspects of the athlete's functioning. As will be discussed, injury and the subsequent acute treatment can result in diminished soft tissue tensile strength, decreased aerobic capacity, cellular and neurological changes, and residual disability even in the absence of symptoms. Rehabilitation needs to address all of these issues, with an initial goal of symptom resolution and an ultimate goal of restored function and continued fitness to minimize the risk of recurrent injury and preserve long-term performance (Herring & Kibler 1998). This concept is important in understanding why rehabilitation is necessary in the first place and why 'rehabilitation' really refers to an ongoing process of training and maintaining the injured athlete.

Injury

Specific tissues respond differently to the stress and strain associated with trauma (see Chapters 3–5). Generally speaking, however, injury occurs when the forces applied to a given anatomical structure exceed the physiological tolerance or reparative capabilities of that structure. As a gross step in assessing injuries, they can be broken down into two major types: macrotraumatic or microtaumatic (Leadbetter 1994; Quillen *et al.* 1996; Herring & Kibler 1998). Macrotrauma refers to acute, extreme forces that overwhelm the tensile or structural properties of a given tissue. This is generally thought of as resulting in the acute deformation or disruption of previously normal structures, such as might occur with an acute ankle fracture or anterior cruciate ligament tear. Microtrauma, on the other hand, refers to smaller forces that cause lesser degrees of cellular or structural disruption and occur at a rate or

severity that exceeds the tissue's ability to enact appropriate repair or maintenance. This can result in weakening of the structural properties of the affected tissue, adaptations of function in adjacent or compensatory structures, pain, impaired performance and, potentially, tissue failure. There is a continuum of injury present between these two mechanisms of 'acute' and 'chronic' injury, however; many apparently acute or macrotraumatic events causing disruption are strongly related to underlying degeneration, weakness or misuse resulting from a lengthier microtraumatic process of tissue degeneration. The vast majority of acute tendon ruptures, in fact, are associated with prior pathological change in the tendon (Leadbetter 1994). This conceptual model reinforces the concept that injury occurrence, prevention and treatment represent ongoing, dynamic processes occurring within the body's structural and cellular balance (Fig. 7.2).

A structural format for approaching the treatment of an athletic injury needs to include a full understanding of the clinical and physiological alterations induced by or associated with injury (Table 7.1). The injured athlete is typically being assessed by medical personnel for complaints of pain, weakness, oedema or dysfunction. The presenting symptoms can be referred to as the *clinical symptom complex*. For a patient with a rotator cuff injury, there may be local complaints of pain, weakness and diminished range of motion

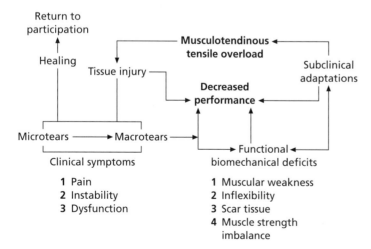

Fig. 7.2 The injury cycle and feedback mechanisms, illustrating the multifactorial nature of athletic injury. (From Kibler *et al.* 1992, with permission.)

Table 7.1 Complete diagnosis of rotator cuff tendonitis/impingement in a baseball pitcher. (Adapted from Herring 1990.)

Clinical symptom complex	Impingement symptom pattern Anterior–superior glenohumeral instability Decreased pitch velocity Prolonged recovery time
Tissue injury complex	Tear in posterior capsule Tear in rotator cuff Glenoid labral attrition
Tissue overload complex	Tensile load on posterior shoulder capsule Tensile load on posterior shoulder muscles Tensile load on scapular stabilizing muscles
Functional biomechanical deficit complex	Internal rotation inflexibility External/internal rotation strength imbalance Lateral scapular slide Alteration of trunk motion with increased passive lumbar lordosis and decreased lateral lumbar flexion Decreased hip mobility
Subclinical adaptation complex	Altered shoulder or elbow positioning Decreased pitch velocity

all affecting the injured shoulder. The actual tissue injury represents the *tissue injury complex*. In the above-mentioned athlete with a rotator cuff injury, this may be a partial tear of the supraspinatus tendon. Frequently, medical assessment focuses on these two components of the injured athlete. The actual symptomatic tissue injury, however, may be accompanied by problems with associated structures that have been overloaded, suboptimally lengthened or otherwise impaired by the acute injury, or that may be contributing to the injury. These related problems are referred to as the *tissue overload complex* (Herring 1990; Herring & Kibler 1998). In the athlete with a shoulder injury, this may include tensile load on the posterior shoulder capsule due to dynamic instability of the glenohumeral joint or excessive load on the rhomboids related to relative lateral translation of the scapula.

In looking beyond local tissue injury, the clinician also has to assess underlying biomechanical or technique issues involved with the performance of an injured athlete. Continuing with the shoulder example, studies of relative isokinetic strength in uninjured elite water polo players and collegiate tennis players have shown signifi-

cant strength imbalance at the shoulder with a relative increase in strength of the shoulder internal rotators compared with the external rotators (McMaster *et al.* 1991; Chandler *et al.* 1992). This relative imbalance has been hypothesized to be related to shoulder injuries in those athletes due to an alteration of the normal mechanics of the glenohumeral joint (McMaster *et al.* 1991; Chandler *et al.* 1992). This is an example of the *functional biomechanical deficit complex* which includes abnormalities in strength or flexibility associated with injury. Finally, alterations in mechanics, motion or task performance may result from injury or functional biomechanical deficits. These associated problems are referred to as the *subclinical adaptation complex*. As this name would imply, these adaptations may not be directly associated with symptoms but can contribute to progression or perpetuation of injury and impaired performance (Herring 1990; Kibler *et al.* 1991; Herring & Kibler 1998). An example of this would be a baseball pitcher who lowers the elbow of his or her throwing arm and changes the release point of the ball due to a combination of shoulder pain, dynamic instability and internal rotation inflexibility.

Viewing injury in the context just described allows medical personnel to fully evaluate all of the contributing biomechanical and physiological factors affecting an athlete's injury, impaired performance and full symptom complex. Once this is assessed, an appropriate strategy for correcting deficits in all relevant areas can be addressed, and an acute injury treatment plan can advance to a full management programme for the athlete.

Tissue damage—the tissue injury complex

Although the general inflammatory cascade is similar in all acute soft tissue injuries, the distinct structural and reparative properties of different tissues impact on how this process affects recovery and performance. The injury and repair processes for specific tissues are well addressed in other chapters in this book (see Chapters 3–5). However, some specific aspects of soft tissue injury and repair will be briefly reviewed in order to more fully develop the underpinnings of rehabilitation treatment.

Ligament injuries frequently occur as a result of acute macrotraumatic forces applied to the ligament causing structural disruption of varying degrees. The amount of force necessary to cause ligamentous disruption is dependent upon the size of the ligament, the age of the individual and the joint position at the time of injury. The healing process results in scar formation with collagen deposition but is frequently inadequate to withstand future load bearing (Frank 1996). Even in the best of circumstances, maximal recovery may take more than 1 year and still result in a decrement of 30–50% in tensile strength (Leadbetter 1994). Immobilization may additionally impair the structural properties of an injured ligament (Frank 1996; Salter 1996). As the functional role of a ligament is to serve as a passive support for joint positioning and to potentially provide proprioceptive feedback, the rehabilitation of ligamentous injuries needs to include work on restoring or improving dynamic joint control through the kinetic chain in order to reinforce the stabilizing properties of an injured ligament. The loss of joint stability associated with an acute ligament injury also needs to be considered during the early phase of rehabilitation in order to avoid further injury to the ligament complex.

Tendon injuries are slightly different from ligamentous injuries and, subsequently, pose different issues in the rehabilitation process. Tendons may also be acutely injured due to macrotraumatic forces applied across the musculotendinous unit. However, tendons are also the structures most frequently involved in overuse, or, perhaps more appropriately termed, chronic overload syndromes, which involve repetitive loading with partial disruption of the tendon structure (Herring & Nilson 1987; Curwin 1996). In overload injuries, the forces applied to an injured tendon may be within a physiological range for the tendon but they occur at a frequency that prohibits adequate recovery or repair processes. This may ultimately lead to failure of the tendon structure (Curwin 1996). Tendon repair mechanisms would imply that progressive loading of the injured structure is necessary to optimize the restoration of the tensile strength. Given the frequency with which extrinsic factors are associated with tendon injuries, it is also important to assess an athlete for issues of flexibility, strength imbalance, equipment and technique in order to minimize deleterious effects that may be associated with external appliances or maladaptive motion patterns. These issues could potentially involve the tissue overload complex, the functional biomechanical deficit complex or the subclinical adaptation complex, and illustrate the importance of recognizing how all of these areas contribute to the problems of an injured athlete.

Muscular injuries are, yet again, distinct from isolated tendinous or ligamentous injuries. Muscle injuries may occur in the midsubstance of the muscle proper, such as in a contusion, or in the region of the myotendinous junction, as in a strain. In considering differences between tendinous and muscular injuries, the region of the musculotendinous junction warrants particular attention. Muscle strain injury is felt to occur during elongation of the muscle, typically during forceful eccentric contraction, and is particularly common in sports involving sprinting or jumping (Noonan & Garrett 1992; Taylor *et al.* 1993; Jonhagen *et al.* 1994; Bennell & Crossley 1996; Garrett 1996; Jarvinen *et al.* 2000). The vast majority of muscular strain injuries have been shown to occur at the region of the musculotendinous junction, generally affecting the muscle immediately adjacent to the junction rather than in the junction itself (Taylor *et al.* 1993; Garrett 1996; Malone *et al.* 1996). 'Two-joint' muscles, such as the rectus femoris, gastrocnemius and hamstrings, are particularly vulnerable to this type of injury (Noonan & Garrett 1992; Mair *et al.* 1996; Jarvinen *et al.* 2000). The tensile forces generated by the muscle during maximal eccentric loading combined with the forces associated with elongation of the static viscoelastic components of the muscle probably contribute to the frequency with which strain injury occurs during moments of forceful eccentric contraction of the muscle (Malone *et al.* 1996). There are, additionally, distinctive properties of the sarcomeres and membranous structures adjacent to the musculotendinous junction that may contribute to this area being particularly vulnerable to strain injury (Noonan & Garrett 1992).

Healing of muscular strain injuries, as well as of disruptions of the muscle more distant to the site of the musculotendinous junction, consists of scar deposition with regeneration and ingrowth of contractile elements and nerves (Jarvinen *et al.* 2000). Acutely, there is a significant decline in contractile strength and peak load tolerance in injured muscle, and the scar is at its weakest point until 10–12 days after injury (Taylor *et al.* 1993; Jarvinen *et al.* 2000). Tensile strength recovery also appears to lag behind the recovery of force-generating capacity (tension generation), making the muscle perhaps more vulnerable to repeat injury than it may appear by tension-generating capacity alone (i.e. gross measures of 'strength') (Garrett 1996). Scar formation may significantly impair the ability of contractile elements in injured muscle to repair, and contractile ability may be reduced by 10–20% long term (Jarvinen & Lehto 1993; Leadbetter

1994). The type of treatment chosen and the length of immobilization may also have a significant impact on the actual reparative processes within injured muscle and the degree to which contractile elements penetrate the connective tissue (Jarvinen & Lehto 1993).

Accurately assessing the nature and severity of the tissue injury in an affected athlete, i.e. the tissue injury complex, is crucial in determining an appropriate rehabilitation approach to the patient. The type of tissue injured, the degree of structural damage, the concurrent structures affected and the potentially deleterious effects of immobilization on adjacent structures all need to be taken into account in treatment. Although different tissues are discussed in isolation above, an injury frequently results in alterations to several different tissue components. For example, a surgically treated acute tear of the anterior cruciate ligament in an athlete may ultimately result in alterations of bone, tendon and ligament with additional components of muscular atrophy, capsular tightness, aerobic deconditioning and alterations in neural control. Understanding each of the individual components associated with an injury allows for a more comprehensive and precise approach to treatment.

Immobilization and rest

Acute injury of soft tissue or bone is frequently managed by a period of immobilization of the injured body part or by rest of the injured area or the athlete as a whole. This is done to allow for adequate healing and restoration of tensile strength so that the injured structure may begin to bear physiological loads with less risk for recurrent injury. Periods of immobilization required for the treatment of different injuries can vary highly. For example, ankle or radial fractures may frequently be immobilized in a rigid cast for 4–6 weeks, acute spinal fractures may be treated with a rigid brace for up to 3 months, and some authors recommend the use of a rigid brace for 6–12 months in the management of spondylolysis (Steiner & Micheli 1985; Tropp & Norlin 1995; McDowell 1997; Byl *et al.*

1999). Although often viewed as a useful tool in the management of musculoskeletal injuries, immobilization and inactivity can have significant deleterious effects on the injured athlete. These changes may affect how an athlete will be able to progress through a rehabilitation programme after injury. Understanding the scope and time course of deficits involved with rest and immobilization allows health care professionals to apply both preventative and restorative care in the course of recovery.

Muscle

At the muscular level, there are significant changes in the function and structural properties of the musculotendinous unit treated with immobilization. These changes include reductions in strength, limb volume, limb weight and the cross-sectional area of muscles as a whole and of individual muscle fibres (Muller 1970; Wills *et al*. 1982; Booth 1987; Veldhuizen *et al*. 1993; Bloomfield 1997; Zarzhevsky *et al*. 1999). There are, additionally, selective changes in enzymatic function and protein synthesis and alterations to the musculotendinous junction with reduced contact area between the muscle cells and tendineal collagen fibres (Wills *et al*. 1982; Appell 1990; Kannus *et al*. 1992; Hortobagyi *et al*. 2000). All of these factors play a role in the functional implications for managing patients with injuries treated with immobilization.

When looking strictly at muscle strength, the losses associated with immobilization can be profound. A recent study by Hortobagyi *et al*. (2000) found that healthy volunteers placed in a fibreglass cast for 3 weeks sustained an average 47% decrease in eccentric, concentric and isometric strength of knee extension. Similar decreases in peak isometric torque of 53% for knee extension and 26% for knee flexion were noted by Veldhuizen *et al*. (1993) after 4 weeks of cast immobilization in healthy volunteers (Fig. 7.3) Geboers *et al*. (2000) found a 28% decrease in dorsiflexion torque for individuals who underwent cast immobilization for 4–6 weeks after ankle fractures. A study of individuals casted for

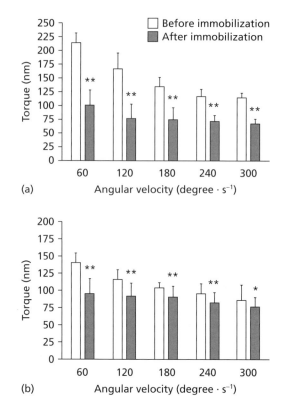

Fig. 7.3 Peak torque of: (a) knee extension and (b) knee flexion before and after 4 weeks of cast immobilization in healthy volunteers. The bars show the medians and 75th percentiles (*n* = 8). *, *P* < 0.05; **, *P* < 0.01. (From Veldhuizen *et al*. 1993, with permission.)

8 weeks after open reduction and internal fixation of an ankle fracture found a reduction of about 50% for ankle plantar flexion peak isometric torque with reductions in isokinetic torque for all angular speeds and positions (Shaffer *et al*. 2000). The strength losses seem to be more dramatic with the use of rigid immobilization than with either limb suspension or bed rest, although these also result in dramatic reductions in strength over a fairly rapid time course (Berg *et al*. 1991; Bloomfield 1997). This may suggest that there is a beneficial effect on relative strength loss by the preservation of some degree of joint mobility, although the true magnitude of any such effect is not clear currently. Declines in muscular strength with immobilization

Fig. 7.4 Magnetic resonance imaging (MRI) of the bilateral thighs (axial view) of an otherwise healthy 36-year-old female 8 weeks after arthroscopic surgery on the right knee. Note the prominent atrophy in the quadriceps musculature on the right. Atrophy in the hamstrings is less pronounced. There was no atrophy noted preoperatively. VL, vastus lateralis; VI, vastus intermedius; RF, rectus femoris; BF, biceps femoris (long head); ST, semitendinosis; SM, semimembranosis.

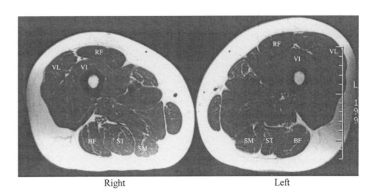

Right   Left

or disuse appear to be most prominent in anti-gravity extensor muscles such as the quadriceps and gastrocnemius/soleus (Appell 1990; Dittmer & Teasell 1993; Veldhuizen *et al.* 1993; Bloomfield 1997; Hortobagyi *et al.* 2000). Overall, the most rapid period of strength loss seems to be early in the course of immobilization with little additional loss occurring after the first week (Muller 1970; Wills *et al.* 1982; Appell 1990).

The losses in strength are paralleled by muscle atrophy and losses in muscle fibre size (Fig. 7.4). Human studies have shown a decrease in fibre size by up to 14–17% after 72 h of immobilization (Lindboe & Platou 1984; Booth 1987). In the study mentioned previously by Veldhuizen *et al.* (1993), healthy subjects who were placed in a long leg cast for 4 weeks were found to have sustained a 21% loss in quadriceps cross-sectional area by computed tomography and a 16% decrease in fibre diameter.

Although the strength losses associated with immobilization occur rapidly, the recovery of strength and mass may take a very long time, and strength may never recover completely in some cases. Rutherford *et al.* (1990) found a marked reduction in strength and cross-sectional area of previously injured and immobilized limbs compared with the contralateral, uninjured limbs in patients assessed 1–5 years after their injuries. Similarly, other authors report prolonged decrements in strength or muscle mass for weeks to months after immobilization (Grimby *et al.* 1980; Wills *et al.* 1982; Appell 1990; Tropp & Norlin 1995; Zarzhevsky *et al.* 1999; Cruz-Martinez *et al.* 2000). The rate and extent of recovery may be dependent upon the type and intensity of retraining applied. Both the effects of immobilization and the response to training appear to be speed and task specific (Grimby *et al.* 1980; Wills *et al.* 1982; Rutherford 1988; Appell 1990; Zarzhevsky *et al.* 1999). These issues clearly have a major bearing upon any rehabilitation plan for an injured athlete who has been treated with rest and/or immobilization.

Neural changes

Loss in muscle mass may not be the only factor affecting muscular performance following rest or immobilization. There appear to be neural changes that affect relative muscular efficiency. This is suggested by changes in the relative electromyograph (EMG) activity per unit of force produced, a decrease in the number of functioning motor units and a decrease in reflex potentiation (Bloomfield 1997). Cruz-Martinez *et al.* (2000) found EMG abnormalities felt to be consistent with quadriceps motor neurone inhibition in patients studied after 1–4 months of knee immobilization after injury. Seki *et al.* (2001a, 2000b) studied the effects of 6 weeks of immobilization on the function of the first dorsal interosseus

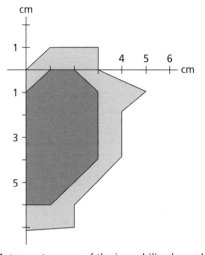

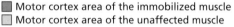

■ Motor cortex area of the immobilized muscle
□ Motor cortex area of the unaffected muscle

Fig. 7.5 Motor cortex areas of both tibialis anterior muscles in a patient with unilateral immobilization of the ankle for 8 weeks. (From Liepert *et al.* 1995, with permission from Elsevier Science.)

muscle of the hand and found that the maximal motor neurone firing rate was decreased transiently. The changes in maximal firing rate were more profoundly affected during the first 3 weeks of immobilization than in the latter 3 weeks and seemed to recover close to normal after 6 weeks following the period of immobilization. The authors felt that changes in the contractile properties of muscle after immobilization can be causally related to the alterations in firing rate of the motor neurones.

In addition to alterations at the spinal cord or muscular level, there is evidence that immobilization affects cortical function as well. A study by Liepert *et al.* (1995) using transcranial magnetic stimulation identified a decrease in the motor cortex area associated with tibialis anterior function in patients immobilized at the ankle (Fig. 7.5). The cortical changes reversed rapidly after voluntary muscular function, but suggest that cortical reorganization may occur with immobilization. This may potentially play a role in reduced muscular efficiency and motor control following injury and disuse.

An additional factor affecting muscular efficiency after injury may be the influence of degenerative changes or joint effusion on muscular function. It has been proposed that the presence of a joint effusion or degenerative joint changes may cause reflex inhibition of certain muscle groups or fibre types (Spencer *et al.* 1984; Young *et al.* 1987; Hurley & Newham 1993; Young 1993; Hopkins *et al.* 2001). This concept is supported, in part, by work showing differential reflex inhibition or relative excitability of selected muscle groups at a joint affected by an effusion (Young *et al.* 1987; Hopkins *et al.* 2001). Spencer *et al.* (1984) studied the effects of progressive instillation of fluid into the knee joints of healthy volunteers in order to assess the effects of an effusion on reflex inhibition. They found that increasing volumes of fluid instilled into the joint were associated with reductions in the H-reflex amplitude recorded from the quadriceps muscles. The H (or Hoffman) reflex is felt to reflect the relative excitability of the motor neurone pool. The degree of change in the amplitude of the evoked response was related to the volume instilled in a linear manner (Fig. 7.6). The changes were not seen in anaesthetized joints, consistent with a mechanism of motor neurone inhibition mediated by afferent receptors in the knee joint or capsule.

The potential inhibitory effect of a joint effusion on motor neurone function may represent a confounding factor when comparing studies that involve individuals treated with immobilization after an injury (in which there may well be an associated effusion) to those that involve the immobilization of healthy volunteers (who probably do not have an effusion present). However, in clinical practice, immobilized joints are very frequently associated with an injury or surgical intervention that may result in an effusion. Understanding the potential for neurological changes seen with either immobilization alone or with an effusion may allow clinicians to better understand the functional properties of the limb of an injured athlete affected by an effusion, a period of immobilization, or both.

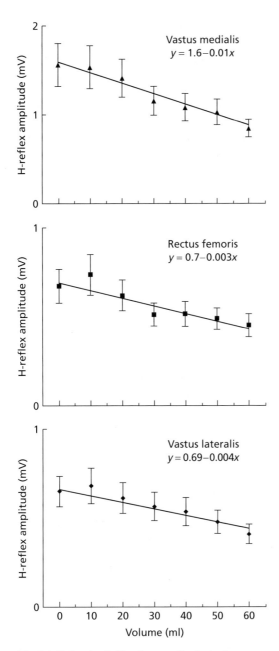

Fig. 7.6 Reduction in H-reflex amplitudes in the quadriceps muscles as a function of the volume of saline introduced into the knee joint. (From Spencer *et al.* 1984, with permission.)

Vascular changes

Along with muscular and neural changes associated with immobilization, there also appear to be significant local vascular changes. Immobilization affects both the vascular density in the muscle and the three-dimensional structure of the vessels themselves (Kvist *et al.* 1995; Oki *et al.* 1998). In a study on the rat gastrocnemius, Kvist *et al.* (1995) found that 3 weeks of immobilization resulted in a 30% reduction in capillary density in the musculotendinous junction of the immobilized muscle. As most of the blood supply to a tendon is felt to come from the muscle vasculature, a decrease in the capillary bed at the musculo-tendinous junction may be a contributing factor to subsequent injury due to loss of tensile strength in the tendon (Kvist *et al.* 1995). The potential for recovery of the vascular system appears to be good with remobilization and occurs much more rapidly in muscles mobilized earlier and in those subjected to progressively increased physical training (Jarvinen & Lehto 1993; Kvist *et al.* 1995).

Joint function

Immobilized joints are subject to multiple potential changes after immobilization, including contracture, adhesions, cartilage atrophy, erosions at areas of bony contact and reduced load tolerance of ligamentous attachments (Akeson *et al.* 1987; Dittmer & Teasell 1993). Loss of joint motion is a significant concern following immobilization for an injury. Human and animal studies have shown significant deficits in motion of affected joints following immobilization (Akeson *et al.* 1987; Tropp & Norlin 1995; Reynolds *et al.* 1996; Salter 1996; Schollmeier *et al.* 1996; Byl *et al.* 1999; Trudel *et al.* 1999; Trudel & Uhthoff 2000). In a rat model using immobilization at the knee, Trudel *et al.* (1999) found that joint contracture occurred as little as 2 weeks after immobilization and progressed at an average rate of $3.8°·week^{-1}$ for 16 weeks with an apparent plateau reached after that point (Fig. 7.7). In a study on the effects of cast immobilization for distal radial fractures treated non-operatively, Byl *et al.* (1999) found

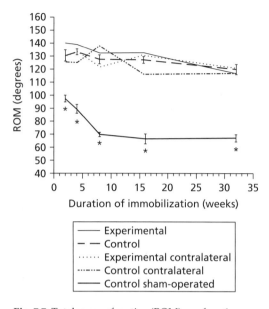

Fig. 7.7 Total range of motion (ROM) as a function of immobilization of the knee (in weeks) in a rat model. By the time of the initial assessment at 2 weeks, there had already been a loss of 29° of motion in the immobilized joints compared with controls. The lines at the upper portion of the graph represent the various controls in the study and a combined comparison group (dashed line) used for statistical comparisons. *, $P < 0.001$. (From Trudel *et al.* 1999, with permission.)

marked reductions in range of motion after cast removal (average cast time = 4.1 weeks). Their results included losses of greater than 50% of expected motion for all planes in the wrist and restriction of pronation and supination to 40% of normal.

Studies on the persistence of joint contracture after immobilization and injury vary, and the actual results in a given case are probably dependent upon multiple issues including the actual nature of the injury and the extent and duration of immobilization. After 4 weeks of immobilization of the knee in a plaster cast in healthy human volunteers, Veldhuizen *et al.* (1993) found that range of motion returned to normal within 3 days after cast removal. In a canine model of shoulder immobilization, Schollmeier *et al.* (1996) found that 12 weeks of cast use resulted in significant losses in passive range of motion initially that

were normalized by 12 weeks after cast removal. In contrast to this, Tropp and Norlin (1995) found significant declines in range of motion at the ankle 10 weeks after surgical treatment for ankle fractures with motion close to normal by 12 months after injury. Significant joint dysfunction well beyond this timeframe following immobilization has also been recognized in the medical literature for well over a century (Salter 1996).

Beyond loss of range of motion, numerous other aspects of joint function and structure are affected by immobilization. It has been proposed that joint function and homeostasis are dependent upon motion and use (Akeson *et al.* 1987; Salter 1996). In the absence of these factors (i.e. with immobilization), the functional and structural properties of the joint cannot be maintained. This leads to a number of documented changes in the joint structure. These include the degradation of articular cartilage, adherence of the synovial membrane to the underlying cartilage and within synovial folds, synovial hyperplasia, destruction of ligamentous attachment sites and proliferation of connective tissue into the joint space (Akeson *et al.* 1987; Salter 1996; Schollmeier *et al.* 1996). Synovial fluid is also affected, with reductions in hyaluronic acid levels noted following immobilization in an animal model (Pitsillides *et al.* 1999). There is, additionally, degradation of the collagen fibre structure of associated ligaments, probably presenting a potential source of recurrent injury (Akeson *et al.* 1987).

Cardiovascular and aerobic capacity

In addition to changes in locally involved structures, immobilization and rest can have profound effects on overall cardiovascular and aerobic capacity. Dramatic declines in $\dot{V}O_{2\,max}$ and maximal exercise performance can occur with extended rest (Neufer 1989; Convertino 1997). The rate of loss of aerobic capacity has been estimated at 0.9% per day for 30 days of bed rest (Convertino 1997). The decline in $\dot{V}O_{2\,max}$ initially appears to be due to a reduction in circulating blood volume and venous return with a subsequent decline in cardiac output and stroke volume (Neufer 1989;

Convertino 1997). Peripheral mechanisms of decreased muscle capillarization, decreased vascular conductance and decreased muscular oxidative enzyme capacity also occur with detraining but do not seem to play a major role in initial declines in $\dot{V}O_{2max}$. These changes may be more important in submaximal exercise tolerance, however (Neufer 1989). Changes in $\dot{V}O_{2max}$ may be more profound in conditioned athletes, in part due to their greater relative level of aerobic fitness compared to untrained individuals (Convertino 1997).

Losses in aerobic fitness are related to the relative duration, frequency and intensity of training levels that are retained during periods of reduced activity that may follow an injury. $\dot{V}O_{2max}$ can be maintained for up to 15 weeks with reductions in training frequency of up to 66% if the training duration is held constant (Neufer 1989). A combined reduction of training frequency and duration that results in a 70% reduction in energy demand can maintain $\dot{V}O_{2max}$ over a period of 4 weeks (Neufer 1989). Maintaining the intensity of exercise training during periods of reduced frequency or duration of activity, however, is crucial to maintaining $\dot{V}O_{2max}$ (Neufer 1989). In the rehabilitation of an injured athlete, attempts to modify exercise patterns, where appropriate, to allow for continued limited training sessions with maintained cardiovascular intensity may be helpful in the acute stage and to potentially reduce the systemic cardiovascular effects of rest for a local tissue injury.

When viewing the changes that occur in aerobic capacity with extended rest or reduced activity in conjunction with the effects of rest and immobilization on joint function, and vascular, neural and muscular functioning, the need to assess the athlete as a whole becomes more apparent. Local tissue injury combined with the wide-ranging effects frequently associated with the required treatment can present significant challenges to obtaining optimal recovery and performance following an athletic injury. Thoroughly understanding these issues and following the approach to rehabilitation outlined previously (Table 7.1) allows a clinician to incorporate a global view of athletic function into a rehabilitation plan from the onset of injury through resumption of play.

The kinetic chain and muscular balance

As noted previously, comprehensive rehabilitation of an injured athlete requires that a clinician assess the entire kinetic chain for problems that may arise from or contribute to injury (Fig. 7.1). Two of the major issues that relate to the mechanics of, and force transmission through, the kinetic chain are relative strength and flexibility across regions of the chain. Determining the optimal degree of flexibility or muscular balance for a given athlete may not necessarily follow uniform parameters, however, and these factors need to be assessed in the context of a given individual and the demands of his or her sport.

The role of abnormalities in relative muscular balance in the occurrence of athletic injuries has been debated in the literature. A review on the topic by Grace (1985) noted that, although muscular imbalance as a causative factor in athletic injury seemed logical, there was little definitive proof of this. Part of the problem arises from the lack of any clear definition of 'imbalance' for a given muscular group. However, there are a number of reports since the date of that review that have identified relative muscular imbalance in studies of athletes postinjury, in screening of uninjured athletes commonly at risk for particular injuries, and as a significant risk factor for injury in prospective studies (Fleck & Falkel 1986; Taimela et al. 1990; Kibler et al. 1991; Knapik et al. 1991; McMaster et al. 1991; Chandler et al. 1992; Jonhagen et al. 1994; Baumhauer et al. 1995; Orchard et al. 1997). Kibler et al. (1991) identified relative ankle inflexibility and deficits in peak plantar flexion torque in the affected legs of runners with plantar fasciitis. A prospective study on the risk of ankle injury in college athletes found that injured and uninjured athletes differed in relative dorsiflexion to plantar flexion and eversion to inversion ratios as measured with isokinetic testing (Baumhauer et al. 1995). Another prospective study on college athletes by Knapik *et al.* (1991) also found that muscular imbalance either across the knee or between sides in a given athlete or imbalance in hip motion between sides was associated with a higher risk of injury. Similarly, Orchard *et al.* (1997) identified low hamstring to quadriceps peak torque ratios as a risk factor for hamstring injury in a prospective study of professional Australian rules footballers. Muscular imbalance about the shoulder has also been described in a variety of 'overhead' athletes, such as tennis players, swimmers and water polo players (Fleck & Falkel 1986; McMaster *et al.* 1991; Chandler *et al.* 1992).

As with muscle imbalance, the role of flexibility in sports injuries remains debated. Issues of flexibility are frequently cited as relating to athletic injury (Keller *et al.* 1987; Taimela *et al.* 1990; Taylor *et al.* 1990; Kibler *et al.* 1991; Knapik *et al.* 1991; Jonhagen *et al.* 1994; Worrell 1994; Baumhauer *et al.* 1995; Stocker *et al.* 1995; Bennell & Crossley 1996; Gleim & McHugh 1997). Several studies have found a positive association between injury and greater overall flexibility or 'ligamentous laxity', although other studies have failed to show an association between the two (Keller *et al.* 1987; Taimela *et al.* 1990; Baumhauer *et al.* 1995; Stocker *et al.* 1995; Bennell & Crossley 1996). Some authors note that relative inflexibility of a particular muscular group may be a predisposing factor to injury, particularly musculotendinous strain (Keller *et al.* 1987; Knapik *et al.* 1991; Jonhagen *et al.* 1994; Worrell 1994). Studies by Kibler *et al.* (1991) and Jonhagen *et al.* (1994) have shown relative decreases in passive range of motion measures compared with controls in athletes with either plantar fasciitis or prior hamstring strains, respectively. In a review of the role of flexibility in sports injury, Gleim and McHugh (1997) noted that, as with muscular imbalance, there is a lack of any standard definition for 'flexibility' and that there are a variety of ways in which flexibility can be assessed (such as static vs dynamic and stretch tolerance vs muscle stiffness). They also noted that specific flexibility patterns are associated with specific sports or even positions within a given sport. In some instances, lesser degrees of flexibility may, in fact, be beneficial in force production associated with rapid muscular contraction (Gleim & McHugh 1997). It is likely that a variety of physiological and anthropomorphic factors allow a given athlete to obtain an elite level of performance in a given task. Traits that are beneficial for some sport-specific tasks may actually be detrimental to the performance of others. The function of an athlete needs to be viewed in the context of that athlete's particular sport and the entire motion chain that allows for the performance of specific skills. Injury and rehabilitation must encompass this view, and deficits in flexibility (or the presence of excessive laxity) need to be assessed in the performance of a given task.

Given the data available on muscular balance, injury and soft tissue physiology, restoration of balanced strength and flexibility along the kinetic chain emerges as an important issue for rehabilitation and injury prevention. The overload process resulting in soft tissue injury and clinical symptoms is multifactorial. Aspects of technique and training clearly play a role, as do aspects of the functional kinetic chain affecting motion across a joint (Chandler & Kibler 1993). Addressing these issues in a comprehensive fashion allows for appropriate interventions to optimize athletic performance. For a detailed description of rehabilitation techniques utilizing this framework, the reader is referred to Chapter 14 in this text that is devoted to this very topic.

Conclusions

Injury and immobilization have wide-ranging physiological effects on the athlete. A comprehensive understanding of these issues is crucial in the management of an injured athlete. The athlete should be assessed not only for the acutely injured tissue but also for underlying biomechanical problems along the kinetic chain and subclinical adaptations. Athletic injuries need to be seen in the context of the entire athlete, including an accurate diagnosis of acute tissue injuries and an understanding of the individual's clinical symptoms. The athlete should be evaluated for other potentially overloaded structures, functional deficits such as strength imbalance, and for alterations in motion or technique that arise from or contribute to injury. Using this type of approach with a detailed knowledge of the issues discussed in other chapters of this text, clinicians can formulate a comprehensive rehabilitation strategy for the injured athlete that can restore function and provide long-term benefits in health and performance.

References

Akeson, W.H., Amiel, D., Ing, D., Abel, M.F., Garfin, S.R. & Woo, S.L.-Y. (1987) Effects of immobilization on joints. *Clinical Orthopaedics and Related Research* **219**, 28–37.

Appell, H.-J. (1990) Muscular atrophy following immobilization: a review. *Sports Medicine* **10** (1), 42–58.

Baumhauer, J.F., Alosa, D.M., Renstrom, P.A.F.H., Trevino, S. & Beynnon, B. (1995) A prospective study of ankle injury risk factors. *American Journal of Sports Medicine* **23** (5), 564–570.

Bennell, K.L. & Crossley, K. (1996) Musculoskeletal injuries in track and field: incidence, distribution and risk factors. *Australian Journal of Science and Medicine in Sport* **28** (3), 69–75.

Berg, H.E., Dudley, G.A., Haggmark, T., Ohlsen, H. & Tesch, P.A. (1991) Effects of lower limb unloading on skeletal muscle mass and function in humans. *Journal of Applied Physiology* **70** (4), 1882–1885.

Bloomfield, S.A. (1997) Changes in musculoskeletal structure and function with prolonged bed rest. *Medicine and Science in Sports and Exercise* **29** (2), 197–206.

Booth, F.W. (1987) Physiologic and biochemical effects of immobilization on muscle. *Clinical Orthopaedics and Related Research* **219**, 15–20.

Braun, B.L. (1999) Effects of ankle sprain in a general medicine clinic population 6–18 months after medical evaluation. *Archives of Family Medicine* **8** (2), 143–148.

Byl, N.N., Kohlhase, W. & Engel, G. (1999) Functional limitation immediately after cast immobilization and closed reduction of distal radius fractures: a preliminary report. *Journal of Hand Therapy* **12**, 201–211.

Chandler, T.J. & Kibler, W.B. (1993) A biomechanical approach to the prevention, treatment and rehabilitation of plantar fasciitis. *Sports Medicine* **15** (5), 344–352.

Chandler, T.J., Kibler, W.B., Stracener, E.C., Zeigler, A.K. & Pace, B. (1992) Shoulder strength, power, and endurance in college tennis players. *American Journal of Sports Medicine* **20** (4), 455–458.

Convertino, V.A. (1997) Cardiovascular consequences of bed rest: effect on maximal oxygen uptake. *Medicine and Science in Sports and Exercise* **29** (2), 191–196.

Cruz-Martinez, A., Ramirez, A. & Arpa, J. (2000) Quadriceps atrophy after knee traumatisms and immobilization: electrophysiological assessment. *European Neurology* **43**, 110–114.

Curwin, S.L. (1996) Tendon injuries: pathophysiology and treatment. In: *Athletic Injuries and Rehabilitation* (Zachazewski, J.E., Magee, D.J. & Quillen, W.S., eds). W.B. Saunders, Philadelphia: 27–53.

DeLee, J.C. & Farney, W.C. (1992) Incidence of injury in Texas high school football. *American Journal of Sports Medicine* **20** (5), 575–580.

Dittmer, D.K. & Teasell, R. (1993) Complications of immobilization and bed rest. Part 1: Musculoskeletal and cardiovascular complications. *Canadian Family Physician* **39**, 1428–1432, 1435–1437.

Fleck, S.J. & Falkel, J.E. (1986) Value of resistance training for the reduction of sports injuries. *Sports Medicine* **3**, 61–68.

Frank, C.B. (1996) Ligament injuries: pathophysiology and healing. In: *Athletic Injuries and Rehabilitation* (Zachazewski, J.E., Magee, D.J. & Quillen, W.S., eds). W.B. Saunders, Philadelphia: 9–25.

Garrett, W.E. (1996) Muscle strain injuries. *American Journal of Sports Medicine* **24** (6), S2–S8.

Geboers, J.F.M., van Tuiji, J.H., Seelen, H.A.M. & Drost, M.R. (2000) Effect of immobilization on ankle dorsiflexion strength. *Scandinavian Journal of Rehabilitation Medicine* **32**, 66–71.

Gleim, G.W. & McHugh, M.P. (1997) Flexibility and its effect on sports injury and performance. *Sports Medicine* **24** (5), 289–299.

Grace, T.G. (1985) Muscle balance and extremity injury: a perplexing balance. *Sports Medicine* **2**, 77–82.

Grimby, G., Gustafsson, E., Peterson, L. & Renstrom, P. (1980) Quadriceps function and training after knee ligament surgery. *Medicine and Science in Sports and Exercise* **12** (1), 70–75.

Henry, J.H., Lareau, B. & Neigut, D. (1982) The injury rate in professional basketball. *American Journal of Sports Medicine* **10** (1), 16–18.

Herring, S.A. (1990) Rehabilitation of muscle injuries. *Medicine and Science in Sports and Exercise* **22** (4), 453–456.

Herring, S.A. & Kibler, W.B. (1998) A framework for rehabilitation. In: *Functional Rehabilitation of Sports and Musculoskeletal Injuries* (Kibler, W.B., Herring, S.A., Press, J.M. & Lee, P.A., eds). Aspen, Gaithersburg: 1–8.

Herring, S.A. & Nilson, K.L. (1987) Introduction to overuse injuries. *Clinics in Sports Medicine* **6** (2), 225–239.

Hopkins, J.T., Ingersoll, C.D., Krause, A., Edwards, J.E. & Cordova, M.L. (2001) Effect of knee joint effusion on quadriceps and soleus motoneuron pool excitability. *Medicine and Science in Sports and Exercise* **33** (1), 123–126.

Hortobagyi, T., Dempsey, L., Fraser, D., Zheng, D., Hamilton, G. & Dohm. L. (2000) Changes in muscle strength, muscle fibre size and myofibrillar gene expression after immobilization and retraining in humans. *Journal of Physiology* **524** (1), 293–304.

Hurley, M.V. & Newham, D.J. (1993) The influence of arthrogenous muscle inhibition on quadriceps rehabilitation of patients with early, unilateral osteoarthritic knees. *British Journal of Rheumatology* **32** (2), 127–131.

Jarvinen, M.J. & Lehto, M.U.K. (1993) The effects of early mobilisation and immobilisation on the healing process following muscle injuries. *Sports Medicine* **15** (2), 78–89.

Jarvinen, T.A.H., Kaariainen, M., Jarvinen, M. & Kalimo, H. (2000) Muscle strain injuries. *Current Opinion in Rheumatology* **12**, 155–161.

Jonhagen, S., Nemeth, G. & Eriksson, E. (1994) Hamstring injuries in sprinters: the role of concentric and eccentric hamstring muscle strength and flexibility. *American Journal of Sports Medicine* **22** (2), 262–266.

Kannus, P., Jozsa, L., Kvist, M., Lehto, M. & Jarvinen, M. (1992) The effect of immobilization on the myotendinous junction: an ultrastructural, histochemical and immunohistochemical study. *Acta Physiologica Scandinavica* **144**, 387–394.

Keller, C.S., Noyes, F.R. & Buncher, R. (1987) The medical aspects of soccer injury epidemiology. *American Journal of Sports Medicine* **15** (3), 230–237.

Kibler, W.B. (1998) Determining the extent of the functional deficit. In: *Functional Rehabilitation of Sports and Musculoskeletal Injuries* (Kibler, W.B., Herring, S.A., Press, J.M., & Lee, P.A., eds). Aspen, Gaithersburg: 1–8.

Kibler, W.B., Goldberg, C. & Chandler, T.J. (1991) Functional biomechanical deficits in running athletes with plantar fasciitis. *American Journal of Sports Medicine* **18** (1), 66–71.

Kibler, W.B., Chandler, T.J. & Pace, B.K. (1992) Principles of rehabilitation after chronic tendon injuries. *Clinics in Sports Medicine* **11**, 63.

Knapik, J.J., Bauman, C.L., Jones, B.H., Harris, J.M. & Vaughan, L. (1991) Preseason strength and flexibility imbalances associated with athletic injuries in female college athletes. *American Journal of Sports Medicine* **19** (1), 76–81.

Kvist, M., Hurme, T., Kannus, P. *et al.* (1995) Vascular density at the myotendinous junction of the rat gastrocnemius muscle after immobilization and remobilization. *American Journal of Sports Medicine* **23** (3), 359–364.

Leadbetter, W.B. (1994) Soft tissue athletic injury. In: *Sports Injuries: Mechanisms, Prevention, Treatment* (Fu, F.H. & Stone, D.A., eds). Williams & Wilkins, Baltimore: 733–780.

Liepert, J., Tegenthoff, M. & Malin, J.P. (1995) Changes of cortical motor area size during immobilization. *Electroencephalography and Clinical Neurophysiology* **97** (6), 382–386.

Lindboe, C.F. & Platou, C.S. (1984) Effect of immobilization of short duration on the muscle fibre size. *Clinical Physiology* **4**, 183–188.

Lorish, T.R., Rizzo, T.D., Ilstrup, D.M. & Scott, S.G. (1992) Injuries in adolescent and preadolescent boys at two large wrestling tournaments. *American Journal of Sports Medicine* **20** (2), 199–202.

Macera, C.A. (1992) Lower extremity injuries in runners: advances in prediction. *Sports Medicine* **13** (1), 50–57.

Mair, S.D., Seaber, A.V., Glisson, R.R. & Garrett, W.E. (1996) The role of fatigue in susceptibility to acute muscle strain injury. *American Journal of Sports Medicine* **24** (2), 137–143.

Malone, T.R., Garrett, W.E. & Zachazewski, J.E. (1996) Muscle: deformation, injury, repair. In: *Athletic Injuries and Rehabilitation* (Zachazewski, J.E., Magee, D.J. & Quillen, W.S., eds). W.B. Saunders, Philadelphia: 71–91.

McDowell, G.S. (1997) Spine. In: *Essentials of Musculoskeletal Care* (Snider, R.K., ed.). American Academy of Orthopedic Surgeons, Rosemont, IL: 492–546.

McMaster, W.C. & Troup, J. (1993) A survey of interfering shoulder pain in United States competitive swimmers. *American Journal of Sports Medicine* **21** (1), 67–70.

McMaster, W.C., Long, S.C. & Caiozzo, V.J. (1991) Isokinetic torque imbalances in the rotator cuff of the elite water polo player. *American Journal of Sports Medicine* **19** (1), 72–75.

Muller, E.A. (1970) Influence of training and of inactivity on muscle strength. *Archives of Physical Medicine and Rehabilitation* **51**, 449–462.

Murtaugh, K. (2001) Injury patterns among female field hockey players. *Medicine and Science in Sports and Exercise* **33** (2), 201–207.

Neufer, P.D. (1989) The effect of detraining and reduced training on the physiological adaptations to aerobic exercise training. *Sports Medicine* **8** (5), 302–321.

Noonan, T.J. & Garrett, W.E. (1992) Injuries at the myotendinous junction. *Clinics in Sports Medicine* **11** (4), 783–806.

Oki, S., Itoh, T., Desaki, J., Matsuda, Y., Okumura, H. & Shibata, T. (1998) Three-dimensional structure of the vascular network in normal and immobilized muscles of the rat. *Archives of Physical Medicine and Rehabilitation* **79**, 31–32.

Orchard, J., Marsden, J., Lord, S. & Garlick, D. (1997) Preseason hamstring muscle weakness associated with hamstring muscle injury in Australian footballers. *American Journal of Sports Medicine* **25** (1), 81–85.

Pitsillides, A.A., Skerry, T.M. & Edwards, J.C.W. (1999) Joint immobilization reduces synovial fluid hyaluronan concentration and is accompanied by changes in the synovial intimal cell populations. *Rheumatology* **38**, 1108–1112.

Quillen, W.S., Magee, D.J. & Zachazewski, J.E. (1996) The process of athletic injury and rehabilitation. In: *Athletic Injuries and Rehabilitation* (Zachazewski, J.E., Magee, D.J. & Quillen, W.S., eds). W.B. Saunders, Philadelphia: 3–8.

Reynolds, C.A., Cummings, G.S., Andrew, P.D. & Tillman, L.J. (1996) The effect of nontraumatic immobilization on ankle dorsiflexion stiffness in rats. *Journal of Orthopaedic and Sports Physical Therapy* **23** (1), 27–33.

Rutherford, O.M. (1988) Muscular coordination and strength training: implications for injury rehabilitation. *Sports Medicine* **5**, 196–202.

Rutherford, O.M., Jones, D.A. & Round, J.M. (1990) Long-lasting unilateral muscle wasting and weakness following injury and immobilization. *Scandinavian Journal of Rehabilitation Medicine* **22**, 33–37.

Saal, J.A. (1991) Common American football injuries. *Sports Medicine* **12** (2), 132–147.

Salter, R.B. (1996) History of rest and motion and the scientific basis for early continuous passive motion. *Hand Clinics* **12** (1), 1–11.

Schollmeier, G., Sarkar, K., Fukuhara, K. & Uhthoff, H.K. (1996) Structural and functional changes in the canine shoulder after cessation of immobilization. *Clinical Orthopaedics and Related Research* **323**, 310–315.

Seki, K., Taniguchi, Y. & Narusawa, M. (2001a) Effects of joint immobilization on firing rate modulation of human motor units. *Journal of Physiology* **530** (3), 507–519.

Seki, K., Taniguchi, Y. & Narusawa, M. (2001b) Alterations in contractile properties of human skeletal muscle induced by joint immobilization. *Journal of Physiology* **530** (3), 521–532.

Shaffer, M.A., Okereke, E., Esterhai, J.L. *et al.* (2000) Effects of immobilization on plantar-flexion torque, fatigue resistance, and functional ability following an ankle fracture. *Physical Therapy* **80** (8), 769–780.

Spencer, J.D., Hayes, K.C. & Alexander, I.J. (1984) Knee joint effusion and quadriceps reflex inhibition in man. *Archives of Physical Medicine and Rehabilitation* **65**, 171–177.

Steiner, M.E. & Micheli, L.J. (1985) Treatment of symptomatic spondylolysis and spondylolisthesis with the modified Boston brace. *Spine* **10**, 937–943.

Stocker, D., Pink, M. & Jobe, F.W. (1995) Comparison of shoulder injury in collegiate- and master's-level swimmers. *Clinical Journal of Sports Medicine* **591**, 4–8.

Taimela, S., Kujala, U.M. & Osterman, K. (1990) Intrinsic risk factors and athletic injuries. *Sports Medicine* **9** (4), 205–215.

Taylor, D.C., Dalton, J.D., Seaber, A.V. & Garrett, W.E. (1990) Viscoelastic properties of muscle–tendon units; the biomechanical effects of stretching. *American Journal of Sports Medicine* **18** (3), 300–309.

Taylor, D.C., Dalton, J.D., Seaber, A.V. & Garrett, W.E. (1993) Experimental muscle strain injury: early functional and structural deficits and the increased risk for reinjury. *American Journal of Sports Medicine* **21** (2), 190–194.

Tropp, H. & Norlin, R. (1995) Ankle performance after ankle fracture: a randomized study of early mobilization. *Foot and Ankle International* **16** (2), 79–83.

Trudel, G. & Uhthoff, H.K. (2000) Contractures secondary to immobility: is the restriction articular or muscular? An experimental longitudinal study in the rat knee. *Archives of Physical Medicine and Rehabilitation* **81**, 6–13.

Trudel, G., Uhthoff, H.K. & Brown, M. (1999) Extent and direction of joint motion limitation after prolonged immobility: an experimental study in the rat. *Archives of Physical Medicine and Rehabilitation* **80**, 1542–1547.

Veldhuizen, J.W., Verstappen, F.T.J., Vroemen, J.P.A.M., Kuipers, H. & Greep, J.M. (1993) Functional and morphological adaptations following four weeks of knee immobilization. *International Journal of Sports Medicine* **14**, 283–287.

Wills, C.A., Caiozzo, V.J., Yasukawa, D.I., Prietto, C.A. & McMaster, W.C. (1982) Effects of immobilization of human skeletal muscle. *Orthopaedic Review* **11** (11), 57–64.

Worrell, T.W. (1994) Factors associated with hamstring injuries: an approach to treatment and preventative measures. *Sports Medicine* **17** (5), 338–345.

Young, A. (1993) Current issues in arthrogenous inhibition. *Annals of the Rheumatic Diseases* **52**, 829–834.

Young, A., Stokes, M. & Iles, J.F. (1987) Effects of joint pathology on muscle. *Clinical Orthopaedics and Related Research* **219**, 21–27.

Zarzhevsky, N., Coleman, R., Volpin, G., Stein, H. & Reznick, A.Z. (1999) Muscle recovery after immobilisation by external fixation. *Journal of Bone and Joint Surgery* **81B** (5), 896–901.

Chapter 8

Psychological Factors in Sports Injury Rehabilitation

BRITTON W. BREWER AND ALLEN E. CORNELIUS

Introduction

Rehabilitation of sports injuries involves more than repairing the physical injury and regaining previous levels of physical performance. Optimizing injury rehabilitation also includes understanding the psychological impact of the injury on the athlete and how psychological factors may interact with the rehabilitation process. The purpose of this chapter is to review the research examining psychological factors related to sports injury rehabilitation.

Major advances have been made in recent years in our understanding of the range of psychological factors associated with sports injury rehabilitation. In the early 1990s, Williams and Roepke et al. (1993) and Brewer (1994) made specific suggestions for improving the quality of psychological research on sports injury rehabilitation. Fortunately, many of these recommendations have been heeded. Specifically, responding to the recommendations made by Williams and Roepke, researchers have: (i) identified cognitive and emotional responses to injury that are characteristic of athlete populations (e.g. Leddy et al. 1994; Quinn & Fallon 1999); (ii) investigated the effects of psychological interventions on sports injury rehabilitation (e.g. Ross & Berger 1996; Theodorakis et al. 1996, 1997a, 1997b; Cupal & Brewer 2001); and (iii) initiated the education of sports medicine practitioners on psychological aspects of injury rehabilitation (e.g. Ford & Gordon 1997, 1998; Gordon et al. 1998).

Following the recommendations of Brewer (1994), researchers have: (i) advanced theory (e.g. Evans & Hardy 1995; Johnston & Carroll 1998a; Wiese-Bjornstal et al. 1998; Brewer et al. 2002); (ii) included both psychological and physical variables in their analyses (e.g. LaMott 1994; Durso-Cupal 1996; Ross & Berger 1996; Theodorakis et al. 1996; Theodorakis et al. 1997a; Theodorakis et al. 1997b; Niedfeldt 1998; Morrey et al. 1999; Brewer et al. 2000c); (iii) assessed the prevalence of clinical levels of psychological distress (Leddy et al. 1994; Brewer & Petrie 1995; Brewer et al. 1995a, 1995b; Perna et al. 1998); (iv) implemented prospective, longitudinal research designs (e.g. Smith et al. 1993; LaMott 1994; Leddy et al. 1994; Ross & Berger 1996; Morrey 1997; Petrie et al. 1997b; Udry 1997a; Perna et al. 1998; Roh et al. 1998; Morrey et al. 1999; Brewer et al. 2000c); (v) conducted qualitative investigations (e.g. Shelley 1994; Gould et al. 1997a, 1997b; Udry et al. 1997a, 1997b; Johnston & Carroll 1998a, 1998b; Bianco et al. 1999b); (vi) used control groups of athletes without injuries (e.g. LaMott 1994; Brewer & Petrie 1995; Petrie et al. 1997a; Perna et al. 1999); and (vii) examined groups of athletes that are homogeneous with respect to injury type, severity and prognosis (e.g. LaMott 1994; Ross & Berger 1996; Theodorakis et al. 1996, 1997a, 1997b; Udry 1997a; Morrey et al. 1999; Brewer et al. 2000a, 2000b, 2000c; Cupal & Brewer 2001); and (viii) used experimental research designs (e.g. Ross & Berger 1996; Theodorakis et al. 1996, 1997a, 1997b; Cupal & Brewer 2001).

To provide some structure for the voluminous amount of research that has been conducted on psychological factors in sports injury rehabilitation, two models are presented that describe the hypothesized relationships among psychological and other key variables in the sports injury rehabilitation process. The first model, the integrated model developed by Wiese-Bjornstal *et al.* (1998), describes many of the psychological factors related to athletes' reactions to injuries. The second model is a biopsychosocial model developed by Brewer *et al.* (2002) that places sports injury rehabilitation in a broad contextual framework. Following descriptions of these models, research examining the relationships predicted by these models is reviewed.

Models of psychological response to sports injury and sports injury rehabilitation

COGNITIVE APPRAISAL MODELS

Cognitive appraisal models view an injury as a stressor or a stimulus, and the response of the individual is dependent upon a variety of factors that influence the interpretation of this stimulus. Several cognitive appraisal models have been developed to explain athletes' reactions to sports injuries (e.g. Gordon 1986; Weiss & Troxel 1986; Grove 1993; Wiese-Bjornstal *et al.* 1998), the most comprehensive of which is the integrated model proposed by Wiese-Bjornstal *et al.* (1998) (Fig. 8.1). This model proposes that many preinjury and postinjury factors are related to how an individual reacts to a sports injury. Preinjury factors are personality, history of stressors, coping resources and interventions. Postinjury factors include personal factors (e.g. type and severity of the injury, general health status, demographic variables) and situational factors (e.g. sport played, social support system, accessibility to rehabilitation). These factors combine to determine the cognitive appraisal of the injury, which in turn affects the emotional and behavioural responses to injury, and, ultimately, the rehabilitation out-

come. For example, if the cognitive response to an injury is one of doubt and thoughts of negative outcomes, a negative emotional response is likely to result. If the appraisal of the injury is more positive, with thoughts of full recovery and confidence in rehabilitation, the model predicts that a positive emotional reaction will be more likely.

There has been considerable empirical support for cognitive appraisal models in general, and the integrated model in particular. Sports injury has been identified as a significant source of stress in several studies (Brewer & Petrie 1995; Gould *et al.* 1997a; Bianco *et al.* 1999; Ford & Gordon 1999; Heniff *et al.* 1999), and numerous personal and situational factors have been associated with psychological responses to sports injury (Brewer 1994, 1998, 1999a). Although some of the more complex mediational relationships predicted by the integrated model have not yet found empirical support (Daly *et al.* 1995; Brewer *et al.* 2000c), there is considerable research supporting the usefulness of this model for understanding the diverse array of reactions to sports injuries. The integrated model (Wiese-Bjornstal *et al.* 1998) also has the benefit of providing theoretical guidance for interventions to improve rehabilitation outcomes, as many of the personal and situational factors are subject to modification (e.g. improving social support systems).

BIOPSYCHOSOCIAL MODEL

The integrated model describes the complex relationships of psychological, situational and cognitive variables to emotional and behavioural responses to sports injury, but it does not take into account the breadth of factors that can be related to sports injury rehabilitation processes and outcomes. Because of the multiplicity of factors that potentially interact during sports injury rehabilitation, a model that is comprehensive, yet conceptually grounded, is required. Borrowing from other health outcome research (Cohen & Rodriguez 1995; Matthews *et al.* 1997) and existing models of sports injury rehabilitation

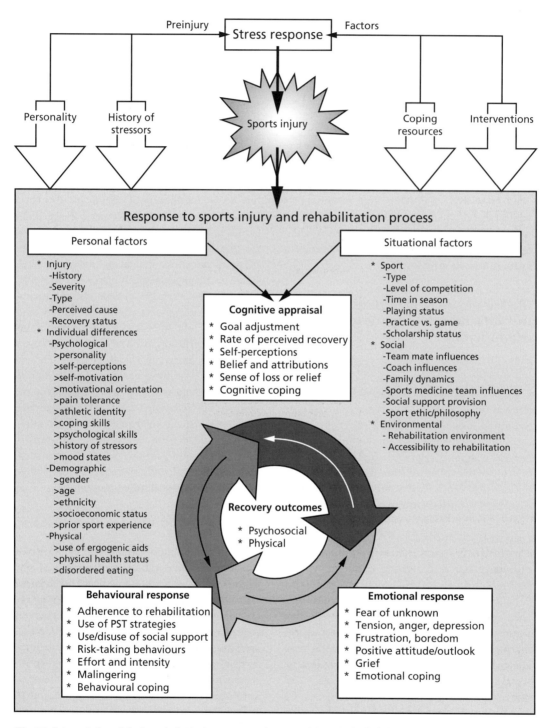

Fig. 8.1 Integrated model of psychological response to the sports injury and rehabilitation process. (From Wiese-Bjornstal *et al.* 1998, with permission. © 1998 by the Association for the Advancement of Applied Sport Psychology.)

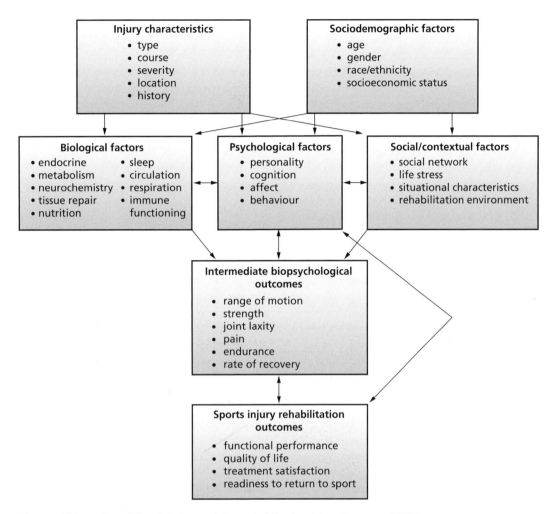

Fig. 8.2 A biopsychosocial model of sports injury rehabilitation. (From Brewer *et al.* 2002)

(Leadbetter 1994; Flint 1998; Wiese-Bjornstal *et al.* 1998), a model incorporating biological, social, medical and psychological factors has been developed (Brewer *et al.* 2002). This biopsychosocial model, as depicted in Fig. 8.2, has seven interacting components: injury characteristics, sociodemographic factors, biological factors, psychological factors, social/contextual factors, intermediate biopsychological outcomes and sports injury rehabilitation outcomes.

The biopsychosocial model proposes that the sports injury rehabilitation process begins with the occurrence of an injury. The specific characteristics of the injury (e.g. type, course, severity, location and history of injury) and sociodemographic factors (e.g. age, gender, race/ethnicity, socioeconomic status) are depicted as influencing biological factors (e.g. nutrition, sleep), psychological factors (e.g. personality, cognition) and social/contextual factors (e.g. social networks, life stress). Psychological factors are the focal point of this model, having reciprocal relationships with both biological and social/contextual factors. Biological, psychological and social/contextual factors are thought to influence intermediate biopsychological outcomes (e.g. strength, rate of recovery), with psychological factors also being reciprocally affected by these outcomes.

The final component of the model, sports injury rehabilitation outcomes, consists of functional performance, quality of life, treatment satisfaction and readiness to return to sport. This phase of the model is reciprocally related to both the intermediate biopsychological outcomes and the psychological factors.

The biopsychosocial model incorporates the various factors that are potentially related to sports injury rehabilitation outcomes, and offers a structure for examining the relationships of these factors in a contextually complete model. Given that the model incorporates findings and concepts from already established models of injury rehabilitation (Leadbetter 1994; Flint 1998; Wiese-Bjornstal et al. 1998), there is already support for many of the hypothesized relationships. However, the broad scope of the model will enable researchers to investigate a wider array of potential influences on the sports rehabilitation process.

Given the centrality of the psychological factors in the integrated model (Wiese-Bjornstal et al. 1998) and the biopsychosocial model (Brewer et al. 2002), and the focus of this chapter, the following sections review the research that examines the relationships between the psychological factors depicted in these models and the other constructs in the models. Specifically, the next section reviews the research findings related to psychological reactions to injury, and the subsequent section examines the literature concerning psychological factors associated with sports injury rehabilitation outcomes.

Psychological responses to sports injury

The subject of psychological disturbance arising from sports injury has been studied extensively since Little (1969) first identified neurotic symptoms in injured athletes. The following sections examine research concerning emotional and behavioural responses to sports injury that has accrued since Little's seminal work. For the purposes of this discussion, sports injuries are defined as physical damage that occurs as the result of an event or process associated with sports participation and disrupts subsequent sports participation. The duration of such disruption of involvement in sports may vary extensively depending on the nature, course and severity of the injury. Emotional responses refer to affective (i.e. feeling) states that are experienced subsequent to injury onset, whereas behavioural responses refer to overt actions that are manifested following the occurrence of injury.

Emotional responses to sports injury

Emotional responses to sports injury have been a widely researched topic within the sports psychology literature. A popular approach has been the application of stage theories that propose that athletes experience an injury as a type of loss. The injury is thought to be perceived by the athlete as a loss of an aspect of the self, and therefore considered to elicit a reaction similar to that exhibited by an individual who has experienced a serious psychological loss (Peretz 1970; Rotella & Heyman 1986). Stage models of grief and loss have proposed that individuals experience a sequence of emotional responses to the loss, leading to eventual adaptation. In perhaps the best known description of these stages, Kubler-Ross 1969) proposed that in response to a major loss, individuals commonly progress through five stages: denial, anger, bargaining, depression and acceptance. Researchers have found that athletes experience many of these same emotions following an injury (Rotella 1985; Astle 1986; Lynch 1988; Silva & Hardy 1991).

Although the five-stage model developed by Kubler-Ross (1969) has been widely discussed by sport psychologists, research investigating athletes' reactions to injury has not fully supported this model. Kubler-Ross's model was derived from her work with terminally ill patients, and the experience of being terminally ill may not be similar enough to having a sports injury to be generalizable (Smith et al. 1990b). There is, however, support for emotional responses to injury being somewhat similar to grief reactions

(Shelley 1994; Macchi & Crossman 1996). In the initial time period following an injury, negative emotions such as depression, frustration, confusion, anger and fear have been documented in several qualitative studies (Gordon & Lindgren 1990; Shelley & Carroll 1996; Shelley & Sherman 1996; Udry *et al.* 1997a; Johnston & Carroll 1998a; Sparkes 1998; Bianco *et al.* 1999b). During the middle phase of rehabilitation, depression and frustration are commonly reported emotions, with the source of these emotions shifting from concerns about the injury to rehabilitation-related issues. As rehabilitation of the injury nears completion, depression and frustration remain prevalent and a fear of reinjury emerges (Johnston & Carroll 1998a; Bianco *et al.* 1999b).

Quantitative studies have also demonstrated that athletes with injuries experience negative emotions to a greater extent than athletes without injuries (Chan & Grossman 1988; Pearson & Jones 1992; Smith *et al.* 1993; Leddy *et al.* 1994; Brewer & Petrie 1995; Johnson 1997, 1998; Petrie *et al.* 1997a, 1997b; Miller 1998; Perna *et al.* 1998; Roh *et al.* 1998; Newcomer *et al.* 1999) and that emotional responses to injury tend to become more adaptive as time progresses (McDonald & Hardy 1990; Smith *et al.* 1990a; Uemukai 1993). There is also evidence that the emotional disturbance of athletes is greater following injury than it is prior to the injury (Dubbels *et al.* 1992; Smith *et al.* 1993; Leddy *et al.* 1994; Miller 1998).

These emotional disturbances are, for the most part, not of a sufficient magnitude or duration to be assigned a clinical diagnosis (Heil 1993). Epidemiological studies, however, have shown that a substantial minority of injured athletes (5–24%) experience clinical levels of emotional disturbance as determined by scores on psychometric instruments and, in some cases, clinical interviews (Leddy *et al.* 1994; Brewer & Petrie 1995; Brewer *et al.* 1995a, 1995b; Perna *et al.* 1998). There are risks of suicide with athletes who experience severe levels of postinjury emotional disturbance, particularly depression (Smith & Milliner 1994).

Stage models suggest that psychological reactions to sports injuries are manifested in a sequential progression of emotions and behaviours. Although most of the emotions identified in stage models (Rotella 1985; Astle 1986; Lynch 1988) are commonly experienced by the majority of athletes with injuries—consistent with the findings on psychological reactions to undesirable events in general (for a review, see Silver & Wortman 1980)—empirical support for a stage-like progression of these emotional states is weak (Brewer 1994). The emotional reactions of athletes with injuries are more varied and less sequential than those postulated by stage models. The only consistent change in emotions over time that has been documented is an overall pattern of decreasing negative emotions and increasing positive emotions as rehabilitation progresses (Grove *et al.* 1990; McDonald & Hardy 1990; Smith *et al.* 1990a; Uemukai 1993; LaMott 1994; Leddy *et al.* 1994; Quackenbush & Crossman 1994; Crossman *et al.* 1995; Macchi & Crossman 1996; Dawes & Roach 1997; Laurence 1997; Morrey 1997; Miller 1998; Quinn & Fallon 1999). A deviation from this pattern, which has been documented in two studies (LaMott 1994; Morrey *et al.* 1999), is a slight increase in negative emotions and a slight decrease in positive emotions as athletes near the end of rehabilitation following reconstructive knee surgery, possibly reflecting athletes' apprehension about returning to sports activity and fear of reinjury (Quinn 1996; Johnston & Carroll 1998a; Bianco *et al.* 1999b). Stage models ignore several important factors related to how athletes respond to an injury, such as their idiosyncratic perceptions of the injury, and situational circumstances such as the severity of the injury and sources of social support (Brewer 1994; Wiese-Bjornstal *et al.* 1998).

The general lack of empirical support for stage models does not mean that they are completely without merit. Recently proposed versions of stage models have evolved from static and rigid stages of previous models to more flexible and dynamic descriptions of psychological responses to sports injury, thereby allowing for more individual variation in how the stages are experienced (Evans & Hardy 1995, 1999). Such modification muddles the simplicity of stage models, but

Table 8.1 Situational factors associated with postinjury emotional disturbance.

Variable	Direction	Reference
Current injury status	+	Alzate *et al.* 1998; Brewer *et al.* 1995a; Quinn 1996
Injury severity	+	Alzate *et al.* 1998; Pargman & Lunt 1989; Perna 1992; Smith *et al.* 1990a, 1993; Uemukai, 1993
Impairment of daily activities	+	Crossman & Jamieson 1985
Life stress	+	Brewer 1993; Petrie *et al.* 1997b; Quinn 1996
Recovery progress	+	Quinn 1996
Impairment of sport activities	–	Brewer *et al.* 1995a
Level of sport involvement	+/–	Crossman *et al.* 1995; Meyers *et al.* 1991
Medical prognosis	–	Gordin *et al.* 1988
Recovery progress	–	McDonald & Hardy 1990; Quinn 1996; Smith *et al.* 1988
Social support for rehabilitation	–	Brewer *et al.* 1995a
Social support satisfaction	–	Green & Weinberg 1998

Direction refers to the positive (+) and negative (–) correlations with postinjury emotional disturbance.

reflects more accurately the dynamic nature of the emotional experience of athletes who have been injured. Stage models have provided impetus for the development of cognitive appraisal models of responses to injury, such as the integrated model (Wiese-Bjornstal *et al.* 1998), which identifies factors that mediate and moderate emotional responses to sports injury.

MEDIATING AND MODERATING FACTORS

The integrated model (Wiese-Bjornstal *et al.* 1998) posits cognitive, personal and situational factors as influences on emotional and behavioural responses to sports injury, with cognitive appraisals mediating the relationships between personal and situational factors and emotional and behavioural responses. However, most of the research in this area has not addressed this mediational effect, but has focused instead on direct associations between various personal and situational factors and emotional and behavioural responses to injury. Therefore, only indirect evidence of the hypothesized mediational role of cognitive appraisals has been obtained.

Personal factors that have been identified as being positively related to postinjury emotional disturbance include self-identification with the athlete role (Brewer 1993; Shelley & Carroll 1996; Sparkes 1998), competitive trait anxiety (Petrie

et al. 1997), investment in playing professional sports (Kleiber & Brock 1992), level of sports involvement (Meyers *et al.* 1991), pessimistic explanatory style (Grove *et al.* 1990) and previous injury experience (Bianco *et al.* 1999b). Athletes with injuries have demonstrated negative relationships between emotional distress and age (Smith *et al.* 1990a; Brewer *et al.* 1995a) and hardiness (Grove *et al.* 1990; Miller 1998). Thus, the individuals most likely to encounter difficulty adjusting emotionally to injury are those who are young, least hardy, most strongly identified with the athlete role, most dispositionally anxious, most invested in having a career as a professional athlete, most experienced in the rigors of sports injury rehabilitation, and most pessimistic. The relationship of emotional distress to age is potentially more complex than a simple linear relationship, as Meyers *et al.* (1991) obtained a curvilinear relationship between age and emotional disturbance for participants recovering from knee surgery. Participants of intermediate age (20–39 years) reported greater levels of emotional disturbance than younger (10–19 years) and older (40–49 years) participants. Injury-related characteristics and aspects of the social and physical environments that can change over time are referred to as situational factors. As shown in Table 8.1, numerous situational factors have been correlated with emotional distress in athletes with injury. In general, research has indicated that athletes are likely to experience greater postinjury emotional disturbance when they perceive their injuries as serious, view themselves as having made little rehabilitative progress, and consider themselves as weakly supported in their rehabilitative pursuits.

According to the integrated model (Wiese-Bjornstal *et al.* 1998), it is cognitive appraisals made concerning the injury that have the most direct effect on emotional and behavioural responses. Numerous types of cognitive appraisals have been correlated with emotional distress in research studies. Greater emotional distress following injury has been associated with the tendencies to interpret pain in a catastrophic manner (Tripp 2000) and to attribute the cause of sports injury to factors residing within oneself (Tedder & Biddle 1998) and pertaining to all areas of one's life (Brewer 1991). Lower levels of postinjury emotional distress have been found for individuals who: (i) think that they will be able to cope with their injuries (Daly *et al.* 1995); (ii) can readily imagine themselves functioning favourably following injury (Fisk & King 1998); (iii) have high general and physical self-esteem (Brewer 1993; Quinn 1996); and (iv) are confident in themselves and their ability to adhere to the rehabilitation protocol, recover fully from injury and succeed in sport (Quinn 1996). Also, in contrast to the findings of Tedder and Biddle, athletes who attribute the cause of their injuries to factors residing within themselves and likely to occur have reported lower levels of postinjury emotional disturbance (Brewer 1999b). Thus, although it is unclear whether taking responsibility for one's injury is adaptive in terms of emotional adjustment, there is little doubt that cognitions indicating confidence in oneself, one's body and one's recovery are associated with more favourable emotional states following sports injury.

Behavioural responses to sports injury

A sports injury can elicit a number of behavioural responses in addition to the emotional responses discussed in the previous section. The two most relevant behaviours, and the most researched, are coping behaviours and adherence to sports injury rehabilitation.

COPING BEHAVIOURS

In an effort to deal effectively with injuries and the related issues that may arise during rehabilitation, athletes may engage in certain behaviours to help them cope with the situation. Specific behavioural strategies that have been identified in athletes with injuries include an aggressive rehabilitation approach, avoiding others, building strength, distracting oneself (e.g. keeping busy, seeking a change of scenery), 'driving through' (e.g. doing things normally, learning about their injuries, resting when tired, working hard to achieve rehabilitation goals), seeking out and using social support networks, trying alternative treatments, and working or training at their own pace (Gould *et al.* 1997b; Bianco *et al.* 1999a). Other studies have examined the use of specific coping strategies, and have found that the most strongly endorsed coping behaviours assessed by the COPE inventory (Carver *et al.* 1989; Scheier *et al.* 1994) were active coping, which involves initiating behaviours to deal directly with a stressor or its effects, and instrumental social support, which pertains to seeking help or information (Grove & Bahnsen 1997; Udry 1997a; Quinn & Fallon 1999).

ADHERENCE TO SPORTS INJURY REHABILITATION

A behavioural response to sports injury that is of central focus to the rehabilitation of the injury is adherence to the recommended rehabilitation protocol, which can involve a number of different behaviours, including: (i) performing clinic-based activities, such as doing exercises designed to increase strength, flexibility and endurance; (ii) modifying physical activity, such as resting and limiting activity; (iii) taking medications; and (iv) completing home-based activities, such as cryotherapy and home rehabilitation exercises

(Brewer 1998, 1999a). This wide range of behaviours requires a correspondingly wide range of assessment techniques for measuring adherence. The most frequently used methods of assessing adherence are documenting patient attendance at clinic-based rehabilitation sessions, recording practitioner ratings of adherence during rehabilitation sessions, and obtaining patient self-reports of home exercise completion (Brewer 1999a). Complicating this diversity of adherence measures is a lack of consistent operationalization of adherence behaviour, with some research reporting a percentage of adherent versus non-adherent individuals, and other research comparing actual adherence behaviour to that recommended by the practitioner.

Recognizing this diversity of adherence measures and conflicting operationalization of the adherence construct, estimates of adherence to sports injury rehabilitation have ranged from 40 to 91% (Brewer 1998, 1999a). Adherence rates tend to be higher for continuous measures of adherence, such as attendance at rehabilitation sessions (e.g. Almekinders & Almekinders 1994; Daly et al. 1995; Laubach et al. 1996) or amount of time spent on home rehabilitation activities (Penpraze & Mutrie 1999), than for more discrete measures of adherence that categorize individuals based on their level of adherence (e.g. Taylor & May 1996). Consistent with a cognitive appraisal approach and the integrated model (Wiese-Bjornstal et al. 1998), researchers have postulated that adherence rates are related to personal and situational factors, as well as cognitive and emotional responses. However, as with emotional responses to sports injury, there is little direct support for the hypothesized mediational role of cognitive appraisals in the relations between personal and situational factors and adherence to sports injury rehabilitation. But researchers have identified many personal, situational and cognitive factors that are associated with sports injury rehabilitation adherence.

Personal factors that have been identified as having a positive relationship with sports injury rehabilitation adherence include: (i) an internal health locus of control (Murphy et al. 1999; Brewer et al. 2000b), which refers to the extent to which a person believes that health outcomes are under their own control; (ii) pain tolerance (Fisher et al. 1988; Byerly et al. 1994; Fields et al. 1995); (iii) self-motivation (Noyes et al. 1983; Fisher et al. 1988; Duda et al. 1989; Brewer et al. 1994a; Fields et al. 1995; Culpepper et al. 1996; Brewer et al. 2000c); (iv) task involvement (Duda et al. 1989), which is the degree to which a person is motivated to improve against their own personal standards; and (v) tough mindedness (Wittig & Schurr 1994). Personal factors that have been shown to be negatively associated with adherence to sports injury rehabilitation are: (i) a chance health locus of control (Brewer et al. 2000b), which refers to the extent to which a person believes that health outcomes are influenced by chance or luck; (ii) ego involvement (Duda et al. 1989), which is the degree to which a person is motivated by comparisons with other individuals; and (iii) trait anxiety (Eichenhofer et al. 1986). Thus, in terms of dispositional characteristics, the athletes most likely to adhere to their rehabilitation programmes are those who are self-motivated, strong-willed and tolerant of discomfort.

As shown in Table 8.2, a diverse array of situational factors has been found to correlate with adherence to sports injury rehabilitation programmes. In general, higher levels of adherence have been associated with: (i) a supportive clinical environment; and (ii) a rehabilitation programme that is convenient, valued and perceived as efficacious.

The integrated model (Wiese-Bjornstal et al. 1998) predicts that, as with personal and situational factors, cognitive variables should be related to behaviours such as adherence to rehabilitation. Research has shown that individuals who have high adherence rates also report a high ability to cope with their injuries (Daly et al. 1995), have high rehabilitation self-efficacy (Taylor & May 1996), perceive little threat to their self-esteem (Lampton et al. 1993), attribute their recovery to stable and personally controllable factors (Laubach et al. 1996), set rehabilitation goals, use imagery and use positive self-talk (Scherzer et al. 1999).

Table 8.2 Situational factors associated with adherence to sports injury rehabilitation.

Variable	Direction	Reference
Academic class status	+	Culpepper *et al.* 1996; Shank 1988
Academic performance level	+	Shank 1988
Belief in the efficacy of the treatment	+	Duda *et al.* 1989; Noyes *et al.* 1983; Taylor & May 1996
Comfort of the clinical environment	+	Brewer *et al.* 1994a; Fields *et al.* 1995; Fisher *et al.* 1988
Convenience of rehabilitation scheduling	+	Fields *et al.* 1995; Fisher *et al.* 1988
Degree of career goal definition	+	Shank 1988
Importance or value of rehabilitation	+	Taylor & May 1996
Injury duration	+	Culpepper *et al.* 1996
Perceived academic load	+	Shank 1988
Perceived sports participation time	+	Shank 1988
Perceived time availability for rehabilitation	+	Shank 1988
Perceived exertion during rehabilitation	+	Brewer *et al.* 1994a; Fisher *et al.* 1988
Perceived susceptibility to further complications without rehabilitation	+	Taylor & May 1996
Postcollegiate sports participation plans	+	Shank 1988
Rehabilitation practitioner expectancy	+	Taylor & May 1995
Social support for rehabilitation	+	Byerly *et al.* 1994; Duda *et al.* 1989; Finnie 1999; Fisher *et al.* 1988

Direction refers to the positive (+) correlations with postinjury emotional disturbance.

Thus, athletes who are confident in their ability to meet the demands of rehabilitation, accept responsibility for their rehabilitation, and allocate mental effort to their rehabilitation tend to exhibit the highest levels of adherence.

One of the few cognitive processes that has received any experimental attention with regard to sports injury rehabilitation adherence is goal setting. Penpraze and Mutrie (1999) assigned athletes with injuries to either a group that was assigned specific rehabilitation goals or a group that received non-specific rehabilitation goals. Athletes in the specific goals group had a greater understanding of, and adherence to, their rehabilitation protocols than athletes in the non-specific goal group. These experimental findings extended earlier qualitative findings that task-orientated goal setting was related to a greater perception of rehabilitation adherence in athletes with injuries (Gilbourne & Taylor 1995, 1998; Gilbourne *et al.* 1996).

The integrated model also predicts that emotional responses and other behavioural responses will be associated with adherence to sports injury rehabilitation, although only a few studies have examined such relationships. Mood disturbance has been negatively related to adherence in three (Daly *et al.* 1995; Brickner 1997; Alzate *et al.* 1998), but a fourth study found no association between adherence levels and psychological disturbance (Brewer *et al.* 2000c). The only behavioural response that has been investigated in association with sports injury rehabilitation adherence has been the use of instrumental coping behaviours, which involve asking for additional information about the injury or the rehabilitation programme (Udry 1997a). Instrumental coping behaviours were positively related to adherence levels for individuals who were undergoing rehabilitation following reconstructive knee surgery designed to facilitate a return to sports participation.

Psychological factors and sports injury rehabilitation outcomes

In addition to psychological responses to sports injury reviewed in the preceding section, the psychological correlates of sports injury rehabilitation outcomes are also of vital interest. Both the integrated model (Wiese-Bjornstal *et al.* 1998) and the biopsychosocial model (Brewer *et al.* 2002) specify relationships between psychological variables and sports injury rehabilitation outcomes. These models predict that the same clusters of personal, situational, cognitive, emotional and behavioural variables associated with psychological responses to sports injury will also be related to sports injury rehabilitation outcomes. Research that has investigated relationships between psychological factors and sports injury rehabilitation outcomes is discussed in the next sections. For the purposes of this discussion, sports injury rehabilitation outcomes refer not only to the variables listed in the category of the same name in the biopsychosocial model shown in Fig. 8.2, but also to the variables listed in the biopsychosocial model (Brewer *et al.* 2002) as 'intermediate biopsychological outcomes', as these variables (e.g. endurance, joint laxity, pain, range of motion, recovery rate, strength) are often used as indices of rehabilitation outcome in research investigations.

PERSONAL FACTORS

Personal factors related to sports injury rehabilitation outcomes have been a topic of interest since Wise *et al.* (1979) discovered that two personality variables (i.e. hysteria and hypochondriasis) were inversely related to recovery following knee surgery. Subsequent studies have shown that being optimistic (LaMott 1994), male (Johnson 1996, 1997) and strongly identified with the athlete role (Brewer *et al.* 2000c) have all been positively related to rehabilitation outcomes following sports injuries. Research has not yet uncovered the mechanisms by which these personal factors may influence outcome, or what other of the myriad personal factors may be related to sports injury rehabilitation outcomes.

SITUATIONAL FACTORS

The situational factor that has received the most amount of research attention with respect to sports injury rehabilitation outcomes has been

social support, which refers to the quantity, quality and type of interactions that athletes have with other people (Udry 1996). Social support is considered to be multidimensional, with the structure proposed by Richman *et al.* (1993) the most widely used in sports injury rehabilitation research (Ford & Gordon 1993; Izzo 1994; LaMott 1994; Bianco & Orlick 1996; Quinn 1996; Ford 1998; Johnston & Carroll 1998b). The Richman structure categorizes social support as one of eight types: listening support, emotional support, emotional challenge, task appreciation, task challenge, reality confirmation, material assistance and personal assistance. These different types of social support may be provided by different members of an athlete's social network, including coaches, friends, relatives, team mates, sports administrators and medical personnel (Lewis & LaMott 1992; Izzo 1994; Bianco & Orlick 1996; Macchi & Crossman 1996; Peterson 1997; Udry 1997b; Udry *et al.* 1997b; Ford 1998; Johnston & Carroll 1998b; Bianco *et al.* 1999a; Udry & Singleton 1999). The needs for particular types of social support and the ability of an athlete's social support network to provide certain types of support may vary during the rehabilitation process (Ford 1998; LaMott 1994; Quinn 1996; Udry 1997a; Johnston & Carroll 1998b).

Given the complexity of social support networks and the changing social support needs of injured athletes over the course of rehabilitation, it is not surprising that research in this area has produced conflicting results. For example, social support has been positively related (Tuffey 1991), not related (Brewer *et al.* 2000c) and negatively related (Quinn & Fallon 2000) to rehabilitation outcome. These inconsistencies are probably due to the way in which social support has been differentially operationalized across different studies. The importance of considering different aspects of social support and their potential different relationships to rehabilitation outcome is highlighted in a study of skiers (Gould *et al.* 1997a). Skiers who experienced successful injury rehabilitation were less likely to perceive a lack of attention/empathy from others and less likely to encounter negative social relationship, yet

Table 8.3 Cognitive factors associated with sports injury rehabilitation outcomes.

Variable	Direction	Reference
Attentional focus on healing	+	Loundagin & Fisher 1993
Attribution of recovery to stable and controllable factors	+	Brewer *et al.* 2000a; Laubach *et al.* 1996
Cognitive appraisal of injury coping ability	+	Niedfeldt 1998
Cognitive appraisal of the injury situation	+	Johnson 1996, 1997
Denial	+/−	Quinn & Fallon 2000; Grove & Bahnsen 1997
Emotional focus/venting	−	Grove & Bahnsen 1997
Emotion-focused coping	+	Quinn 1996
Expected recovery rate	+	Laurence 1997
Management of thoughts and emotions	+	Gould *et al.* 1997b
Mental disengagement	-	Grove & Bahnsen 1997
Number of rehabilitation goals	+	Johnson 1996, 1997
Pain catastrophizing	+	Tripp 2000
Positive attitude toward rehabilitation	+	Johnson 1996, 1997
Positive reinterpretation	−	Grove & Bahnsen 1997
Recovery confidence	+	Niedfeldt 1998; Quinn & Fallon 2000
Rehabilitation self-efficacy	+	Shaffer 1992
Self-confidence	+	Johnson 1996, 1997
Use of goal setting	+	Gould *et al.* 1997b; Ievleva & Orlick 1991; Loundagin & Fisher 1993
Use of healing/recovery imagery	+	Ievleva & Orlick 1991; Loundagin & Fisher 1993
Use of imagery/visualization	+	Gould *et al.* 1997b

Direction refers to the positive (+) and negative (−) correlations with sports injury rehabilitation outcomes.

were *more* likely to indicate feeling socially isolated than skiers who experienced unsuccessful injury rehabilitation. Thus, when examining the relationships between rehabilitation outcome and social support, it is imperative that that the specific type of social support is considered. Further research is needed to better understand the roles of the different types of social support in the injury rehabilitation process.

COGNITIVE FACTORS

As indicated in Table 8.3, research has identified many cognitive factors that are associated with sports injury rehabilitation outcomes. Overall, the research in this area suggests that positive cognitions and the use of psychological skills will enhance the rehabilitation process. Some of the findings, however, such as those for denial and emotion-focused coping/emotional focus (Quinn 1996; Grove & Bahnsen 1997; Quinn & Fallon

2000), are equivocal. These inconsistencies, along with the retrospective and correlational nature of the majority of studies on cognitive factors associated with sports injury rehabilitation outcomes, indicate that more research (especially prospective and experimental research) is needed in this area to better understand the role of cognition in influencing rehabilitation outcomes.

EMOTIONAL FACTORS

Only a few studies have examined relationships between emotional variables and sport rehabilitation outcomes. Positive relationships to have been found between rehabilitation outcomes and general well-being (Johnson 1996, 1997) and vigour (Quinn 1996), whereas negative associations have been documented for anger (LaMott 1994; Alzate *et al.* 1998), anxiety (Johnson 1996, 1997), fear, frustration, relief (LaMott 1994), mood disturbance, depression (Alzate *et al.* 1998; Tripp

2000), fatigue, tension (Alzate *et al.* 1998) and psychological distress (Brewer *et al.* 2000c). Although all of the findings regarding the relationship between emotions and sports injury rehabilitation outcomes are purely correlational in nature, most of the studies cited (i.e. Johnson 1996, 1997; Alzate *et al.* 1998; Brewer *et al.* 2000c; Quinn & Fallon 2000) were prospective in that emotions were measured at one point in time (e.g. prior to surgery, at the beginning of rehabilitation) and sports injury rehabilitation outcomes were measured at a later point in time (e.g. at the end of rehabilitation). Consequently, there is evidence that for reasons not currently understood, positive emotions may often precede favourable rehabilitation outcomes.

BEHAVIOURAL FACTORS

The behavioural factor examined most frequently in reference to sports injury rehabilitation outcomes has been adherence to rehabilitation. One would assume that greater adherence to rehabilitation would be associated with better outcome, but this has not always been the case. The relationship between adherence to rehabilitation and rehabilitation outcome has been found to be positive (Meani *et al.* 1986; Derscheid & Feiring 1987; Hawkins 1989; Satterfield *et al.* 1990; Tuffey

1991; Treacy *et al.* 1997; Alzate *et al.* 1998; Brewer *et al.* 2000c; Quinn & Fallon 2000), non-significant (Noyes *et al.* 1983; Brewer *et al.* 2000c; Quinn & Fallon 2000) and, surprisingly, negative (Shelbourne & Wilckens 1990; Quinn & Fallon 2000). These discrepant findings are probably due to a variety of factors, including the nature of the injury studied, the specifics of the rehabilitation protocol, the phase of rehabilitation that was the focus of study, and the particular measures of adherence and outcome (Brewer 1999a).

Only a few behaviours other than adherence to rehabilitation have received any empirical investigation. Better sports injury rehabilitation outcomes have been found to be associated with higher levels of active coping (Quinn & Fallon 1999), lower levels of physical activity (Gould *et al.* 1997b) and higher levels of seeking social support (Johnson 1996, 1997; Gould *et al.* 1997b).

PSYCHOLOGICAL INTERVENTIONS TO ENHANCE REHABILITATION OUTCOMES

Support for the influence of a wide variety of psychological factors on sports injury rehabilitation outcomes can be inferred from the results of experimental studies in which psychological interventions have been applied to athletes with injuries. As shown in Table 8.4, a number of

Table 8.4 Controlled studies examining the effects of psychological interventions on physical and psychological rehabilitation outcomes.

Reference	Intervention	Effect(s) of intervention
Krebs 1981	Biofeedback	Greater strength and EMG output
Draper 1990	Biofeedback	Greater strength and ROM
Draper & Ballard 1991	Biofeedback	Greater strength
Levitt *et al.* 1995	Biofeedback	Greater extensor torque and quadriceps fibre recruitment
Theodorakis *et al.* 1996	Goal setting	Greater strength
Theodorakis *et al.* 1997b	Goal setting	Greater strength and self-efficacy
Ross & Berger 1996	Stress inoculation training	Greater physical functioning, less pain, less reinjury anxiety
Theodorakis *et al.* 1997b	Self-talk	Greater strength
Johnson 2000	Multimodal	Greater positive mood and readiness for competition
Cupal & Brewer 2001	Relaxation/guided imagery	Greater strength, less pain, less reinjury anxiety

interventions have been investigated experimentally for their effects on physical and psychological rehabilitation outcomes, including biofeedback (Krebs 1981; Draper 1990; Draper & Ballard 1991; Levitt *et al.* 1995), goal setting (Theodorakis *et al.* 1996, 1997b), imagery/relaxation (Cupal & Brewer 2001), self-talk (Theodorakis *et al.* 1997a), stress inoculation training (Ross & Berger 1996) and a multimodal intervention consisting of goal setting, imagery, relaxation and stress management (Johnson 2000). Case study data have also supported the efficacy of interventions such as counselling, goal setting, hypnosis, positive self-talk, relaxation and systematic desensitization for positively effecting rehabilitation outcome variables such as confidence, motivation, perception of pain, physical recovery, psychological adjustment, reinjury anxiety and range of motion (Rotella & Campbell 1983; Nicol 1993; Sthalekar 1993; Potter 1995; Brewer & Helledy 1998; Hartman & Finch 1999; Evans *et al.* 2000; Jevon & O'Donovan 2000).

Without exception, the psychological interventions that have been documented in the scientific literature as having been used successfully in sports injury rehabilitation are cognitive–behavioural in nature and involve athletes learning new skills or behaviours to cope more effectively with the rehabilitation process, both physically and psychologically. Biofeedback, for example, involves furnishing patients with physiological information (e.g. electromyographic activity in the quadriceps muscle group) and is thought to produce therapeutic gains by enhancing motivation for rehabilitation activities and enhancing proprioceptive information processing (Levitt *et al.* 1995). Similarly, goal setting, which involves generating (short- and long-term) personal standards of achievement in rehabilitation activities, is posited to provide direction to the athlete's rehabilitation efforts, enhance persistence in rehabilitation and facilitate the development of new rehabilitation strategies (Locke & Latham 1990). Although they are conceptually distinct interventions, relaxation and imagery are often used in conjunction to treat athletes with injuries. Relaxation protocols, which are typically aimed at calming the muscles and the mind, are frequently implemented just prior to the use of imagery procedures, which generally feature mental rehearsal of motivational, healing and performance aspects of rehabilitation. Combining relaxation and imagery techniques is thought to affect rehabilitation outcomes by enhancing rehabilitation motivation and boosting physiological processes such as tissue regeneration/repair and immune/inflammatory responses (Cupal & Brewer 2001). Self-talk (or cognitive restructuring) interventions are designed to alter athletes' thoughts and, ultimately, feelings and behaviours, regarding their rehabilitation.

Because research on psychological interventions in sports injury rehabilitation has focused primarily on documenting the effectiveness of such interventions, the processes by which these interventions exert their effect are not well understood. Referring to the biopsychosocial model, it is postulated that psychological interventions may affect rehabilitation outcome through a variety of mechanisms, including a direct effect, indirect effects through intermediate biopsychological outcomes, and indirect effects through relationships with biological factors and social/contextual factors. The complexities of these possible relationships have yet to be adequately explored by researchers, but it is likely that psychological interventions affect outcomes through a variety of pathways.

Implications for clinical practice

The percentage of athletes who experience difficulties adjusting emotionally or behaviourally to injury furnishes evidence of the need to consider psychological factors in planning, implementing and evaluating sports injury rehabilitation protocols. Further rationale for incorporating psychological aspects into the treatment of sports injuries is provided by the abundance of psychological factors associated with sports injury rehabilitation outcomes and the demonstrated efficacy of psychological interventions in producing desirable sports injury rehabilitation outcomes. Although the value of taking psychological factors into account in sports injury rehabilitation is recognized, the ways in which psychology should be included in the rehabilitation process and by whom is less clearly delineated. Potential opportunities for clinical application of the research on psychological factors in sports injury rehabilitation exist for both sports injury rehabilitation practitioners and sport psychology professionals.

SPORTS INJURY REHABILITATION PRACTITIONERS

A variety of medical professionals provide clinical services to athletes with injuries, including physicians, physiotherapists and athletic trainers. Depending on the frequency of their contact with athletes during the injury rehabilitation process, sports injury rehabilitation practitioners can be in a strategic position to enhance the adjustment of athletes to injury and promote adherence to the treatment protocol. Indeed, sports injury rehabilitation practitioners, in constituting an important situational factor in the integrated model (Wiese-Bjornstal *et al.* 1998) and social/contextual variable in the biopsychosocial model (Brewer *et al.* 2002), have the potential to affect the psychological state of their patients regardless of their intent to do so.

Surveys of sports injury rehabilitation practitioners (e.g. Brewer *et al.* 1991; Gordon *et al.* 1991; Ford & Gordon 1993, 1997; Larson *et al.* 1996; Ninedek & Kolt 2000) have indicated a general awareness of, and interest in, psychological aspects of rehabilitation. Despite this interest and awareness, sports injury practitioners may not feel comfortable or qualified to make judgements or initiate interventions of a psychological nature. Research has indicated that sports injury rehabilitation practitioners may have difficulty recognizing psychological distress among their patients (Brewer *et al.* 1995b; Maniar *et al.* 1999). With appropriate training (Ford & Gordon 1998; Gordon *et al.* 1998), however, rehabilitation professionals can increase their knowledge, skills

and comfort in identifying the warning signs of athletes who are experiencing problems in adjusting psychologically to their injuries.

In some cases, such as when high levels of depression or anxiety are detected, referral to a mental health practitioner is warranted (Brewer *et al.* 1999b). In most circumstances, though, sports injury rehabilitation practitioners can facilitate a smooth navigation of the rehabilitation process by educating athletes about their injuries and likely challenges to be encountered during rehabilitation and, when appropriate, applying a simple psychological intervention such as goal setting (Gilbourne & Taylor 1995, 1998; Gilbourne *et al.* 1996; Theodorakis *et al.* 1996, 1997b; Penpraze & Mutrie 1999) to motivate and focus the rehabilitation efforts of athletes. The importance of patient education and clear patient–practitioner communication is underscored by research demonstrating that athletes with injuries often misperceive their interactions with rehabilitation practitioners (Kahanov & Fairchild 1994) and misunderstand at least some portion of their prescribed rehabilitation regime (Webborn *et al.* 1997).

SPORT PSYCHOLOGY PROFESSIONALS

Despite the growing body of literature documenting the role of psychological factors in influencing sports injury rehabilitation processes and outcomes, only rarely are sport psychology professionals fully fledged members of the sports medicine treatment team (Cerny *et al.* 1992; Larson *et al.* 1996). The low level of involvement of sport psychology professionals in the rehabilitation of athletes with injuries may be due, in part, to: (i) the structure and restrictions of the health care systems in which athletes receive rehabilitation for their injuries; (ii) the lack of standard procedures for rehabilitation practitioners to refer athletes with injuries for counselling or psychotherapy (Larson *et al.* 1996); and (iii) the reluctance of athletes with injuries to participate in 'extra' therapeutic activity beyond their physical rehabilitation even if they find the interventions sufficiently credible (Brewer *et al.* 1994b).

In circumstances where a sport psychology professional is not involved in the day-to-day assessment of athletes with injuries and in the initiation of psychological interventions such as imagery and relaxation, as seems to be the norm, sports injury rehabilitation practitioners are encouraged to identify sport psychology professionals to serve as consultants, referral targets and resources on psychological aspects of rehabilitation. Some sport psychology professionals have clinical training and can work with athletes who show signs of mental disorders or severe adjustment reactions. Unfortunately, when sport psychology professionals are not integral members of the sports medicine treatment team, they are more likely to be contacted regarding difficult patients than regarding routine ways that psychology can be applied to enhance the rehabilitation of athletes with injuries. Further research documenting the role of psychological factors and the efficacy of psychological interventions in sports injury rehabilitation is needed to advance the standing of sport psychology professionals in the enterprise of sports injury rehabilitation.

Future research directions

The proliferation of, and progress in, research concerning psychological correlates of sports injury rehabilitation parameters since the recommendations made by Williams and Roepke (1993) and Brewer (1994) has been heartening. However, this body of research has only scratched the surface of the potential questions still in need of answers. The two models used as a framework for the review of literature in this chapter, the integrated model (Wiese-Bjornstal et al. 1998) and the biopsychosocial model (Brewer et al. 2002), have provided not only a structure for examining the literature to date, but offer many suggestions for future research. As demonstrated by the research reviewed in this chapter, many of the postulated direct pathways of both models have been supported, but many have yet to be examined. In particular, although both models predict that psychological factors

will influence emotions, behaviour, cognitions and, ultimately, rehabilitation outcome, most studies have focused on highly specific psychological factors and only one of these types of variables. This has led to a hodgepotch of direct relationships, with little comparability of the psychological factors studied across the different outcome measures. Both models also propose that many psychological factors are related to injury and injury rehabilitation processes as mediating variables, and these mediating relationships have yet to be sufficiently investigated. To examine these relationships, studies will have to become more integrated, including measures of the multiple constructs of both the integrated model and the biopsychosocial model. It must also be recognized that the rehabilitation process is a dynamic one, and more frequent assessments of the psychological factors (as in time series analysis) and intraindividual analyses are needed to examine the fluid and diverse nature of the constructs involved (Evans & Hardy 1999).

One area of research vital to ensure progress in this area of enquiry is the development and standardization of adequate measures of the specific constructs involved. Diversity in measurement methods and inconsistent operationalization of constructs has led to difficulty in making comparisons across studies. Increased standardization of instruments and definitions of the constructs are likely to lead to a more consistent and unified body of research (Evans & Hardy 1999). However, the development of adequate instruments is a difficult and time-consuming endeavour, and research on psychological aspects of sports injury rehabilitation has suffered from instruments that have not demonstrated good psychometric properties (Brewer et al. 1999a; Slattery 1999). Only with adequately designed and validated measures can the various constructs involved in the psychological aspects of sports injury be effectively examined.

A further area of enquiry on which future research should focus is the specific processes and effectiveness of psychological interventions in sports injury rehabilitation. Although a variety of interventions have been found to be related to better sports injury rehabilitation outcomes (Cupal 1998), the specifics of the mechanisms through which these interventions operate are not well understood. Only by clearly understanding *how* these interventions work can the interventions be tailored effectively to the multiplicity of personal variables, situational variables and psychological variables implicated in the sports injury rehabilitation process.

It will also be important to examine ways in which psychological interventions interact with medical interventions (e.g. immobilization, medications, physical therapy, surgery, therapeutic exercise) to influence emotional and behavioural functioning during injury rehabilitation. Given that, from a biopsychosocial perspective (Brewer *et al.* 2002), medical interventions may directly affect both biological factors and intermediate biopsychosocial outcomes, it would not be surprising if certain psychological interventions were found to be especially effective for some injuries and in conjunction with particular medical treatments. For example, a psychological intervention designed to enhance motivation might be more appropriate for injury rehabilitation protocols that have heavy behavioural demands (e.g. extensive rehabilitation exercises) than for those with more passive features (e.g. activity restriction, immobilization). Unquestionably, the agenda for further research on psychological interventions in sports injury rehabilitation should include randomized controlled clinical trials comparing frequently advocated psychological interventions (e.g. cognitive restructuring, counselling, goal setting, imagery, relaxation) separately and in combination. Such research can help provide practitioners with more detailed information on what interventions, administered in which ways and by whom at which frequencies, are likely to be most effective for which athletes under what circumstances.

A paradoxical direction for future research is to explore the potential *benefits* of sports injury (Udry 1999). Some recent qualitative studies have documented that some athletes with injuries have reported experiencing higher levels of life satisfaction, performance enhancement, personal growth, psychosocial development and academic performance as a result of their injuries (Rose & Jevne 1993; Udry *et al.* 1997a; Ford 1998; Niedfeldt 1998; Ford & Gordon 1999). However, again, the specific personal, situational and psychological variables that are related to these benefits have not been identified, and further studies, both qualitative and quantitative, are needed to expand our knowledge of this fascinating counter-intuitive line of research.

From a theoretical standpoint, explanatory models for psychological aspects of sports injury are in their infancy. The integrated model (Wiese-Bjornstal *et al.* 1998) and the biopychosocial model (Brewer *et al.* 2002) described in this chapter have been proposed only recently, and although supported by a growing body of research, there are still many predictions derived from these models that have not yet received empirical support. Further data gathered within the contexts of these models will probably inspire modification to the models as they currently exist. Additionally, there is evidence indicating that psychological factors are related to the *occurrence* of injury (Meeuwisse & Fowler 1988; Williams & Andersen 1998) and these relationships could be incorporated into a model that could cover the entire spectrum of the injury process, from biopsychosocial factors related to the likelihood of experiencing an injury to the implications of these factors for the outcome of sports injury rehabilitation.

Conclusions

The proliferation of research investigating the psychological factors related to sports injury rehabilitation has demonstrated the importance of these factors to rehabilitation outcome. Descriptive, correlational, experimental, quantitative and qualitative research has shown that a variety of behavioural, cognitive, emotional and situational factors are involved in the sports injury rehabilitation process. Only through an adequate understanding of these factors and their interrelationships can well-designed interventions be proposed to enhance the rehabilitation process and, potentially, speed up or improve the outcome of sports injury rehabilitation.

Author note

Preparation of this chapter was supported in part by grant number R29 AR44484 from the National Institute of Arthritis and Musculoskeletal and Skin Diseases. Its contents are solely the responsibility of the authors and do not represent the official views of the National Institute of Arthritis and Musculoskeletal and Skin Diseases.

References

Almekinders, L.C. & Almekinders, S.V. (1994) Outcome in the treatment of chronic overuse sports injuries: a retrospective study. *Journal of Orthopaedic and Sports Physical Therapy* **19**, 157–161.

Alzate, R., Ramirez, A. & Lazaro, I. (1998) Psychological aspect of athletic injury. Paper presented at the 24th International Congress of Applied Psychology, San Francisco, CA.

Astle, S.J. (1986) The experience of loss in athletes. *Journal of Sports Medicine and Physical Fitness* **26**, 279–284.

Bianco, T.M. & Orlick, T. (1996) Social support influences on recovery from sports injury [Abstract]. *Journal of Applied Sport Psychology* **8** (Suppl.), S57.

Bianco, T., Eklund, R.C. & Gordon, S. (1999a) Coach support of injured athletes: coaches and athletes share their views. Paper presented at the annual meeting of the Association for the Advancement of Applied Sport Psychology, Banff, Alberta, Canada.

Bianco, T., Malo, S. & Orlick, T. (1999b) Sports injury and illness: elite skiers describe their experiences. *Research Quarterly for Exercise and Sport* **70**, 157–169.

Brewer, B.W. (1991) Causal attributions and adjustment to athletic injury. Paper presented at the annual meeting of the North American Society for the Psychology of Sport and Physical Activity, Pacific Grove, CA.

Brewer, B.W. (1993) Self-identity and specific vulnerability to depressed mood. *Journal of Personality* **61**, 343–364.

Brewer, B.W. (1994) Review and critique of models of psychological adjustment to athletic injury. *Journal of Applied Sport Psychology* **6**, 87–100.

Brewer, B.W. (1998) Adherence to sports injury rehabilitation programs. *Journal of Applied Sport Psychology* **10**, 70–82.

Brewer, B.W. (1999a) Adherence to sports injury rehabilitation regimens. In: *Adherence Issues in Sport and Exercise* (Bull, S.J., ed.). Wiley, Chichester: 145–168.

Brewer, B.W. (1999b) Causal attribution dimensions and adjustment to sports injury. *Journal of Personal and Interpersonal Loss* **4**, 215–224.

Brewer, B.W. & Helledy, K.I. (1998) Off (to) the deep end: psychological skills training and water running. *Applied Research in Coaching and Athletics Annual* **13**, 99–118.

Brewer, B.W. & Petrie, T.A. (1995) A comparison between injured and uninjured football players on selected psychosocial variables. *Academic Athletic Journal* **10**, 11–18.

Brewer, B.W., Van Raalte, J.L. & Linder, D.E. (1991) Role of the sport psychologist in treating injured athletes: a survey of sports medicine providers. *Journal of Applied Sport Psychology* **3**, 183–190.

Brewer, B.W., Daly, J.M., Van Raalte, J.L., Petitpas, A.J. & Sklar, J.H. (1994a) A psychometric evaluation of the Rehabilitation Adherence Questionnaire [Abstract]. *Journal of Sport and Exercise Psychology* **16** (Suppl.), S34.

Brewer, B.W., Jeffers, K.E., Petitpas, A.J. & Van Raalte, J.L. (1994b) Perceptions of psychological interventions in the context of sports injury rehabilitation. *Sport Psychologist* **8**, 176–188.

Brewer, B.W., Linder, D.E. & Phelps, C.M. (1995a) Situational correlates of emotional adjustment to athletic injury. *Clinical Journal of Sport Medicine* **5**, 241–245.

Brewer, B.W., Petitpas, A.J., Van Raalte, J.L., Sklar, J.H. & Ditmar, T.D. (1995b) Prevalence of psychological distress among patients at a physical therapy clinic specializing in sports medicine. *Sports Medicine, Training and Rehabilitation* **6**, 138–145.

Brewer, B.W., Daly, J.M., Van Raalte, J.L., Petitpas, A.J. & Sklar, J.H. (1999a) A psychometric evaluation of the Rehabilitation Adherence Questionnaire. *Journal of Sport and Exercise Psychology* **21**, 167–173.

Brewer, B.W., Petitpas, A.J. & Van Raalte, J.L. (1999b) Referral of injured athletes for counseling and psychotherapy. In: *Counseling in Sports Medicine* (Ray, R. & Wiese-Bjornstal, D.M., eds). Human Kinetics, Champaign, IL: 127–141.

Brewer, B.W., Cornelius, A.E., Van Raalte, J.L. *et al.* (2000a) Attributions for recovery and adherence to rehabilitiation following anterior cruciate ligament reconstruction: a prospective analysis. *Psychology and Health* **15**, 283–291.

Brewer, B.W., Cornelius, A.E., Van Raalte, J.L. *et al.* (2000b) Health locus of control and adherence to rehabilitation following anterior cruciate ligament (ACL) reconstruction. Paper presented at the Annual Meeting of the Association for the Advancement of Applied Sport Psychology, Nashville, TN.

Brewer, B.W., Van Raalte, J.L., Cornelius, A.E. *et al.* (2000c) Psychological factors, rehabilitation adherence, and rehabilitation outcome after anterior cruciate ligament reconstruction. *Rehabilitation Psychology* **45**, 20–37.

Brewer, B.W., Andersen, M.B. & Van Raalte, J.L. (2002) Psychological aspects of sports injury rehabilitation: toward a biopsychosocial approach. In: *Medical Aspects of Sport and Exercise* (Mostofsky, D.I. & Zaichkowsky, L.D., eds). Fitness Information Technology, Morgantown, WV: 41–54.

Brickner, J.C. (1997) *Mood states and compliance of patients with orthopedic rehabilitation*. Master's thesis, Springfield College, MA.

Byerly, P.N., Worrell, T., Gahimer, J. & Domholdt, E. (1994) Rehabilitation compliance in an athletic training environment. *Journal of Athletic Training* **29**, 352–355.

Carver, C.S., Scheier, M.F. & Weintraub, J.K. (1989) Assessing coping strategies: a theoretically based approach. *Journal of Personality and Social Psychology* **56**, 267–283.

Cerny, F.J., Patton, D.C., Whieldon, T.J. & Roehrig, S. (1992) An organizational model of sports medicine facilities in the United States. *Journal of Orthopaedic and Sports Physical Therapy* **15**, 80–86.

Chan, C.S. & Grossman, H.Y. (1988) Psychological effects of running loss on consistent runners. *Perceptual and Motor Skills* **66**, 875–883.

Cohen, S. & Rodriguez, M.S. (1995) Pathways linking affective disturbance and physical disorders. *Health Psychology* **14**, 374–380.

Crossman, J. & Jamieson, J. (1985) Differences in perceptions of seriousness and disrupting effects of athletic injury as viewed by athletes and their trainer. *Perceptual and Motor Skills* **61**, 1131–1134.

Crossman, J., Gluck, L. & Jamieson, J. (1995) The emotional responses of injured athletes. *New Zealand Journal of Sports Medicine* **23**, 1–2.

Culpepper, W.L., Masters, K.S. & Wittig, A.F. (1996) Factors influencing injured athletes' adherence to rehabilitation. Paper presented at the Annual Meeting of the American Psychological Association, Toronto, Canada.

Cupal, D.D. (1998) Psychological interventions in sports injury prevention and rehabilitation. *Journal of Applied Sport Psychology* **10**, 103–123.

Cupal, D.D. & Brewer, B.W. (2001) Effects of relaxation and guided imagery on knee strength, reinjury anxiety, and pain following anterior cruciate ligament reconstruction. *Rehabilitation Psychology* **46**, 28–43.

Daly, J.M., Brewer, B.W., Van Raalte, J.L., Petitpas, A.J. & Sklar, J.H. (1995) Cognitive appraisal, emotional adjustment, and adherence to rehabilitation following knee surgery. *Journal of Sport Rehabilitation* **4**, 23–30.

Dawes, H. & Roach, N.K. (1997) Emotional responses of athletes to injury and treatment. *Physiotherapy* **83**, 243–247.

Derscheid, G.L. & Feiring, D.C. (1987) A statistical analysis to characterize treatment adherence of the 18 most common diagnoses seen at a sports medicine clinic. *Journal of Orthopaedic and Sports Physical Therapy* **9**, 40–46.

Draper, V. (1990) Electromyographic biofeedback and recovery of quadriceps femoris muscle function following anterior cruciate ligament reconstruction. *Physical Therapy* **70**, 11–17.

Draper, V. & Ballard, L. (1991) Electrical stimulation versus electromyographic biofeedback in the recovery of quadriceps femoris muscle function following anterior cruciate ligament surgery. *Physical Therapy* **71**, 455–464.

Dubbels, T.K., Klein, J.M., Ihle, K. & Wittrock, D.A. (1992) The psychological effects of injury on college athletes. Paper presented at the 7th Annual Red River Psychology Conference, Fargo, ND.

Duda, J.L., Smart, A.E. & Tappe, M.K. (1989) Predictors of adherence in rehabilitation of athletic injuries: an application of personal investment theory. *Journal of Sport and Exercise Psychology* **11**, 367–381.

Durso-Cupal, D.D. (1996) *The efficacy of guided imagery on recovery for individuals with anterior cruciate ligament (ACL) replacement*. Doctoral dissertation, Utah State University.

Eichenhofer, R.B., Wittig, A.F., Balogh, D.W. & Pisano, M.D. (1986) Personality indicants of adherence to rehabilitation treatment by injured athletes. Paper presented at the Annual Meeting of the Midwestern Psychological Association, Chicago.

Evans, L. & Hardy, L. (1995) Sports injury and grief responses: a review. *Journal of Sport and Exercise Psychology* **17**, 227–245.

Evans, L. & Hardy, L. (1999) Psychological and emotional response to athletic injury: measurement issues. In: *Psychological Bases of Sports Injuries*, 2nd edn (Pargman, D., ed.). Fitness Information Technology, Morgantown: 49–64.

Evans, L., Hardy, L. & Fleming, S. (2000) Intervention strategies with injured athletes: an action research study. *Sport Psychologist* **14**, 188–206.

Fields, J., Murphey, M., Horodyski, M. & Stopka, C. (1995) Factors associated with adherence to sports injury rehabilitation in college-age recreational athletes. *Journal of Sport Rehabilitation* **4**, 172–180.

Finnie, S.B. (1999) The rehabilitation support team: using social support to aid compliance to sports injury rehabilitation programs. Paper presented at the Annual Meeting of the Association for the Advancement of Applied Sport Psychology, Banff, Alberta, Canada.

Fisher, A.C., Domm, M.A. & Wuest, D.A. (1988) Adherence to sports-injury rehabilitation programs. *Physician and Sportsmedicine* **16** (7), 47–52.

Fisk, L.M. & King, L.A. (1998) Predictors of loss of identity among injured athletes. Paper presented at the Annual Meeting of the American Psychological Association, San Francisco, CA.

Flint, F.A. (1998) Integrating sport psychology and sports medicine in research: the dilemmas. *Journal of Applied Sport Psychology* **10**, 83–102.

Ford, I.W. (1998) *Psychosocial processes in sports injury occurrence and rehabilitation.* Doctoral thesis, University of Western Australia, Nedlands.

Ford, I.W. & Gordon, S. (1993) Social support and athletic injury: the perspective of sport physiotherapists. *Australian Journal of Science and Medicine in Sport* **25**, 17–25.

Ford, I.W. & Gordon, S. (1997) Perspectives of sport physiotherapists on the frequency and significance of psychological factors in professional practice: implications for curriculum design in professional training. *Australian Journal of Science and Medicine in Sport* **29**, 34–40.

Ford, I.W. & Gordon, S. (1998) Perspectives of sport trainers and athletic therapists on the psychological content of their practice and training. *Journal of Sport Rehabilitation* **7**, 79–94.

Ford, I.W. & Gordon, S. (1999) Coping with sports injury: resource loss and the role of social support. *Journal of Personal and Interpersonal Loss* **4**, 243–256.

Gilbourne, D. & Taylor, A.H. (1995) Rehabilitation experiences of injured athletes and their perceptions of a task-oriented goal-setting program: the application of an action research design. *Journal of Sports Sciences* **13**, 54–55.

Gilbourne, D. & Taylor, A.H. (1998) From theory to practice: the integration of goal perspective theory and life development approaches within an injury-specific goal-setting program. *Journal of Applied Sport Psychology* **10**, 124–139.

Gilbourne, D., Taylor, A.H., Downie, G. & Newton, P. (1996) Goal-setting during sports injury rehabilitation: a presentation of underlying theory, administration procedure, and an athlete case study. *Sports Exercise and Injury* **2**, 192–201.

Gordin, R., Albert, N.J., McShane, D. & Dobson, W. (1988) The emotional effects of injury on female collegiate gymnasts. Paper presented at the Seoul Olympic Scientific Congress, Seoul, South Korea.

Gordon, S. (1986) Sport psychology and the injured athlete: a cognitive–behavioral approach to injury response and injury rehabilitation. *Science Periodical on Research and Technology in Sport* **BU-1**, 1–10.

Gordon, S. & Lindgren, S. (1990) Psycho-physical rehabilitation from a serious sports injury: case study of an elite fast bowler. *Australian Journal of Science and Medicine in Sport* **22**, 71–76.

Gordon, S., Milios, D. & Grove, J.R. (1991) Psychological aspects of the recovery process from sports injury: the perspective of sport physiotherapists. *Australian Journal of Science and Medicine in Sport* **23**, 53–60.

Gordon, S., Potter, M. & Ford, I. (1998) Toward a psychoeducational curriculum for training sport-injury rehabilitation personnel. *Journal of Applied Sport Psychology* **10**, 140–156.

Gould, D., Udry, E., Bridges, D. & Beck, L. (1997a) Stress sources encountered when rehabilitating from season-ending ski injuries. *Sport Psychologist* **11**, 361–378.

Gould, D., Udry, E., Bridges, D. & Beck, L. (1997b) Coping with season-ending injuries. *Sport Psychologist* **11**, 379–399.

Green, S.L. & Weinberg, R.S. (1998) The relationship between athletic identity, coping skills, social support, and the psychological impact of injury [Abstract]. *Journal of Applied Sport Psychology* **10** (Suppl.), S127.

Grove, J.R. (1993) Personality and injury rehabilitation among sport performers. In: *Psychological Bases of Sports Injuries* (Pargman, D., ed.). Fitness Information Technology, Morgantown: 99–120.

Grove, J.R. & Bahnsen, A. (1997) *Personality, injury severity, and coping with rehabilitation.* Unpublished manuscript, University of Western Australia, Nedlands.

Grove, J.R., Stewart, R.M.L. & Gordon, S. (1990) Emotional reactions of athletes to knee rehabilitation. Paper presented at the Annual Meeting of the Australian Sports Medicine Federation, Alice Springs, Australia.

Hartman, A. & Finch, L. (1999) A case study to examine the use of goal setting in facilitating social support for injured athletes rehabilitating from injury. Paper presented at the Annual Meeting of the Association for the Advancement of Applied Sport Psychology, Banff, Alberta, Canada.

Hawkins, R.B. (1989) Arthroscopic stapling repair for shoulder instability: a retrospective study of 50 cases. *Arthroscopy: Journal of Arthroscopic and Related Surgery* **2**, 122–128.

Heil, J. (1993) Sport psychology, the athlete at risk, and the sports medicine team. In: *Psychology of Sports Injury* (Heil, J., ed.). Human Kinetics, Champaign, IL: 1–13.

Heniff, C.B., Wiese-Bjornstal, D.M., Henert, S.E., Schwenz, S., Shaffer, S.M. & Gardetto, D. (1999) A comparison between injured and uninjured NCAA division I female athletes on life event stress, weekly hassles and uplifts, and mood state. Paper presented at the Annual Meeting of the Association for the Advancement of Applied Sport Psychology, Banff, Alberta, Canada.

Ievleva, L. & Orlick, T. (1991) Mental links to enhanced healing: an exploratory study. *Sport Psychologist* **5**, 25–40.

Izzo, C.M. (1994) *The relationship between social support and adherence to sports injury rehabilitation.* Master's thesis, Springfield College, MA.

Jevon, S.M. & O'Donovan, S.M. (2000) Psychological support delivery through the primary care provider in a sports medicine clinic: a case study of a British Championship motorcycle racer. *Physical Therapy in Sport* **1**, 85–90.

Johnson, U. (1996) Quality of experience of long-term injury in athletic sports predicts return after rehabilitation. In: *Aktuell Beteendevetenskaplig Idrottsforskning* (Patriksson, G., ed.). SVEBI, Lund: 110–117.

Johnson, U. (1997) A three-year follow-up of long-term injured competitive athletes: influence of psychological risk factors on rehabilitation. *Journal of Sport Rehabilitation* **6**, 256–271.

Johnson, U. (1998) Psychological risk factors during the rehabilitation of competitive male soccer players with serious knee injuries [Abstract]. *Journal of Sports Sciences* **16**, 391–392.

Johnson, U. (2000) Short-term psychological intervention: a study of long-term-injured competitive athletes. *Journal of Sport Rehabilitation* **9**, 207–218.

Johnston, L.H. & Carroll, D. (1998a) The context of emotional responses to athletic injury: a qualitative analysis. *Journal of Sport Rehabilitation* **7**, 206–220.

Johnston, L.H. & Carroll, D. (1998b) The provision of social support to injured athletes: a qualitative analysis. *Journal of Sport Rehabilitation* **7**, 267–284.

Kahanov, L. & Fairchild, P.C. (1994) Discrepancies in perceptions held by injured athletes and athletic trainers during the initial evaluation. *Journal of Athletic Training* **29**, 70–75.

Kleiber, D.A. & Brock, S.C. (1992) The effect of career-ending injuries on the subsequent well-being of elite college athletes. *Sociology of Sport Journal* **9**, 70–75.

Krebs, D.E. (1981) Clinical EMG feedback following meniscectomy: a multiple regression experimental analysis. *Physical Therapy* **61**, 1017–1021.

Kubler-Ross, E. (1969) *On Death and Dying.* Macmillan, New York.

LaMott, E.E. (1994) *The anterior cruciate ligament injured athlete: the psychological process.* Doctoral dissertation, University of Minnesota, Minneapolis.

Lampton, C.C., Lambert, M.E. & Yost, R. (1993) The effects of psychological factors in sports medicine rehabilitation adherence. *Journal of Sports Medicine and Physical Fitness* **33**, 292–299.

Larson, G.A., Starkey, C.A. & Zaichkowsky, L.D. (1996) Psychological aspects of athletic injuries as perceived by athletic trainers. *Sport Psychologist* **10**, 37–47.

Laubach, W.J., Brewer, B.W., Van Raalte, J.L. & Petitpas, A.J. (1996) Attributions for recovery and adherence to sports injury rehabilitation. *Australian Journal of Science and Medicine in Sport* **28**, 30–34.

Laurence, C. (1997) Attributional, affective and perceptual processes during injury and rehabilitation in active people. Paper presented at the 14th World Congress on Psychosomatic Medicine, Cairns, Australia.

Leadbetter, W.B. (1994) Soft tissue athletic injury. In: *Sports Injuries: Mechanisms, Prevention, and Treatment* (Fu, F.H. & Stone, D.A., eds). Williams & Wilkins, Baltimore: 733–780.

Leddy, M.H., Lambert, M.J. & Ogles, B.M. (1994) Psychological consequences of athletic injury among high-level competitors. *Research Quarterly for Exercise and Sport* **65**, 347–354.

Levitt, R., Deisinger, J.A., Wall, J.R., Ford, L. & Cassisi, J.E. (1995) EMG feedback-assisted postoperative rehabilitation of minor arthroscopic knee surgeries. *Journal of Sports Medicine and Physical Fitness* **35**, 218–223.

Lewis, L. & LaMott, E.E. (1992) Psychosocial aspects of the injury response in the pro football: an exploratory study. Paper presented at the Annual Meeting of the Association for the Advancement of Applied Sport Psychology, Colorado Springs, CO.

Little, J.C. (1969) The athlete's neurosis—a deprivation crisis. *Acta Psychiatrica Scandinavica* **45**, 187–197.

Locke, E. & Latham, G. (1990) *A Theory of Goal Setting and Task Performance.* Prentice Hall. Englewood Cliffs, NJ.

Loundagin, C. & Fisher, L. (1993) The relationship between mental skills and enhanced athletic injury rehabilitation. Poster presented at the Annual Meeting of the Association for the Advancement of Applied Sport Psychology and the Canadian Society for Psychomotor Learning and Sport Psychology, Montreal, Canada.

Lynch, G.P. (1988) Athletic injuries and the practicing sport psychologist: practical guidelines for assisting athletes. *Sport Psychologist* **2**, 161–167.

Macchi, R. & Crossman, J. (1996) After the fall: reflections of injured classical ballet dancers. *Journal of Sport Behavior* **19**, 221–234.

Maniar, S., Perna, F., Newcomer, R., Roh, J. & Stilger, V. (1999a) Athletic trainers' recognition of psychological distress following athletic injury: implications for referral. In: *Pre-Injury Screening and Post-Injury Assessment: Interactions Between Sport Psychologists and the Sports Medicine Team* (Perna, F., chair). Symposium conducted at the Annual Meeting of the Association for the Advancement of Applied Sport Psychology, Banff, Alberta, Canada.

Matthews, K.A., Shumaker, S.A., Bowen, D.J. *et al.* (1997) Women's health initiative: why now? What is it? What's new? *American Psychologist* **52**, 101–116.

McDonald, S.A. & Hardy, C.J. (1990) Affective response patterns of the injured athlete: an exploratory analysis. *Sport Psychologist* **4**, 261–274.

Meani, E., Migliorini, S. & Tinti, G. (1986) La patologia de sovraccarico sportivo dei nuclei di accrescimento apofisari. [The pathology of apophyseal growth centres caused by overstrain during sports]. *Italian Journal of Sports Traumatology* **8**, 29–38.

Meeuwisse, W.H. & Fowler, P.J. (1988) Frequency and predictability of sports injuries in intercollegiate athletes. *Canadian Journal of Sport Sciences* **13**, 35–42.

Meyers, M.C., Sterling, J.C., Calvo, R.D., Marley, R. & Duhon, T.K. (1991) Mood state of athletes undergoing orthopaedic surgery and rehabilitation: a preliminary report. *Medicine and Science in Sports and Exercise* **23** (Suppl.), S138.

Miller, W.N. (1998) Athletic injury: mood disturbances and hardiness of intercollegiate athletes [Abstract]. *Journal of Applied Sport Psychology* **10** (Suppl.), S127–S128.

Morrey, M.A. (1997) *A longitudinal examination of emotional response, cognitive coping, and physical recovery among athletes undergoing anterior cruciate ligament reconstructive surgery.* Doctoral dissertation, University of Minnesota, Minneapolis.

Morrey, M.A., Stuart, M.J., Smith, A.M. & Wiese-Bjornstal, D.M. (1999) A longitudinal examination of athletes' emotional and cognitive responses to anterior cruciate ligament injury. *Clinical Journal of Sport Medicine* **9**, 63–69.

Murphy, G.C., Foreman, P.E., Simpson, C.A., Molloy, G.N. & Molloy, E.K. (1999) The development of a locus of control measure predictive of injured athletes' adherence to treatment. *Journal of Science and Medicine in Sport* **2**, 145–152.

Newcomer, R., Perna, F., Maniar, S., Roh, J. & Stilger, V. (1999) Depressive symptomatology distinguishing injured from non-injured athletes. In: *Pre-Injury Screening and Post-Injury Assessment: Interactions Between Sport Psychologists and the Sports Medicine Team* (Perna, F., chair). Symposium conducted at the Annual Meeting of the Association for the Advancement of Applied Sport Psychology, Banff, Alberta, Canada.

Nicol, M. (1993) Hypnosis in the treatment of repetitive strain injury. *Australian Journal of Clinical and Experimental Hypnosis* **21**, 121–126.

Niedfeldt, C.E. (1998) *The integration of physical factors into the cognitive appraisal process of injury rehabilitation.* Master's thesis, University of New Orleans, LA.

Ninedek, A. & Kolt, G.S. (2000) Sport physiotherapists' perceptions of psychological strategies in sport rehabilitation. *Journal of Sport Rehabilitation* **9**, 191–206.

Noyes, F.R., Matthews, D.S., Mooar, P.A. & Grood, E.S. (1983) The symptomatic anterior cruciate-deficient knee. Part II: the results of rehabilitation, activity modification, and counseling on functional disability. *Journal of Bone and Joint Surgery* **65A**, 163–174.

Pargman, D. & Lunt, S.D. (1989) The relationship of self-concept and locus of control to the severity of injury in freshmen collegiate football players. *Sports Training, Medicine and Rehabilitation* **1**, 203–208.

Pearson, L. & Jones, G. (1992) Emotional effects of sports injuries: implications for physiotherapists. *Physiotherapy* **78**, 762–770.

Penpraze, P. & Mutrie, N. (1999) Effectiveness of goal setting in an injury rehabilitation programme for increasing patient understanding and compliance [Abstract]. *British Journal of Sports Medicine* **33**, 60.

Peretz, D. (1970) Development, object-relationships, and loss. In: *Loss and Grief: Psychological Management in Medical Practice* (Schoenberg, B., Carr, A.C., Peretz D. & Kutscher, A.H., eds). Columbia University Press, New York: 3–19.

Perna, F. (1992) A re-examination of injury and post-athletic career adjustment. Paper presented at the Annual Meeting of the Association for the Advancement of Applied Sport Psychology, Colorado Springs, CO.

Perna, F.M., Roh, J., Newcomer, R.R. & Etzel, E.F. (1998) Clinical depression among injured athletes: an empirical assessment [Abstract]. *Journal of Applied Sport Psychology* **10** (Suppl.), S54–S55.

Perna, F.M., Ahlgren, R.L. & Zaichkowsky, L. (1999) The influence of career planning, race, and athletic injury on life satisfaction among recently retired collegiate male athletes. *Journal of Applied Sport Psychology* **13**, 144–156.

Peterson, K. (1997) Role of social support in coping with athletic injury rehabilitation: a longitudinal qualitative investigation [Abstract]. *Journal of Applied Sport Psychology* **9** (Suppl.), S33.

Petrie, T.A., Brewer, B. & Buntrock, C. (1997a) A comparison between injured and uninjured NCAA division I male and female athletes on selected psychosocial variables [Abstract]. *Journal of Applied Sport Psychology* **9** (Suppl.), S144.

Petrie, T.A., Falkstein, D.L. & Brewer, B.W. (1997b) Predictors of psychological response to injury in female collegiate athletes. Paper presented at the Annual Meeting of the American Psychological Association, Chicago.

Potter, M.J. (1995) *Psychological intervention during rehabilitation case studies of injured athletes.* Master's thesis, University of Western Australia, Nedlands.

Quackenbush, N. & Crossman, J. (1994) Injured athletes: a study of emotional response. *Journal of Sport Behavior* **17**, 178–187.

Quinn, A.M. (1996) *The psychological factors involved in the recovery of elite athletes from long term injuries.* Doctoral dissertation, University of Melbourne, Melbourne.

Quinn, A.M. & Fallon, B.J. (1999) The changes in psychological characteristics and reactions of elite athletes from injury onset until full recovery. *Journal of Applied Sport Psychology* **11**, 210–229.

Quinn, A.M. & Fallon, B.J. (2000) Predictors of recovery time. *Journal of Sport Rehabilitation* **9**, 62–76.

Richman, J.M., Rosenfeld, L.B. & Hardy, C.J. (1993) The social support survey: a validation study of a clinical measure of the social support process. *Research on Social Work Practice* **3**, 288–311.

Roh, J., Newcomer, R.R., Perna, F.M. & Etzel, E.F. (1998) Depressive mood states among college athletes: pre- and post-injury [Abstract]. *Journal of Applied Sport Psychology* **10** (Suppl.), S54.

Rose, J. & Jevne, R.F.J. (1993) Psychosocial processes associated with sports injuries. *Sport Psychologist* **7**, 309–328.

Ross, M.J. & Berger, R.S. (1996) Effects of stress inoculation on athletes' postsurgical pain and rehabilitation after orthopedic injury. *Journal of Consulting and Clinical Psychology* **64**, 406–410.

Rotella, B. (1985) The psychological care of the injured athlete. In: *Sport Psychology: Psychological Considerations in Maximizing Sport Performance* (Bunker, L.K., Rotella R.J. & Reilly, A.S., eds). Mouvement, Ann Arbor: 273–287

Rotella, R.J. & Campbell, M.S. (1983) Systematic desensitization: psychological rehabilitation of injured athletes. *Athletic Training* **18**, 140–142, 151.

Rotella, R.J. & Heyman, S.R. (1986) Stress, injury, and the psychological rehabilitation of athletes. In: *Applied Sport Psychology: Personal Growth to Peak Performance* (Williams, J.M., ed.). Mayfield. Palo Alto: 343–364.

Satterfield, M.J., Dowden, D. & Yasamura, K. (1990) Patient compliance for successful stress fracture rehabilitation. *Journal of Orthopaedic and Sports Physical Therapy* **11**, 321–324.

Scheier, M.F., Carver, C.S. & Bridges, M.W. (1994) Distinguishing optimism from neuroticism (and trait anxiety, self-mastery, and self-esteem): a reevaluation of the life orientation test. *Journal of Personality and Social Psychology* **67**, 1063–1078.

Scherzer, C.B., Brewer, B.W., Cornelius, A.E. *et al.* (1999) Self-reported use of psychological skills and adherence to rehabilitation following anterior cruciate ligament reconstruction. Paper presented at the Annual Meeting of the Association for the Advancement of Applied Sport Psychology, Banff, Alberta, Canada.

Shaffer, S.M. (1992) *Attributions and self-efficacy as predictors of rehabilitative success.* Master's thesis, University of Illinois, Champaign.

Shank, R.H. (1988) *Academic and athletic factors related to predicting compliance by athletes to treatments.* Doctoral dissertation, University of Virginia, Charlottesville.

Shelbourne, K.D. & Wilckens, J.H. (1990) Current concepts in anterior cruciate ligament rehabilitation. *Orthopaedic Review* **19**, 957–964.

Shelley, G.A. (1994) Athletic injuries: the psychological perspectives of high school athletes. Poster presented at the Annual Meeting of the Association for the Advancement of Applied Sport Psychology, Incline Village, NV.

Shelley, G.A. & Carroll, S.A. (1996) Athletic injury: a qualitative, retrospective case study [Abstract]. *Journal of Applied Sport Psychology* **8** (Suppl.), S162.

Shelley, G.A. & Sherman, C.P. (1996) The sports injury experience: a qualitative case study [Abstract]. *Journal of Applied Sport Psychology* **8** (Suppl.), S164.

Silva, J.M. & Hardy, C.J. (1991) The sport psychologist: psychological aspects of injury in sport. In: *The Sportsmedicine Team and Athletic Injury Prevention* (Mueller, F.O. & Ryan, A., eds). Davis, Philadelphia: 114–132.

Silver, R.L. & Wortman, C.B. (1980) Coping with undesirable events. In: *Human Helplessness: Theory and Applications* (Garber, J. & Seligman, M.E.P., eds). Academic Press, New York: 279–375.

Slattery, M.M. (1999) Construction of an instrument designed to measure alienation in sport of the injured athlete [Abstract]. *Research Quarterly for Exercise and Sport* **70** (Suppl.), A114.

Smith, A.M. & Milliner, E.K. (1994) Injured athletes and the risk of suicide. *Journal of Athletic Training* **29**, 337–341.

Smith, A.M., Young, M.L. & Scott, S.G. (1988) The emotional responses of athletes to injury. *Canadian Journal of Sport Sciences* **13** (Suppl.), 84P–85P.

Smith, A.M., Scott, S.G., O'Fallon, W.M. & Young, M.L. (1990a) Emotional responses of athletes to injury. *Mayo Clinic Proceedings* **65**, 38–50.

Smith, A.M., Scott, S.G. & Wiese, D.M. (1990b) The psychological effects of sports injuries. Coping. *Sports Medicine* **9**, 352–369.

Smith, A.M., Stuart, M.J., Wiese-Bjornstal, D.M., Milliner, E.K., O'Fallon, W.M. & Crowson, C.S. (1993) Competitive athletes: preinjury and postinjury mood state and self-esteem. *Mayo Clinic Proceedings* **68**, 939–947.

Sparkes, A.C. (1998) An Achilles heel to the survival of self. *Qualitative Health Research* **8**, 644–664.

Sthalekar, H.A. (1993) Hypnosis for relief of chronic phantom limb pain in a paralysed limb: a case study. *Australian Journal of Clinical Hypnotherapy and Hypnosis* **14**, 75–80.

Taylor, A.H. & May, S. (1995) Physiotherapist's expectations and their influence on compliance to sports injury rehabilitation. In: *Ninth European Congress on Sport Psychology Proceedings: Part II* (Vanfraechem-Raway, R. & Vanden Auweele, Y., eds). European Federation of Sports Psychology, Brussels: 619–625.

Taylor, A.H. & May, S. (1996) Threat and coping appraisal as determinants of compliance to sports injury rehabilitation: an application of protection motivation theory. *Journal of Sports Sciences* **14**, 471–482.

Tedder, S. & Biddle, S.J.H. (1998) Psychological processes involved during sports injury rehabilitation: an attribution-emotion investigation [Abstract]. *Journal of Sports Sciences* **16**, 106–107.

Theodorakis, Y., Malliou, P., Papaioannou, A., Beneca, A. & Filactakidou, A. (1996) The effect of personal goals, self-efficacy, and self-satisfaction on injury rehabilitation. *Journal of Sport Rehabilitation* **5**, 214–223.

Theodorakis, Y., Beneca, A., Malliou, P., Antoniou, P., Goudas, M. & Laparidis, K. (1997a) The effect of a self-talk technique on injury rehabilitation [Abstract]. *Journal of Applied Sport Psychology* **9** (Suppl.), S164.

Theodorakis, Y., Beneca, A., Malliou, P. & Goudas, M. (1997b) Examining psychological factors during injury rehabilitation. *Journal of Sport Rehabilitation* **6**, 355–363.

Treacy, S.H., Barron, O.A., Brunet, M.E. & Barrack, R.L. (1997) Assessing the need for extensive supervised rehabilitation following arthroscopic surgery. *American Journal of Orthopedics* **26**, 25–29.

Tripp, D.A. (2000) *Pain catastrophizing in athletic individuals: scale validation and clinical application.* Doctoral thesis, Dalhousie University, Halifax, Canada.

Tuffey, S. (1991) *The use of psychological skills to facilitate recovery from athletic injury.* Master's thesis, University of North Carolina, Greensboro.

Udry, E. (1996) Social support: exploring its role in the context of athletic injuries. *Journal of Sport Rehabilitation* **5**, 151–163.

Udry, E. (1997a) Coping and social support among injured athletes following surgery. *Journal of Sport and Exercise Psychology* **19**, 71–90.

Udry, E. (1997b) Support providers and injured athletes: a specificity approach [Abstract]. *Journal of Applied Sport Psychology* **9** (Suppl.), S34.

Udry, E. (1999) The paradox of injuries: unexpected positive consequences. In: *Psychological Bases of Sports Injuries,* 2nd edn (Pargman, D., ed.). Fitness Information Technology, Morgantown: 79–88.

Udry, E. & Singleton, M. (1999) Views of social support during injuries: congruence among athletes and coaches? Paper presented at the Annual Meeting of the Association for the Advancement of Applied Sport Psychology, Banff, Alberta, Canada.

Udry, E., Gould, D., Bridges, D. & Beck, L. (1997a) Down but not out: athlete responses to season-ending injuries. *Journal of Sport and Exercise Psychology* **19**, 229–248.

Udry, E., Gould, D., Bridges, D. & Tuffey, S. (1997b) People helping people? Examining the social ties of athletes coping with burnout and injury stress. *Journal of Sport and Exercise Psychology* **19**, 368–395.

Uemukai, K. (1993) Affective responses and the changes in athletes due to injury. In: *Proceedings of the 8th World Congress of Sport Psychology* (Serpa, S., Alves, J., Ferreira, V. & Paula-Brito, A., eds). International Society of Sport Psychology, Lisbon: 500–503.

Webborn, A.D.J., Carbon, R.J. & Miller, B.P. (1997) Injury rehabilitation programs: 'what are we talking about?'. *Journal of Sport Rehabilitation* **6**, 54–61.

Weiss, M.R. & Troxel, R.K. (1986) Psychology of the injured athlete. *Athletic Training* **21**, 104–109, 154.

Wiese-Bjornstal, D.M., Smith, A.M., Shaffer, S.M. & Morrey, M.A. (1998) An integrated model of response to sports injury: psychological and sociological dimensions. *Journal of Applied Sport Psychology* **10**, 46–69.

Williams, J.M. & Andersen, M.B. (1998) Psychosocial antecedents of sports injury: review and critique of the stress and injury model. *Journal of Applied Sport Psychology* **10**, 5–25.

Williams, J.M. & Roepke, N. (1993) Psychology of injury and injury rehabilitation. In: *Handbook of Research on Sport Psychology* (Singer, R.N., Murphey, M. & Tennant, L.K., eds). Macmillan, New York: 815–839.

Wise, A., Jackson, D.W. & Rocchio, P. (1979) Preoperative psychologic testing as a predictor of success in knee surgery. *American Journal of Sports Medicine* **7**, 287–292.

Wittig, A.F. & Schurr, K.T. (1994) Psychological characteristics of women volleyball players: relationships with injuries, rehabilitation, and team success. *Personality and Social Psychology Bulletin* **20**, 322–330.

PART 4

CLINICAL REHABILITATION INTERVENTIONS

Chapter 9

Pharmacological Agents and Acupuncture in Rehabilitation

JULIE K. SILVER AND JOSEPH AUDETTE

Introduction

Medications are a mainstay of treatment in the injured athlete—both for their pain relief and healing properties. Yet, despite the widespread use and acceptance of many medications, more often than not there is little research to endorse their use. In this chapter, we will focus on the primary medication classes that are used in sports medicine, especially during the first stage of rehabilitation. However, the reader is cautioned to recognize that the evidence that we rely so heavily on is sparse in this area. Therefore, it is recommended that all medications in athletes be used judiciously with a distinct regard for the risks and side effects as well as the potential benefits, which include pain relief and early return to play.

Non-steroidal anti-inflammatory drugs

A brief history

Inflammation has been around longer than doctors have known how to treat it. But since the very first physicians began to record what makes up the basis of our current medical knowledge, they have described inflammation. In the oldest known medical textbook, the *Edwin Smith papyrus* that was written by Egyptian healers 17 centuries before the birth of Christ, the body's reaction to injury was called '*shememet*'. The term *shememet* is always followed by a hieroglyph for 'fire' that symbolizes the hallmarks of acute inflammation (Vertosick 2000). One thousand years later, the Greek physician Hippocrates coined the term '*phlegmone*' which means 'the burning thing'. Then, in the first century after the death of Christ, the Roman author Cornelius Celsus provided what is the basis for our description of inflammation today: *rubor et tumour cum calore et dolore* (redness and swelling with heat and pain) (Vertosick 2000).

It is not surprising that since our ancestral healers were so cognizant of inflammation that they would also have found ways to treat it. Indeed, ancient Egyptians and Assyrians used willow extract to reduce the redness and pain of inflamed joints; however, the first description of salicylate therapy did not come until several thousand years later. One historian notes that the 'story begins in modern times with a letter from the Reverend Edward Stone of Chipping Norton to the Royal Society in 1763. He wrote: "There is a bark of an English tree which I have found by experience to be a powerful astringent and very efficacious in curing anguish and intermitting disorders"' (Wall 2000).

Although there were various historical attempts to use willow bark and its derivatives, it was not until Hermann Kolbe, a professor of chemistry at Marburg University, succeeded in synthesizing salicylic acid (the precursor to modern aspirin) that it became widely used. In what is described as 'a strange twist of history' (Vertosick 2000), one patient who was disgusted with Kolbe's concoction of salicylic acid that caused severe gastrointestinal upset, approached his son, a chemist for the German manufacturer of chemical dyes, Fredrich Bayer & Company, and together they synthesized acetylsalicylic acid. They called this new drug Aspirin. Today there are more than 30 000 tons of aspirin sold worldwide, and aspirin and its cohorts in the non-steroidal anti-inflammatory drug (NSAID) class are universally used to control both pain and inflammation.

Chemical properties and mechanism of action

Today there are dozens of NSAIDs available commercially, which all have a common mechanism of action (Huff & Prentice 1999). Some of the more common NSAIDs are listed in Table 9.1. NSAIDs are widely used as first-line agents in sports injuries, particularly in soft tissue injuries that involve muscles, tendons and ligaments. These medications are used primarily for two reasons: (i) to decrease inflammation, and (ii) to reduce pain. NSAIDs also have antipyretic effects,

but this is not usually a factor in their use for sports injuries. Because some of the NSAIDs are easily available without a prescription, they are often used haphazardly and improperly. Moreover, the literature has not clearly defined when NSAIDs should be used, what dose is most appropriate and for what period of time they should be used after an injury. Thus, even when they are prescribed by skilled clinicians, NSAIDs may cause more harm than good.

Inflammation is the normal response in tissue to any trauma—whether it is acute (macrotruama) or chronic (microtrauma, generally due to repetitive motion). The purpose of the inflammatory response (see Chapter 2 for a more detailed discussion) is to contain the injury, remove the irreparably injured (necrotic) tissue and restore function by re-establishing structural integrity. The acute inflammatory response occurs most significantly in the first 48 h after injury. During this period of time, the inflammatory response is mediated by local vasoactive products such as histamine, bradykinin and serotonin, which are

Table 9.1 Dosage of currently available NSAIDs.

Generic name	Common dose (mg)	Usual dosing frequency
Aspirin	325	Q 2–4 h
Celecoxib	100	BID
Diclofenac	75	BID
Diflunisal	500	BID
Etodolac	400	BID
Fenoprofen	600	QID
Flurbiprofen	100	TID
Ibuprofen	800	QID
Indomethacin	25–50	TID
Ketoprofen	75	TID
Ketorolac	10	QID
Meclofenamate	100	TID
Nabumetone	500	2 QD
Naproxen	500	BID
Oxaprozin	600	2 QD
Piroxicam	20	QD
Rofecoxib	25	QD
Salicylsalicylic acid	750	QID
Sodium salicylate	650	Q 4 h
Sulindac	200	BID
Tolmetin	400	TID

BID, twice a day; Q 2–4 h, every 2–4 h; QD, each day; 2 QD, two once a day; Q 4 h, every 4 h; QID, four times a day; TID, three times a day.

released from mast cells in order to increase blood flow and permeability. Their effects predominate in the first hour after injury.

The acute inflammatory response is then partially maintained by a class of mediators called the *eicosanoids*, which leads to the formation of prostaglandins and leukotrienes. The primary focus of medications to control inflammation (in particular NSAIDs) has been to control prostaglandin synthesis, which is in large part responsible for the increased vascular permeability and vasodilatation at the site of injury. What happens in chronic injuries or those without a significant initial inflammatory phase is not well elucidated. For example, lateral epicondylitis or 'tennis elbow' was long thought to be a 'tendinitis' that was caused by an inflammatory condition. Not surprisingly, NSAIDs have been a first-line treatment for this condition. However, more recent studies reveal that microscopically the process is more consistent with a tendinosis—demonstrating angiofibroblastic hyperplasia, hyaline degeneration, fibrinoid necrosis and granulation tissue with very few inflammatory cells (Nirschl 1992).

After the initial 24–48 h, the cellular inflammatory response begins the 'clean-up' process. This marks the beginning of the reparatory phase. The cells most involved in this process are macrophages and neutrophils that are responsible for digesting and clearing away unusable products in order to promote healthy tissue healing. It is in this phase that much of the controversy over NSAIDs occurs. The question that remains unanswered to date is whether NSAIDs retard this important phase of healing and whether this in fact might delay or impair the healing process (Leadbetter 1990).

Since the inflammatory response consists of vasodilatation with extravasation of blood that carries blood cells and other products into the area of injury, and this initial response is followed by the recruitment of inflammatory cells such as leucocytes and macrophages, then part of this process involves clearing the injured area of debris such as necrotic muscle tissue and disrupted connective tissues (Almekinders 1993). If the clean-up process is halted or impaired, it is not clear whether the healing process will suffer.

There are studies that have tried to address this, although the answer is not yet clear. For example, in one study 24 white rabbits sustained injury to the medial collateral ligament of one hindleg (Moorman *et al*. 1999). The rabbits were treated orally, twice daily, with a 2-week course of either ibuprofen or placebo. The ligaments were tested and there was no statistically significant difference in the values of the mechanical properties of the ligaments in the rabbits treated with ibuprofen versus placebo. The authors concluded that, under the conditions of the study, there was no deleterious effect of a short course of ibuprofen on the mechanical properties of medial collateral ligaments. However, in contradistinction to this study, another study was done on male rats where they underwent surgical transection of the medial collateral ligament (Elder *et al*. 2001). Postoperatively, half the rats were treated with celecoxib and the others were not. This study found that ligaments in the celecoxib-treated rats had a 32% lower load to failure than the untreated ligaments. Needless to say a reduced ligamentous strength is an unacceptable outcome in athletes eager to return to training and competition as early as possible.

Additionally, NSAIDs are known to affect the clotting process, and it is not clear in acute injury what impact this has on the tissues and the healing process. Unfortunately, studies have not been done to clearly delineate: (i) whether NSAIDs truly help to heal sports injuries or merely act as suppressers of the initial immune response as well as pain modulators; (ii) if they do help initially, then at what point do they become ineffective or even detrimental; and (iii) if they help for all injuries or just injuries in which one would anticipate a lot of inflammation such as an acute contusion or sprain/strain injury. There is a paucity of literature that illustrates when and how to use NSAIDs for sports-related injuries.

Regardless of the injury, NSAIDs have two main functions in the treatment of sports injuries: (i) to modify the inflammatory process; and (ii) to provide analgesia (Huff & Prentice 1999). The primary mechanism of action of NSAIDs in the inflammatory process is to inhibit prostaglandin production. Prostaglandins are a group of fatty acids that help to mediate the inflammatory response. A decrease in prostaglandin synthesis through the inhibition of cyclooxygenase (COX) is believed to significantly inhibit the inflammatory response (Vane 1971). There are at least two forms of COX inhibitors present in humans (Huskisson *et al.* 1973; Polisson 1996). These enzymes act differently in the body and their actions in large part determine the side effects of NSAIDs. There has been increasing interest in NSAIDs that selectively promote COX-1 while inhibiting COX-2 (DeWitt *et al.* 1993). Examples of NSAIDs that selectively inhibit COX-2 are celecoxib and rofecoxib (see Table 9.1 for dosing).

This fairly straightforward explanation of how NSAIDs work is probably more complex in reality and has been challenged by a number of studies. Some investigators have suggested that NSAIDs may act directly on the inflammatory cells (Wahl *et al.* 1977; Ceuppens *et al.* 1986) and that perhaps some NSAIDs are fairly weak inhibitors of prostaglandin synthesis but appear to have a more pronounced analgesic effect (McCormack & Brune 1991). It is interesting to note that aspirin is the only NSAID that irreversibly inhibits COX; the other effects of other NSAIDs are reversible.

The mechanism by which NSAIDs produce analgesia appears to be multifactorial. Aspirin can interfere with the transmission of painful impulses in the thalamus (Moncada & Vane 1979). Blocking the inflammatory response is also probably a factor in decreasing pain. Both effects on pain and inflammation are thought to be due to the blocking of proinflammatory prostaglandins in the soft tissues.

Despite numerous studies elaborating on the mechanism of action of NSAIDs, it is not entirely clear whether they influence the outcome after sports injuries. Clearly, they attenuate the classic inflammatory response that consists of pain (dolor), heat (calor), redness (rubor), swelling (tumour) and loss of function (*functio laesa*) (Leadbetter 1990). But the degree to which they affect healing is not clear. In fact, they may actually slow healing in some instances. Moreover, in some injuries in which there is a marked inflammatory response, such as an acute contusion or sprain/strain injury, the effect of NSAIDs (either good or bad) may be more significant than in injuries where there is less of an inflammatory response (e.g. chronic repetitive strain injuries or delayed-onset muscle soreness, DOMS). Yet, despite the fact that compelling studies, which would support the use of NSAIDs in athletes, are lacking, there are studies that suggest a definite role for their use. For example, in one study where 364 Australian Army recruits with ankle sprains sustained during training were treated with placebo or piroxicam, the latter group had less pain and were able to resume training more rapidly than the placebo group (Slatyer *et al.* 1997). Two other studies revealed that NSAIDs in young adult males and in healthy older individuals attenuated the exercise-induced inflammation, strength loss and soreness associated with eccentric exercise (DOMS) (Dudley *et al.* 1997; Baldwin *et al.* 2001).

Dosing

Table 9.1 lists the common NSAIDs and their doses. When taken orally, NSAIDs typically reach steady-state concentrations in the serum after three to five half-lives (Stankus 1999). The clearance of these agents (usually via the liver) is variable, which accounts for the wide spectrum of elimination times. Thus, typically NSAIDs are prescribed for 2–3 weeks and monitored for their effectiveness. The use of multiple NSAIDs has not been shown to be more effective than monotherapy and increases the risk of adverse side effects (Stankus 1999). However, NSAIDs can be used safely with other analgesics if pain control is an issue (e.g. acetaminophen or opioids).

Topical preparations of NSAIDs have been shown to have a more reduced blood concentration than after oral or intramuscular administration (Doogan 1989; Heynemann 1995; Dominkus *et al.* 1996). However, they do appear to reach their target tissues and have been found in muscle and subcutaneous tissue after topical use (Dominkus *et al.* 1996). Topical preparations of NSAIDs are gaining favour in sports medicine due to a number of promising studies that suggest objective and subjective improvement of symptoms (Akermark & Forsskahl 1990; Thorling *et al.* 1990; Russell 1991; Airaksinen *et al.* 1993).

Side effects

The side effects of NSAIDs result primarily from the inhibition of prostaglandin synthesis and occur in the following systems (in order of decreasing relative frequency): (i) gastrointestinal (e.g. gastritis or ulceration); (ii) renal (interstitial nephritis); (iii) dermatological (rash); and (iv) central nervous system (CNS) changes (Mortensen 1989).

By far the most notable side effect of NSAIDs is the toxicity to the gastrointestinal tract. Typical symptoms of gastric toxicity include heartburn or dyspepsia, gastritis and, potentially, ulceration. One-third to one-half of all patients who die of ulcer-related complications have recently been on NSAID therapy (Hollander 1994). Studies have demonstrated a markedly increased (4–30-fold) risk of developing ulcer disease associated with NSAID use (Soll *et al.* 1991; Griffith *et al.* 1991). Although the risk of gastrointestinal side effects is significant, it is important to note that most of the literature regarding this topic does not reflect its use in young, healthy athletes. Both topical NSAIDs and the oral selective COX-2 inhibitors may be safer alternatives regarding gastrointestinal toxicity than traditional oral NSAIDs (Dominkus *et al.* 1996; DeWitt *et al.* 1993). Additionally, medications used concurrently with NSAIDs, such as omeprazole, may provide some protection (Goodman & Simon 1994).

Renal toxicity is also an important consideration when using NSAIDs. Although serious renal complications are uncommon, there are examples of severe renal toxicity that have resulted from NSAID use. In one case report a 20-year-old female athlete developed end-stage renal failure that was attributed to 'regular use of anti-inflammatory analgesic medication for minor

sports injuries' (Griffiths 1992). This occurred when she was in a stressful situation in a different country and was playing tennis for 4 h a day in a hot climate. Thus, it is likely that dehydration also contributed to her condition. There is also some evidence to suggest that in runners NSAIDs may be harmful due to a reduction in renal blood flow (Walker *et al.* 1994). It is important to remember that renal blood flow is reduced during exercise in healthy athletes and that proteinuria and haematuria have been reported after long-distance running and cycling (Eichner 1990; Mittleman & Zambraski 1992). Future studies are needed to investigate the possible interactions of exercise and NSAIDs.

Rashes have been noted with both oral and topical NSAIDs. Typically these are benign urticarial rashes that resolve when the medication is discontinued. But more severe dermatological rashes have been described, e.g. Stevens–Johnson syndrome and erythema multiforme (Stankus 1999). It is important to note that the triad of nasal polyposis, asthma and rhinitis may be an indication of increased risk of NSAID-induced hypersensitivity reaction (Stankus 1999).

Central nervous system side effects are uncommon but may include headache, tinnitus, depression, aseptic meningitis, mental status changes and coma (Stankus 1999). NSAIDs may alter blood pressure control or decrease the effectiveness of antihypertensive medications. NSAIDs also impair the normal function of platelets and may increase the bleeding time. Of note is that NSAIDs are not recommended in the pregnant athlete.

Steroidal medications

A brief history and forms of administration

Both corticosteroids and anabolic steroids have been used in the treatment of sports injuries. However, since the International Olympic Committee (IOC) (see doping issues, p. 200) and most other agencies governing the use of drugs in athletes ban anabolic steroids, this section will be primarily devoted to corticosteroid use—both oral and injectable forms. Local anaesthetic medications that are often used in conjunction with corticosteroid injections (but may be used alone) will also be covered. The relevant restrictions on the use of local anaesthetics and glucocorticoids are discussed in the section on doping (p. 200).

The use of corticosteroids has a much more recent history than that of NSAIDs. It was not until the 1920s that Dr Philip Hench noted that patients with hypoadrenalism had many of the same symptoms as people with rheumatoid arthritis. Dr Hench concluded that rheumatoid arthritis must have a component of adrenal hormone insufficiency and could be cured with hormone replacement. Hench's theory could not be tested until the 1930s when pure preparations of adrenal hormones became available. However, the hormone product that came from human adrenal glands (called compound E) was still not readily available. Years later, in 1948, Hench conducted the first clinical trial and the results were just as he suspected—patients with rheumatoid arthritis reacted miraculously to cortisone (compound E). Hench and his co-worker won the Nobel prize for medicine in 1950 and his Nobel address was titled, 'The reversibility of certain rheumatic and non-rheumatic conditions by the use of cortisone' (Vertosick 2000).

Although this finding was an important one, it was not what many people had hoped—a cure for rheumatoid arthritis and other medical conditions that involve inflammation. In fact, further studies revealed that cortisone had very serious side effects and could not be taken in large quantities for long periods of time. It is now common knowledge in the medical community and even in the public domain that corticosteroids produce significant deleterious side effects when taken orally.

In the injectable forms, although there are fewer systemic side effects, there are some potential hazards that mandate that these medications be prescribed with caution. It is critical that steroids used in injectable forms are properly delivered to the target site. Imaging techniques such as fluoroscopy are sometimes used to help guide the practitioner (Micheli & Solomon 1997).

Injections also have the advantage of being both diagnostic and therapeutic. Favourable results are common with injectable steroids (Kapetanos 1982; Wiggins *et al.* 1994; Holt *et al.* 1995). Iontophoresis (using electrical stimulation) and phonophoresis (using ultrasound) are other methods of delivering corticosteroids locally and may prove to have some benefit (Franklin *et al.* 1995; Breen 1996).

Chemical properties and mechanism of action

The exact mechanism by which glucocorticoids work to mitigate inflammation is not entirely understood. Glucocorticoids are adrenocortical steroids that occur naturally and can be manufactured synthetically (*Physicians' Desk Refererence* 2002). These drugs are readily absorbed from the gastrointestinal tract. Prednisone is the most commonly prescribed synthetic oral glucocorticoid and will be the model for this discussion. In athletes, prednisone and the other glucocorticoids are prescribed primarily for their powerful anti-inflammatory properties.

Anabolic steroids are synthetic derivatives of the hormone testosterone. The actions of anabolic steroids are therefore similar to that of testosterone. In spite of the widespread use of adrenergic steroids by bodybuilders and other athletes, the effects of these drugs are poorly understood. Testosterone is known to increase muscle mass, but it is not known whether testosterone truly improves physical function and health-related quality of life (Bhasin *et al.* 2001). Anabolic steroids are banned in Olympic competitions. However, in clinical medicine there are some legitimate uses for these drugs including the promotion of weight gain after weight loss following extensive surgery, burns or severe trauma, to offset the side effects associated with prolonged corticosteroid use and for the relief of bone pain accompanying osteoporosis (*Physicians' Desk Reference* 2002). More recently, there has been increased interest in the effect of male hormones and the synthetic derivatives on the healing of skeletal muscle (Beiner *et al.* 1999; Bhasin *et al.* 2001).

Table 9.2 Common sites of injection in athletes. One per cent lidocaine or 0.25% bupivicaine should be used with long-acting, insoluble steroid salts such as triamcinalone acetate or betamethasone acetate.

Injection sites	Needle	Volume (cm^3)	Comments
Joints			
Ulnocarpal	No. 25, 1.5 in	1–3	Steroid volume to anaesthetic ratio 1 : 1
Radiocarpal			
Carpometacarpal			
Elbow	No. 25, 1.5 in	2–3	Steroid volume to anaesthetic ratio 1 : 2
Ankle			
Shoulder	No. 25, 1.5 in	7–10	Steroid volume to anaesthetic ratio 1 : 6–9
Knee			
Sacroiliac joint			
Bone–tendon			
Med/lat epicondyle	No. 27, 1.25 in	2–3	Steroid volume to anaesthetic ratio 1 : 1
Plantar fascia			
Patellar tendon			
Achilles tendon			
Pubic symphysis	No. 25, 1.5 in	3–5	Steroid volume to anaesthetic ratio 1 : 2–4
Hamstrings			
Adductors			
Tendon sheaths			
Thumb extensor	No. 27, 1.25 in	1–3	Steroid volume to anaesthetic ratio 1 : 1
Finger flexors			
Posterior tibial	No. 27, 1.25 in	3–5	Steroid volume to anaesthetic ratio 1 : 2–4
Biceps (long head)			
Bursae			If aspirating, will need No. 18–20 needle first
Prepatellar	No. 25, 1.5 in	2–3	Steroid volume to anaesthetic ratio 1 : 1
Pes anserine			
Olecranon			
Subacromial	No. 25, 1.5 in	7–10	Steroid volume to anaesthetic ratio 1 : 6–9
Greater trochanter			
Perineural			
Carpal tunnel	No. 27, 1.25 in	2–5	Steroid volume to anaesthetic ratio 2 : 1
Tarsal tunnel			
Suprascapular notch			
Cubital tunnel			

Dosing

Systemic corticosteroids are dosed in a variety of ways and the literature does not support a 'best way' approach. Often in an acute injury, corticosteroids are prescribed in a weaning fashion with the highest dose taken on the first few days and then tapering off the medication altogether within 1–2 weeks. There are commercially available 'dose packs' that are used for just this purpose. Longer term steroid use typically involves a more constant dose (e.g. 5 or 10 mg of prednisone daily), but is really practitioner-dependent. This approach is rarely used, if ever, in sports injuries and the systemic use of gluco-corticoids is banned by the IOC (see doping issues, p. 200).

Injections can be done with corticosteroid alone or mixed with a local anaesthetic, at a number of sites (Table 9.2). In joints or bursae, aspiration of fluid may be done prior to injecting the medication. The dose and amount of injected material depends on the medication used and the structure that is being injected. There are no hard and fast rules on dosing, but some general guidelines advocated in the literature include: using 2.5–10 mg of prednisolone tebutate suspension in small joints (e.g. hand and foot), 10–25 mg in medium-sized joints (e.g. wrist and elbow) and 20–40 mg in large joints (e.g. knee and shoulder) (Swain & Kaplan 1995).

Side effects

The side effects associated with systemic corticosteroid use are many and often are associated with long-term use. Some of the more serious side effects include fluid and electrolyte disturbances, steroid myopathy, osteoporosis, aseptic necrosis of the femoral and humeral heads, peptic ulcer, pancreatitis, impaired wound healing, headaches, convulsions, suppression of growth in children, Cushingoid state, cataracts and glaucoma (*Physicians' Desk Reference* 2002).

Injections carry the risk of injury to a blood vessel, nerve or other important structure. The deleterious effects on articular cartilage, tendons and the plantar fascia are somewhat disputed (Read & Motto 1992; Shrier *et al.* 1996), but there is the possibility of tendon or plantar fascial rupture following corticosteroid injection (Acevedo & Beskin 1998; Smith *et al.* 1999). An allergic reaction to the medication used, vasovagal syncope and infection are also important considerations (Table 9.3). Injectable steroids may also cause subcutaneous tissue atrophy and skin depigmentation, which are both usually just cosmetic concerns for the patient. When used by a skilled clinician, side effects are rare. Postinjection pain is rather common, however, and patients should be cautioned that they may experience a slight increase in pain for 1–2 days following the injection.

Muscle relaxants

The literature on the use of muscle relaxants in athletes in practically non-existent. It is mentioned here only because, anecdotally, physicians often do prescribe muscle relaxants for sprain/strain-type injuries. Whether muscle relaxants help or hinder healing is unclear. Equally unknown is whether muscle relaxants provide any pain relief effect or whether they allow athletes to return to their sport at an earlier date. What is known is that there are many different types of muscle relaxants that work by different pathways. Many of these have CNS side effects and at best cause fatigue or dry mouth and at worst can cause serious illness or even death (Linden *et al.* 1983; Kovac 1999; Olcina & Simonart 1999).

Opioids and inflammation

The use of opioids to treat athletic injuries is a controversial area. The reluctance of physicians to use these agents in the arena of sports injuries is due to a number of concerns that are both clinically and behaviourally motivated (Stanley & Weaver 1998). From a clinical point of view, opioids, as potent analgesics, may prevent the normal interpretation of pain signals by athletes and thereby allow too quick a resumption of aggressive training following injury. This could

Table 9.3 Local and systemic complications with local injections of corticosteroids.

Local	Systemic
Subcutaneous atrophy	Transient hyperglycaemia in diabetics
Pigmentation abnormalities	Vasovagal symptoms with syncope
Tendon/ligament rupture	Cognitive effects, 'steroid psychosis'
Accelerated joint destruction	Allergic reactions
Local sterile abscess	Systemic infection
Peripheral nerve injury	Suppression of pituitary–adrenal axis
Muscle necrosis/vascular injury	Avascular necrosis of hip

potentially lead to reinjury and further impairment. From a biobehavioural point of view, treating physicians must also be concerned about the inappropriate use of opioids to enhance performance. In addition, prolonged use of opioids to treat a more persistent injury can cause physical dependence and in rare cases psychological dependence, making cessation of the medication problematic.

Opioids or 'narcotics' are on the IOC list of prohibited substances (see p. 200) (Catlin & Murray 1996). However, given the need for more potent analgesics in treating acute injuries in sports, physicians lobbied the IOC to change its policy regarding opioids. As a result, in 1992, the IOC removed both codeine and dihydrocodeine bitartrate from the list of banned substances. It is interesting to note that codeine is a prodrug and is converted by the liver to morphine, which is the active form of the drug. However, approximately 8–10% of the population are genetically deficient in the hepatic enzyme needed to make this conversion and thus receive no analgesic benefit from codeine (Gourlay 1999). As we learn more about opioid physiology, especially with regard to pain and inflammation, it is likely that in the future selective use of opioids will be approved to treat athletic injuries.

There is increased appreciation of the role that both endogenous and exogenous opioids play in controlling not just pain, but inflammation following injury. The pharmacological actions of opioids have long been thought to reside exclusively within the CNS. Over the last 10 years, a growing understanding of the peripheral effect of opioid medications has developed. All three opioid receptor subtypes (mu, delta and kappa) have been isolated on peripheral axon terminals of small-diameter, unmyelinated sensory neurones (nociceptors or C-fibres). The opiate receptors are manufactured in the dorsal root ganglion and then transported both centrally into the dorsal horn and peripherally to the axon terminal. With inflammation, increased axonal transport of receptor proteins occurs with up-regulation of the expression of the receptors on the C-fibre nerve terminals (Stein *et al*. 2001).

In addition, inflammation causes the perineural barrier to become more permeable, presumably exposing more opioid receptors on the sensory axon to both exogenous and endogenous opioids (Coggeshall *et al*. 1997). This increased receptor expression is stimulated by the release of endogenous opioid peptides such as β-endorphin from CD4+ lymphocytes within inflamed tissue (Mousa *et al*. 2001). The source of the endogenous opioid seems to not be from pituitary secretion, but rather from circulating immune cells that accumulate at the site of acute inflammation. In particular, β-endorphin and met-enkephalin have been found by radioimmunoassay in immunocytes at the site of injury in a rat paw model of acute inflammation (Cabot *et al*. 2001).

In animal models, the evidence suggests that part of the anti-inflammatory action of opioids is to reduce the release of proinflammatory mediators by the axon terminals. Peripheral nociceptors are now understood to not only signal tissue injury centrally, but they also act to release peptides in the periphery, such as substance P and calcitonin gene-related peptide which promote inflammatory cell activity at the site of injury. This axonal reflex to injury is referred to as *neurogenic inflammation* and is also believed to be responsible for tissue swelling and pain outside the area of direct tissue injury. Excessive release of these proinflammatory substances can lead to peripheral sensitization of sensory afferents, which is in part due to an increase in the expression of sodium channels (Fig. 9.1) (Julius & Basbaum 2001). This in turn leads clinically to hyperalgesia or an exaggerated response to minimally painful stimulation (Woolf & Salter 2000). By diminishing the release of these proinflammatory peptides from the C-fibre terminals, opioids may be important in limiting the volume and extent of such sensitization. In addition, opioid receptors have been found on immune cells suggesting a mechanism for the effect of morphine on suppressing lymphocyte proliferation and diminishing the production of various cytokines including interleukin-1β, an important immune modulator (House *et al*. 2001).

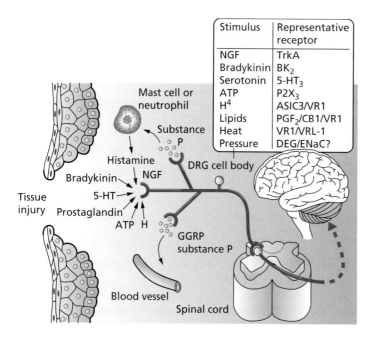

Stimulus	Representative receptor
NGF	TrkA
Bradykinin	BK$_2$
Serotonin	5-HT$_3$
ATP	P2X$_3$
H^4	ASIC3/VR1
Lipids	PGF$_2$/CB1/VR1
Heat	VR1/VRL-1
Pressure	DEG/ENaC?

Fig. 9.1 Schematic diagram of the response of nociceptors to tissue injury. ASIC3, proton receptor; ATP, adenosine triphosphate; BK$_2$, bradykinin receptor 2; CB1, cannabinoid receptor 1; CGRP, calcitonin-gene related peptide; DEG, pressure receptors; DRG, dorsal root ganglion; ENaC, putative pressure receptor; H, protons; 5-HT, serotonin (5-hydroxy-tryptophan; 5-HT$_3$-serotonin receptor 3; NGF, nerve growth factor; PGF$_2$, prostaglandin F-2 receptor; P2X$_3$, purinergic receptor; TrkA, tyrosine kinase receptor A; VR1, vanilloid receptor 1; VRL-1, vanilloid receptor like protein. (From Julius & Basbaum 2001, with permission.)

Clinical applications

Use of intra-articular, preservative-free morphine sulphate has become more prevalent after joint operations such as knee meniscectomy. The goal is to reduce postoperative pain and inflammation and speed recovery. With meniscectomy, the usual recovery time course can last up to 10 weeks before resumption of athletic competition. In general, the more pain and swelling following surgery or injury, the longer the time to recovery. In a recent study that had as outcome measures (i) time to being pain free, (ii) time before cessation of crutches, and (iii) time before return to work, the use of intra-articular morphine with bupivicaine allowed a more than 50% reduction in average time necessary to reach these endpoints when compared to intra-articular saline injection (Rasmussen et al. 1998). The addition of methylprednisolone to bupivicaine and free morphine sulphate led to even greater shortening of the duration before full recovery. Similar findings have been reported following ankle surgery in athletes (Rasmussen & Kehlet 2000). In comparing intra-articular morphine (3 mg in 3 cm^3 saline) with dexamethasone (4 mg in 3 cm^3 saline) in chronic arthritis patients, both produced a significant reduction of pain when compared with saline, and the morphine group had significantly lower synovial leucocyte counts when compared with the dexamethasone group (Stein et al. 1999).

In a review by Kalso et al. (1997), 33 randomized, controlled trials studying 1500 patients were found comparing intra-articular morphine following knee surgery with placebo treatments. Dose ranges of the morphine ranged from 0.5 to 5 mg and no additional benefit was seen with doses above 1 mg per knee. Overall, the studies suggest that there is a prolonged analgesic effect and reduction in consumption of pain medications. However, various methodological problems with the study designs make it difficult to conclude that the use of intra-articular morphine has a significant, clinically relevant effect on post-surgical outcomes.

Side effects

Side effects associated with short-term opioid use mainly involve cognition and the gastrointestinal system. The side effects for all of the commonly

Table 9.4 Dosage of currently available opioids.

Generic name	Morphine equivalent dose, oral (mg)	Starting dose	Usual dosing frequency
Pentazocine (agonist/antagonist)	50–200	50 mg	QID
Propoxyphene	65	50–100 mg	QID
Codeine	30–200	30–60 mg	QID
Morphine	30	15 mg	Q 4 h
Hydrocodone	10	5–7.5 mg	Q 4 h
Meperidine	200	50 mg	Q 4 h
Hydromorphone	2–4	1–2 mg	Q 3–4 h
Fentanyl patch		25 µg/h	72 h
Oxycodone	30	5–10 mg	Q 4 h
Methadone	8–10	2.5–5 mg	Q 8–12 h
Levorphanol	4	2 mg	Q 6–8 h

Q 3–4 h, every 3–4 h; Q 4 h , every 4 h; Q 8–12 h, every 8–12 h; Q 6–8 h, every 6–8 h; QID, four times a day.

prescribed opioid medications (Table 9.4) are essentially similar, although there is a great degree of variation in the side effects caused by various opioid agents for a particular individual. So whereas codeine may cause severe nausea and cognitive disorientation for a particular person, hydrocodone may not.

Cognitively, opioid-naïve individuals may feel disinhibited, with loss of cognitive acuity and mild to moderate sedation when first taking a potent narcotic. Usually these cognitive side effects dissipate with continued use. Associated with the cognitive side of sedation is respiratory depression, especially in the postoperative setting. This is associated with a shift in the responsiveness of the respiratory drive to the carbon dioxide concentration in the lungs, an important mechanism of respiratory regulation during exercise. Although pain is a potent stimulus to overcome this opioid effect, use of other agents to relieve pain, including spinally administered anaesthetics, can at times lead to the sudden relief of pain and the rapid onset of respiratory depression if the dose of opioid medication is not reduced. Other medications can act synergistically with opioids to cause respiratory depression, especially agents in the benzodiazepine and barbiturate class. Carisoprodol is often used as a muscle relaxant for acute pain and can be a

particularly bad combination with opioid medications, as it metabolizes to meprobamate, which is a barbiturate.

Some individuals experience a mild euphoria with the consumption of an opioid medication. This response to opioids may be predictive of an individual being prone to develop addictive behaviours around the use of opioid medications; however, there is no well designed study to make a definitive statement regarding this issue. Of note is the fact that a small percentage of individuals will experience extreme dysphoria, to the point of depression, with the consumption of opioids. Often this will be accompanied by some degree of agitation, both of which resolve with cessation of the agent. Finally, prolonged use of opioid medications can cause reduced libido, but this is not usually a major issue with short-term use (Evans 1999).

Gastrointestinal side-effects are extremely common. Mild to severe nausea can occur, but the most common problem that uniformly affects individuals taking opioids is constipation. Appropriate measures to increase water and fibre intake can usually overcome this problem, but bowel obstruction can occur if left unattended. Less common problems include excessive sweating, pruritis and urinary retention. Extremely high doses of any opioid, but particularly found with meperidine, can lower seizure threshold and can occasionally cause cardiac arrhythmias. However, this is usually not important with short-term use in the setting of injury (Bowdle 1998). Often, the most serious physiological side effect in the outpatient setting from the use of high-dose opioids is hepatitis due to excessive acetaminophen intake found in the combination of short-acting opioids such as oxycodone and hydrocodone.

Finally, the issue of addiction versus tolerance must be raised when discussing the use of opioids in pain. Tolerance occurs with prolonged use of opioids uniformly in all patients and is due to physiological changes in the CNS. Clinically, this is expressed as the need to increase the dose of opioid medication to achieve continued analgesia. Addiction is a biobehavioural phenomenon and is described as a maladaptive, self-destructive activity to continue to obtain and seek more opioid medications despite progressive deterioration in function and social status. Surveys in the acute pain population, such as those with postoperative pain, show that it is extremely rare to see the onset of addictive behaviours with the appropriate use of opioid medications. In the chronic pain population, estimates of the incidence varies from 3.2 to 18.9% (Fishbain *et al.* 1992).

In the future, as we learn more about the effect of opioids on peripheral pain and the inflammatory transduction system of tissue injury, novel methods of treating the pain and inflammation associated with athletic injuries will probably include agents that act on these opioid receptors. Ideally, agents that do not have a significant CNS effect could be used to modulate the immuno-inflammatory response to injury.

Acupuncture in acute pain and inflammation

Discussion of the peripheral effects of endogenous and exogenous opioids would be incomplete without some mention of the effect of acupuncture on pain and tissue injury. The use of acupuncture by athletes to treat acute injuries is very common in Asia and Eastern Europe and is increasingly becoming an option in many Western nations. At the Winter Olympics in Japan in 1998, international exposure came when the acupuncturist in Nagano offered free treatments to Olympic athletes and officials, emphasizing that it is a drug-free way to treat injuries. Even more stunning was the near miraculous recovery in response to acupuncture by the Austrian, Hermann Maier. Maier won gold medals in the giant slalom and super G, 3 days following a dramatic fall and injury that occurred during the downhill competition. Maier mentioned to the press that the use of acupuncture to treat his shoulder and knee injuries following the fall helped him to recover so quickly.

Over the last 30 years, a great deal of scientific evidence has accumulated to substantiate that acupuncture stimulation (AP) and electroacupuncture stimulation (EA) have physiological effects that strongly influence the neurohumoral systems that modulate pain. The evidence for the release of endogenous opioids with AP and EA goes back to the seminal work of Pomeranz in animals and Mayer in humans in the early 1970s (Pomeranz & Chiu 1976; Mayer *et al.* 1977). We now know that acupuncture causes the release of endorphins and enkephalins in the CNS and that these neuropeptides play a significant role in its analgesic efficacy. There is growing evidence that the descending inhibitory control system also plays a role in acupuncture analgesia. This involves the activation of serotonergic neurones in the midbrain, that in turn act to inhibit the transmission of nociceptive information at the level of the dorsal horn (Fig. 9.2). Release of 5-hydroxy tryptamine (5-HTP) in the raphe nucleus of the midbrain has been shown with both EA and AP, and acupuncture analgesia is attenuated with the injection of a serotonin antagonist such as para-cholorophenylalanine (Debreceni 1993).

Acupuncture has been shown in animal models to strongly influence the pituitary–hypothalamic system as well. The arcuate nucleus of the ventromedial hypothalamus contains the β-endorphin-producing cells and lesions of this nucleus abolishes acupuncture analgesia in rats (Debreceni 1993). The hypothalamus secretes

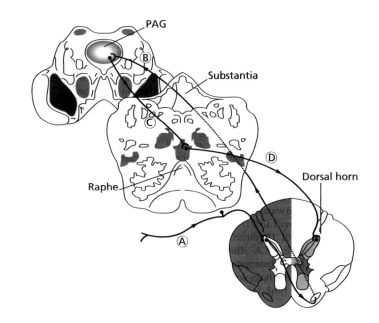

Fig. 9.2 Schematic diagram of pain transmission and modulation in the central nervous system. A, nociceptive input into the dorsal horn. B, ascending pain pathway via the spinothalamic tract with synapse in the periaquaductal grey area (PAG) in the mesencephalon. C, descending, excitatory pathway to the raphe magnus in the rostral medulla. D, the serotonergic, descending, pain-modulating tract has an inhibitory action on the dorsal horn.

β-endorphin into the blood, consistent with the elevated blood levels of endorphin found with both AP and EA. Concurrent with the release of β-endorphin, is the secretion of adrenocorticotrophic hormone with acupuncture, which in turn stimulates adrenal secretion of cortisol causing a general anti-inflammatory effect (Pomeranz 1998). Given the previous discussion relative to the presence of peripheral opioid receptors on C-fibres in inflammatory conditions, the elevation of systemic β-endorphin with acupuncture may exert both an analgesic and an anti-inflammatory effect in sports injuries.

Recent studies indicate that acupuncture also influences the release of immune-modulating cytokines from the hypothalamus such as interleukin 1β and 6 during experimental models of fever (Son *et al.* 2002). The rise of blood β-endorphin with acupuncture also influences peripheral cytokine production in the spleen by causing increases in interferon-γ and reduction of natural killer cell activity (Yu *et al.* 1998). These early data suggest that acupuncture has physiological effects that go far beyond the release of endorphins in the CNS, and has important immune-modulating effects that may prove to be important in the recovery from injury.

Clinical applications

The use of acupuncture for acute injuries has not been studied extensively in athletes. However, a recent study of rotator cuff tendinitis in subjects with sports-related injuries found that true acupuncture needling was significantly superior when looking at both its analgesic effects as well as strength, range of motion and functional scores when compared to a placebo needling control group (Kleinhenz *et al.* 1999). Treatment consisted of using a combination of points in the feet and hands, based on Chinese acupuncture principles, together with meridian-based local points around the shoulder based on tenderness. Subjects received two 22 min treatments per week for 4 weeks and had follow-up assessments at the end of the treatment period and again at 4 months. Acupuncture has also shown efficacy in providing acute pain relief with a single 20 min treatment for chronic lateral epicondylitis (tennis elbow) when compared with placebo. A single treatment was given using only one point near the fibular head (gallbladder 34) on the leg ipsilateral to the elbow pain (Molsberger & Hille 1994). Both of these studies used a placebo needle device for the control group, where a blunt needle presses on the point, but does not pene-trate the skin.

In a randomized trial of acupuncture for osteoarthritis of the knee, significant improve-ment in scores of pain and function were noted when compared with standard treatment on oral NSAIDs (Berman *et al.* 1999). In this study, subjects received 20 min sessions of electroacu-puncture at 2.4–4 Hz for 8 weeks with outcome assessments at 4, 8 and 12 weeks. Finally, in a meta-analysis of randomized controlled trials of acupuncture for low back pain, it was concluded that acupuncture is superior to the various con-trol treatments, but insufficient evidence was available to state whether it was better than placebo needling methods (Ernst & White 1998).

In conclusion, acupuncture appears to be a safe and potentially effective method of treating the pain and inflammation of sports-related injuries. There is sufficient evidence to suggest a physiological mechanism of action that involves neurohumoral processes that have both a central and peripheral effect. Better designed and more specific studies are needed to assess the clinical efficacy of acupuncture in various sports injuries. It is also important to understand how acupunc-ture might affect human performance in athletic competitions.

Doping issues

It is very important for every sports medicine practitioner to become familiar with the list of prohibited substances of the IOC (Table 9.5). Relevant to this chapter are sections IB, IC, IIIC and IIID.

Narcotics such as diamorphine (heroin), meth-adone, morphine and related substances are pro-hibited in Olympic sports competitions. On the other hand, codeine, dextromethorphan, dextro-propoxyphene, dihydrocodeine, diphenoxylate, ethylmorphine, propoxyphene and tramadol are permitted. The sports physician must know the content of various medications to avoid using prohibited substances. Clearly, the doping rules do not apply in an emergency when the life of an athlete may be at risk.

Table 9.5 List of prohibited substances and methods in sports according to the International Olympic Committee.

I Prohibited classes of substances
A. Stimulants
B. Narcotics
C. Anabolic agents
   1. Anabolic androgenic steroids
   2. β_2-agonists
D. Diuretics
E. Peptide hormones, mimetics and analogues

II Prohibited methods
A. Blood doping
B. Artificial oxygen carriers or plasma expanders
C. Pharmacological, chemical and physical manipulation

III Classes of prohibited substances in certain circumstances
A. Alcohol
B. Cannabinoids
C. Local anaesthetics
D. Glucocorticosteroids
E. β-blockers

Anabolic androgenic steroids are prohibited in Olympic sports and there is no indication or exemption to this rule. Since the β_2-agonists have anabolic properties they have been included in the list of prohibited substances. Some β_2-agonists like formoterol, salbutamol, salmeterol and terbutaline are permitted by inhaler only to prevent and/or treat asthma and exercise-induced asthma. Written notification by a respiratory or team physician that the athlete has asthma and/or exercise-induced asthma, is necessary to the relevant medical authority prior to competition. At the Olympic Games, athletes who request permission to inhale a permitted β-agonist will be assessed by an independent medical panel.

Local anaesthetics are permitted under certain conditions. Bupivacaine, lidocaine, mepivacaine, procaine and related substances can be used, but not cocaine. Vasoconstrictor agents may be used in conjunction with local anaesthetics but only local or intra-articular injections may be administered, and only when medically justified. Notification of administration may be necessary where the rules of a responsible authority so provide.

The systemic use of glucocorticoids is prohibited when administered orally, rectally or by intravenous or intramuscular injection. When medically necessary, local and intra-articular injections of glucocorticoids are permitted. Notification of administration may be necessary where the rules of a responsible authority so provide.

References

Acevedo, J.I. & Beskin, J.L. (1998) Complications of plantar fascia rupture associated with corticosteroid injection. *Foot and Ankle International* **19** (2), 91–97.

Airaksinen, O., Venalainen, J. & Pietilainen, T. (1993) Ketoprofen 2.5% gel versus placebo gel in the treatment of acute soft tissue injuries. *International Journal of Clinical Pharmacology, Therapy and Toxicology* **31**, 561–563.

Akermark, C. & Forsskahl, B. (1990) Topical indomethacin in overuse injuries in athletes: a randomized double blind study comparing Elmetacin with oral indomethacin and placebo. *International Journal of Sports Medicine* **11**, 393–396.

Almekinders, L.C. (1993) Anti-inflammatory treatment of muscular injuries in sports. *Sports Medicine* **15** (3), 139–145.

Baldwin, A.C., Stevenson, S.W. & Dudley, G.A. (2001) Nonsteroidal anti-inflammatory therapy after eccentric exercise in healthy older individuals. *Journal of Gerontology* **56A** (8), M510–M513.

Beiner, J.M., Jokl, P., Cholewicki, J. & Panjabi, M.M. (1999) The effect of anabolic steroids and corticosteroids on healing of muscle contusion injury. *American Journal of Sports Medicine* **27** (1), 2–9.

Berman, B.M., Singh, B.B., Lao, L. *et al.* (1999) A randomized trial of acupuncture as an adjunctive therapy in osteoarthritis of the knee. *Rheumatology* **38**, 346–354.

Bhasin, S., Woodhouse, L. & Storer, T.W. (2001) Proof of the effect of testosterone on skeletal muscle. *Journal of Endocrinology* **170**, 27–38.

Bowdle, T.A. (1998) Adverse effects of opioid agonists and agonist–antagonists in anaesthesia. *Drug Safety* **19** (3), 173–189.

Breen, P. (1996) Physiological principles of transdermal iontophoresis. *Athletic Therapy Today* September, 27.

Cabot, P.J., Carter, L., Schafer, M. & Stein, C. (2001) Methionine-enkephalin and dynorphin A release from immune cells and control of inflammatory pain. *Pain* **93** (3), 207–212.

Catlin, D.H. & Murray, T.H. (1996) Performance-enhancing drugs, fair competition, and Olympic sport. *Journal of the American Medical Association* **276** (3), 231–237.

Ceuppens, J.L., Rodriquez, M.A. & Goodwin, J.S. (1982) Non-steroidal anti-inflammatory agents inhibit synthesis of IgM rheumatoid factor *in vitro*. *Lancet* **1**, 52–58.

Coggeshall, R.E., Zhou, S. & Carlton, S.M. (1997) Opioid receptors on peripheral sensory axons. *Brain Research* **764** (1–2), 126–132.

Debreceni, L. (1993) Chemical releases associated with acupuncture and electric stimulation. *Critical Reviews in Physical Rehabilitation Medicine* **5** (3), 247–275.

DeWitt, D.L., Meado, E.A. & Smith, W.L. (1993) PGH synthetase isoenzyme selectivity: the potential for safer nonsteroidal anti-inflammatory drugs. *American Journal of Medicine* **95**, 405–445.

Dominkus, M., Nicolakis, M. & Kotz, R. (1996) Comparison of tissue and plasma levels of ibuprofen after oral and topical administration. *Arzneimihelforschung* **46**, 1138–1143.

Doogan, D.P. (1989) Topical nonsteroidal anti-inflammatory drugs. *Lancet* **2**, 1270–1271.

Dudley, G.A., Czerkawski, J., Meinrod, A., Gillis, G., Baldwin, A. & Scarpone, M. (1997) Efficacy of naproxen sodium for exercise-induced dysfunction muscle injury and soreness. *Clinical Journal of Sports Medicine* **7**, 3–10.

Eichner, E.R. (1990) Hematuria—a diagnostic challenge. *Physician and Sportsmedicine* **18** (11), 53–63.

Elder, C.L., Dahners, L.E. & Weinhold, P.S. (2001) A cyclooxygenase-2 inhibitor impairs ligament healing in the rat. *American Journal of Sports Medicine* **29** (6), 801–805.

Ernst, E. & White, A.R. (1998) Acupuncture for back pain. *Archives of Internal Medicine* **158**, 2235–2241.

Evans, P.J.D. (1999) Opioids for chronic musculoskeletal pain. In: *Opioid Sensitivity of Chronic Noncancer Pain, Progress in Pain Research and Management*, Vol. 14 (Kalso, E., McQuay, H.J. & Wiesenfeld-Hallin, Z., eds). IASP Press, Seattle: 349–365.

Fishbain, D.A., Rosomoff, H.L. & Rosmoff, R.S. (1992) Drug abuse, dependence and addiction in chronic pain patients. *Clinical Journal of Pain* **8**, 77–85.

Franklin, M.E., Smith, S.T., Chenier, T.C. & Franklin, R.C. (1995) Effect of phonophoresis with dexamethasone on adrenal function. *Journal of Orthopaedic and Sports Physical Therapy* **22** (3), 103–107.

Goodman, T.A. & Simon, L.S. (1994) Minimizing the complications of nonsteroidal anti-inflammatory drug therapy. *Journal of Musculoskeletal Medicine* **11**, 33–46.

Gourlay, G.K. (1999) Different opioids—same actions? In: *Opioid Sensitivity of Chronic Noncancer Pain, Progress in Pain Research and Management*, Vol. 14 (Kalso, E., McQuay, H.J. & Wiesenfeld-Hallin, Z., eds). IASP Press, Seattle: 97–115.

Griffith, M.R., Piper, J.M., Daugherty, J.R. *et al.* (1991) Nonsteroidal anti-inflammatory drugs use and increased risk of peptic ulcer disease in elderly patients. *Annals of Internal Medicine* **114**, 257–263.

Griffiths, M.L. (1992) End-stage renal failure caused by regular use of anti-inflammatory analgesic medication for minor sports injuries: a case report. *South African Medical Journal* **81**, 377–378.

Heynemann, C.A. (1995) Topical nonsteroidal anti-inflammatory drugs for acute soft tissue injuries. *Annals of Pharmacotherpy* **29**, 780–782.

Hollander, D. (1994) Gastrointestinal complications of nonsteroidal anti-inflammatory drugs: prophylactic and therapeutic strategies. *American Journal of Medicine* **96**, 274–281.

Holt, M.A., Keene, J.S. & Graf, B.K. (1995) Treatment of osteitis pubis in athletes. *American Journal of Sports Medicine* **23** (5), 601–606.

House, S.D., Mao, X., Wu, G., Espinelli, D., Li, W.X. & Chang, S.L. (2001) Chronic morphine potentiates the inflammatory response by disrupting interleukin-1beta modulation of the hypothalamic–pituitary–adrenal axis. *Journal of Neuroimmunology* **118** (2), 277–285.

Huff, P. & Prentice, W.E. (1999) Using pharmacological agents in a rehabilitation program. In: *Rehabilitation Techniques in Sports Medicine* (Prentice, W.E., ed.). WCB/McGraw-Hill, Boston: 244–265.

Huskisson, E.C., Berry, H., Street, F.G. *et al.* (1973) Indomethacin for soft tissue injuries: a double blind study in football players. *Rheumatology and Rehabilitation* **12**, 159–160.

Julius, D. & Basbaum, A.I. (2001) Molecular mechanisms of nociception. *Nature* **413** (6852), 203–210.

Kalso, E., Tramer, M.R., Carroll, D., McQuay, H.J. & Moore, R.A. (1997) Pain relief from intra-articular morphine after knee surgery: a qualitative systematic review. *Pain* **71** (2), 127–134.

Kapetanos, G. (1982) The effect of the local corticosteroids on the healing and biomechanical properties of the partially injured tendon. *Clinical Orthopaedics* **163**, 170–179.

Kleinhenz, J., Streitberger, K., Windeler, J. *et al.* (1999) Randomized clinical trial comparing the effects of acupuncture and a newly designed placebo needle in rotator cuff tendinitis. *Pain* **83**, 235–241.

Kovac, C. (1999) Airline passenger dies after being sedated by doctor. *British Medical Journal* **318** (7175), 12.

Leadbetter, W.B. (1990) An introduction to sports-induced soft tissue inflammation. In: *Sports Induced Inflammation* (Leadbetter, W.B., Buckwalter, J.B. & Gordon, S.L., eds). American Academy of Orthopedic Surgeons, Park Ridge, IL: 3–23.

Leadbetter, W.B. (1995) Anti-inflammatory therapy in sports injury: the role of nonsteroidal drugs and corticosteroid injection. *Clinics Sports Medicine* **14** (2), 353–410.

Linden, C.H., Mitchiner, J.C., Lindzon, R.D. & Rumack, B.H. (1983) Cyclobenzaprine overdosage. *Journal of Toxicology: Clinical Toxicology* **20** (3), 281–288.

Mayer, D.J., Price, D.D. & Raffii, A. (1977) Antagonism of acupuncture analgesia in man by narcotic antagonist naloxone. *Brain Research* **121**, 368.

McCormack, K. & Brune, K. (1991) Dissociation between antinociceptive and anti-inflammatory effects of nonsteroidal anti-inflammatory drugs: a survey of their analgesic efficacy. *Drugs* **41**, 533–547.

Micheli, L.J. & Solomon, R. (1997) Treatment of recalcitrant iliopsoas tendinitis in athletes and dancers with corticosteroid injection under fluoroscopy. *Journal of Dance Medicine and Science* **1** (1), 7–11.

Mittleman, K.D. & Zambraski, E.J. (1992) Exercise-induced proteinuria is attenuated by indomethacin. *Medicine and Science in Sports and Exercise* **24** (10), 1069–1074.

Molsberger, A. & Hille, E. (1994) The analgesic effect of acupuncture in chronic elbow pain. *British Journal of Rheumatology* **33**, 1162–1165.

Moncada, S. & Vane, J. (1979) Mode of action of aspirin-like drugs. *Advances in Internal Medicine* **24**, 1.

Moorman, C.T., Kukreti, U., Fenton, D.C. & Belkoff, S.M. (1999) The early effect of ibuprofen on the mechanical properties of healing medial collateral ligament. *American Journal of Sports Medicine* **27** (6), 738–741.

Mortensen, M.E. & Rennebohm, R.M. (1989) Clinical pharmacology and use of nonsteroidal anti-inflammatory drugs. *Pediatric Clinics of North America* **36**, 1113–1139.

Mousa, S.A., Zhang, Q., Sitte, N., Ji, R. & Stein, C. (2001) Beta-endorphin-containing memory-cells and mu-opioid receptors undergo transport to peripheral inflamed tissue. *Journal of Neuroimmunology* **115** (1–2), 71–78.

Nirschl, R.P. (1992) Elbow tendinosis/tennis elbow. *Clinics in Sports Medicine* **11**, 851–870.

Olcina, G.M. & Simonart, T. (1999) Severe vasculitis after therapy with diazepam. *American Journal of Psychiatry* **56** (6), 972–973.

Physicians Desk Reference. (2002) Medical Economics Co., Montvale NJ: 1153, 3064.

Polisson, R. (1996) NSAIDs: practical and therapeutical considerations in their selection. *American Journal of Medicine* **100**, 315–365.

Pomeranz, B. (1998) Scientific basis of acupuncture. In: *Basics of Acupuncture*, 4th edn (Stux, G. & Pomeranz, B., eds). Springer-Verlag, Berlin: 4–37.

Pomeranz, B. & Chiu, D. (1976) Naloxone blockade of acupuncture analgesia: endorphins implicated. *Life Science* **19**, 1757.

Rasmussen, S. & Kehlet, H. (2000) Intraarticular glucocorticoid, morphine and bupivacaine reduces pain and convalescence after arthroscopic ankle surgery:

a randomized study of 36 patients. *Acta Orthopaedica Scandinavica* **71** (3), 301–304.

Rasmussen, S., Larsen, A.S., Thomsen, S.T. & Kehlet, H. (1998) Intra-articular glucocorticoid, bupivacaine and morphine reduces pain, inflammatory response and convalescence after arthroscopic meniscectomy. *Pain* **78** (2), 131–134.

Read, M.T.F. & Motto, S.G. (1992) Tendo achillis pain: steroids and outcome. *British Journal of Sports Medicine* **26** (1), 15–21.

Russell, A.L. (1991) Piroxicam 0.5% topical gel compared to placebo in the treatment of acute soft tissue injuries: a double blind study comparing efficacy and safety. *Clinical Investigations in Medicine* **14**, 35–43.

Scott, W.A. (1996) Injection techniques and use in the treatment of sports injuries. *Sports Medicine* **22** (6), 406–416.

Shrier, I., Matheson, G.O. & Kohl, H.W. (1996) Achilles tendonitis: are corticosteroid injections useful or harmful. *Clinical Journal of Sports Medicine* **6**, 245–250.

Slatyer, M.A., Hensley, M.J. & Lopert, R. (1997) A randomized controlled trial of piroxicam in the management of acute ankle sprain in Australian regular army recruits: the kapooka ankle sprain study. *American Journal of Sports Medicine* **25** (4), 544–553.

Smith, A.G., Kosygan, K., Williams, H. & Newman, R.J. (1999) Common extensor tendon rupture following corticosteroid injection for lateral tendinosis of the elbow. *British Journal of Sports Medicine* **33**, 423–425.

Soll, A.H., Weinstein, W.M., Durata, J. *et al.* (1991) Nonsteroidal anti-inflammatory drugs and peptic ulcer disease. *Annals of Internal Medicine* **114**, 307–319.

Son, Y.S., Park, H.J., Kwon, O.B. *et al.* (2002) Antipyretic effects of acupuncture on the lipopolysaccharide-induced fever and expression of interleukin-6 and interleukin-1β mRNAs in the hypothalamus of rats. *Neuroscience Letters* **319**, 45–48.

Stankus, S.J. (1999) Inflammation and the role of anti-inflammatory medications. In: *Handbook of Sports Medicine: A Symptom-Oriented Approach* (Lillegard, W.A., Butcher, J.D. & Rucker, K.S., eds). Butterworth-Heinemann, Boston: 15.

Stanley, K.L. & Weaver, J.E. (1998) Pharmacologic management of pain and inflammation in athletes. *Sports Pharmacology* **17** (2), 375–392.

Stein, C., Machelska, H., Binder, W. & Schafer, M. (2001) Peripheral opioid analgesia. *Current Opinions in Pharmacology* **1** (1), 62–65.

Stein, A., Yassouridis, A., Szopko, C., Helmke, K. & Stein, C. (1999) Intraarticular morphine versus dexamethasone in chronic arthritis. *Pain* **83** (3), 525–532.

Swain, R.A. & Kaplan, B. (1995) Practices and pitfalls of corticosteroid injection. *Physician and Sportsmedicine* **23** (3), 27–40.

Thorling, J., Linden, B., Berg, R. *et al.* (1990) A double blind comparison of naproxen gel and placebo in the treatment of soft tissue injuries. *Current Medical Research Opinions* **12**, 242–248.

Vane, J.R. (1971) Inhibition of prostaglandin synthesis as a mechanism for aspirin-like drugs. *Nature: New Biology* **231**, 232–235.

Vertosick, F.T. (2000) *Why We Hurt: the Natural History of Pain*. Harcourt Inc., New York.

Wahl, L.M., Olsen, C.E., Sandberg, L.E., Margen, P.D. & Ragen, S.E. (1977) Prostaglandin regulation of macrophage collagenase production. *Proceedings of the National Academy of Sciences of the USA* **74**, 4955–4958.

Walker, R.J., Fawcett, J.P., Flannery, E.M. & Gerrard, D.F. (1994) Indomethacin potentiates exercise-induced reduction in renal hemodynamics in athletes. *Medicine and Science in Sports and Exercise* **26** (11), 1302–1306.

Wall, P. (2000) *Pain: the Science of Suffering*. Columbia University Press, New York.

Wiggins, M.E., Fadale, P.D. & Barrach, M. (1994) Healing characteristics of a type 1 collagenous structure treated with corticosteroids. *American Journal of Sports Medicine* **22** (2), 279–288.

Woolf, C.J. & Salter, M. (2000) Neuronal plasticity; increasing the gain in pain. *Science* **288** (5472), 1765–1768.

Yu, Y., Kasahara, T., Sato, T. *et al.* (1998) Role of endogenous interferon-γ on the enhancement of splenic NK cell activity by electroacupuncture stimulation in mice. *Journal of Neuroimmunology* **90**, 176–186.

Chapter 10

Physical Modalities and Pain Management

JOEL M. PRESS, CHRISTOPHER T. PLASTARAS AND
STEVEN L. WIESNER

Introduction

This chapter provides the reader with the fundamentals of various modalities used in the treatment of sports-related injuries. Heat, cold and the use of electrical stimulation may be useful adjunctive components of the rehabilitation programme. By understanding the physiological basis of these modalities, a safe and appropriate treatment choice can be made. One must remember, however, that the most effective modality used will ultimately depend upon the patient's individualized and subjective response to treatment. Lastly, and most importantly, the use of therapeutic modalities is only one component of a comprehensive rehabilitation programme.

Cryotherapy (cold therapy)

As with heat, in order to safely apply and more effectively utilize cryotherapy in the treatment of sports-related injuries, an understanding of the physiological effects is necessary. In comparison with heat, cold produces vasoconstriction with vasodilatation following reflexively; it causes decreased local metabolism; and it minimizes enzymatic activity and the subsequent demand for oxygen (Lehmann & de Lateur 1982a; Ork 1982). Cold diminishes muscle spindle activity as well as slowing nerve conduction velocity. As a result, cold is commonly used for pain control and decreasing muscle spasticity and muscle guarding (Chambers 1969; Mennell 1975; McMaster 1982). Cryotherapy, in comparison to

therapeutic heat, has the opposite effect on collagen extensibility. Cold increases connective tissue stiffness and muscle viscosity, thereby diminishing flexibility.

Based on these various physiological effects, cryotherapy is most commonly used during the first 48 h of acute musculoskeletal injuries such as sprains, strains and contusions (Grana *et al.* 1986). Use beyond the acute phase is justified for continued pain control, muscle re-education and control of swelling when utilized with compression (Quillen & Rouillier 1982; Sloan *et al.* 1988). Contraindications for cryotherapy include ischaemia, cold intolerance, Raynaud's phenomenon, cold allergy, inability to communicate and insensate skin (Basford 1998). Care must be taken when using cold therapy over nerves due to the potential development of neuropraxia (conduction block). Recommendations to minimize this complication include limiting ice application to less than 30 min and protecting any peripheral nerves in the region (Drez *et al.* 1981).

Techniques of application

Ice packs, iced compression wraps, slushes, ice massage, ice whirlpools and vapocoolant sprays are some methods of cold application (Basford 1998). Regardless of the method used, there is a rapid drop in skin temperature with a delayed effect on muscle. This depends on the amount of overlying subcutaneous tissue, with maximum cooling occurring to a muscle depth of 1–2 cm (Halvorson 1989). Ice continues to be the safest and most effective method of application. Care must be taken when using chemical or gel packs due to the poor control of temperature and risk of skin irritation should the envelope break and the chemical come in contact with the individual's skin (Grant 1964; McMaster *et al.* 1978; Lehmann & de Lateur 1982a). Cryostretch and cryokinetics refer to the use of cryotherapy to facilitate joint movement. Decreasing pain and muscle guarding may lead to improved flexibility and muscle function (Roy & Irvin 1983; Halvorson 1989). An additional method of cryotherapy involves the use of vapocoolant sprays (fluori-methane and ethyl chloride), which provide very effective cutaneous local anaesthesia and are commonly used to treat myofascial trigger points. The use of cryotherapy in this context promotes normal muscle resting length by a 'spray and stretch' technique rather than by cooling the muscle itself (Mennell 1975). Fluori-Methane is less explosive, less flammable and produces less cooling than ethyl chloride (Travell & Simons 1983). Concerns, however, have been raised regarding the destruction of the ozone layer by the use of vapocoolant sprays, some of which are considered to be chlorofluorocarbons (Vallentyne & Vallentyne 1988; Simons *et al.* 1990).

Schaubel (1946) showed that the use of ice in 345 patients decreased the need for analgesic medication following assorted orthopaedic operations, as compared with controls. In a study using both clinical and basic science models, Ohkoshi *et al.* (1999) showed that cryotherapy is helpful with pain scores and analgesic use in postoperative anterior cruciate ligament reconstruction patients. Twenty-one patients undergoing reconstructive anterior cruciate ligament reconstruction were randomized into three groups: cryotherapy at 5°C, cryotherapy at 10°C and no cryotherapy for the first 48 postoperative hours. A temperature probe was placed intraoperatively in the suprapatellar pouch and the intercondylar notch through arthroscopic portals. The cryotherapy groups reached 120° of knee flexion 4 days sooner than controls. The 10°C group had significantly lower pain scores and analgesic use as compared with the control

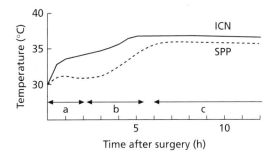

Fig. 10.1 Time–course plot of the change in intra-articular temperature after anterior cruciate ligament reconstruction in the 5°C group. a, low-temperature phase; b, temperature-rising phase; c, thermostatic phase; ICN, intercondylar notch; SPP, suprapatellar pouch. (From Ohkoshi *et al.* 1999, with permission.)

group. Both the cryotherapy groups showed a triphasic temperature curve with a low temperature phase occurring immediately postoperatively and lasting about 2 h; followed by a temperature rising phase; then finally a thermostatic phase. The control group, however, went immediately to a thermostatic phase. During the low temperature phase the cryotherapy groups' suprapatellar pouch temperatures were significantly lower than the intercondylar notch temperatures—both sites being significantly lower than body temperature. Only the suprapatellar pouch temperature remained significantly lower than body temperature during the thermostatic phase. Although the numbers were not large in this interesting study, it helps link the objective intra-articular temperature changes to clinical outcomes (Fig. 10.1). Martin *et al.* (2001) also found reduced intra-articular knee temperatures with ice application with compression.

In a randomized, controlled study, Konrath *et al.* (1996) did *not* find significant differences in medication usage or range of motion in 100 postoperative anterior cruciate ligament reconstruction patients treated with cryotherapy; unfortunately, pain scores were not recorded. Levy and Marmar (1993) reported less swelling, less pain and better range of motion with the use of cryotherapy in patients following total knee arthroplasty.

Levy *et al.* (1997) studied the effect of cryotherapy on temperatures in the glenohumeral joint and the subacromial space following shoulder arthroscopy in 15 patients. They found no significant differences in temperatures as compared with controls; however, clinical information on pain scores was not reported. Pain scores *were* reported in a randomized, controlled study of cryotherapy in 50 postoperative shoulder patients done by Speer *et al.* (1996). The cryotherapy group reported decreased pain frequency and intensity, less need to use medication, better sleep, less swelling and less pain with shoulder movement. Karlsson *et al.* (1994) found significantly improved pain scores with cryotherapy following arthroscopic anterior cruciate ligament reconstruction. Similarly, Lessard *et al.* (1997) also showed decreased pain scores and analgesic use following arthroscopic knee surgery in a randomized, blinded, controlled study of 45 patients.

Cryotherapy has been shown to help patients with sprained ankles return to activity an average of 5.1 days more quickly (Basur *et al.* 1976). Hocutt (1981) found that early cryotherapy returned patients with sprained ankles back to activity an average of 15 days earlier when compared with late cryotherapy or heat therapy.

Paddon-Jones and Quigley (1997) and Yackzan *et al.* (1984) did not find cryotherapy to be effective in treating delayed onset muscle soreness. In a study of rats, Fu *et al.* (1997) found that post-endurance training cryotherapy may actually be deleterious by causing histological myofibril damage.

Merrick *et al.* (1999) found that 5 h of continuous cryotherapy after a crush injury to the triceps surae of rats reduced biochemical secondary injury compared with no treatment. Ho *et al.* (1994) showed that 20 min of cryotherapy on the knees was enough to reduce arterial blood flow, soft tissue blood flow and bone uptake. MacAuley (2001) reviewed 45 textbooks and found considerable variation in the recommended duration and frequency of the use of ice. Although there is no definitive recommendation regarding the duration of treatment, cryotherapy is typically used for a period of 20–30 min at a time. There is more risk of frostbite if ice is used directly on the skin. In a review of cryotherapy in sports medicine, Swenson *et al.* (1996) deemed cryotherapy as 'effective and harmless', as few complications are reported.

Contrast baths

Contrast baths, which alternate the use of heat and cold, have been described as a form of 'vascular exercise' due to alternating dilatation and constriction of blood vessels. By alternating cycles of heat and cold, a hyperaemic response may by created, thereby improving circulation and assisting in the healing response. Specific indications would include improving range of motion, controlling swelling and providing pain control. Contraindications include those already discussed for therapeutic heat and cold, particularly active bleeding and vascular insufficiency. A protocol commonly used is as follows (Lehmann & de Lateur 1982a; Halvorson 1989):

1 The affected region is submerged in a warm bath of 38–43°C for 10 min.

2 This is followed by a cold bath of half ice/half water at 13–18°C for 1 min.

3 A warm bath is then used for 4 min.

4 This is followed by a cold bath for 1 min.

5 Steps 3 and 4 are then alternated for a total treatment cycle of 20–30 min.

6 The sequence ends with a cold bath.

Exercising the area may occur during the heating phase with rest during the cooling phase. A somewhat different protocol is described by Roy and Irvin (1983) in which the treatment begins and ends with cold immersion. However, it is not clear that this technique works better than cold alone.

Therapeutic heat modalities

In order to better understand the appropriate role for heat therapy, one needs to be aware of the various modes available. Heat can be transferred to tissue by three methods.

1 *Conduction*: Direct heat transfer from one surface to another due to direct contact. This

Table 10.1 Physiological effects of heat.

• Vasodilatation of arterioles and capillaries	Improved oxygen delivery to tissues
• Increased diffusion across membranes	Oedema formation
• Hyperaemia	Removal of inflammatory substances
• Increased metabolic tissue demands	Decreases muscle spindle sensitivity, thereby encouraging muscle relaxation

is a form of superficial heat. Examples would include hydrocollator packs and paraffin baths. The penetration depth depends on the thickness of the subcutaneous tissue.

2 *Convection*: Heat transfer due to the movement of air or water across a body surface. This, too, is a form of superficial heat. Examples would include hydrotherapy and fluidotherapy.

3 *Conversion*: Transfer of heat due to a change in the form of energy. Examples of superficial heat conversion would include radiant energy such as that produced by infrared lamps. Deep heating, also known as diathermy, is due to conversion through the use of short waves, electromagnetic microwaves and ultrasound.

To best utilize therapeutic heat modalities, an understanding of the physiological effects is necessary (Table 10.1). Heating can create changes which are both local and distant, with the far-field effects being less pronounced. A consensual response may also be seen whereby heating one part of the body creates an increase in blood flow in other regions. As heat is applied to a body surface, circulatory changes occur which include vasodilatation of the arterioles and capillaries. As a result of increased metabolic tissue demands, there is a subsequent increase in blood flow with the arrival of various leucocytes, improved delivery of oxygen, increased capillary permeablity and hyperaemia. Due to the increased blood flow, diffusion across membranes occurs more effectively leading to oedema formation, especially during the acute process (Cox *et al.* 1986).

Additional physiological effects include pain control through vasodilatation, which, when applied during the later stages of healing, leads to improved blood flow through the removal of pain-causing inflammatory substances such as bradykinins, prostaglandin and histamine

substrates. Heat also acts directly on free nerve endings and provides muscle relaxation by decreasing the muscle spindle's sensitivity to stretch via the gamma system (Lehmann & de Lateur 1990). Inhibitory pathways can be activated by the use of heat modalities with subsequent muscle relaxation. Central processes may also provide for sedation and decreased pain awareness. Thus, therapeutic heat assists in altering the pain–muscle guarding (spasm) cycle (Fountain *et al.* 1960).

One of the most useful therapeutic effects of heat includes improved collagen flexibility, especially when accompanied by prolonged stretching, as well as a subjective decrease in joint stiffness. Lehmann *et al.* (1970) showed that lengthening of the tendon and decreasing tendon tension occurred most effectively when the tendon was loaded in an elevated temperature bath of 45°C as compared with one at 25°C. Furthermore, only when stretch was applied in conjunction with heat did lengthening occur (Warren *et al.* 1971, 1976b). There are some studies, however, that do not support this. In a small study of 24 subjects, Taylor *et al.* (1995) showed that heat or cold modality made no significant difference in hamstring length when used in conjunction with a sustained hamstring stretch.

Based on the physiological effects of therapeutic heat, indications for heat modalities with specific attention to the injured athlete include pain, muscle spasm, contracture, bursitis and tenosynovitis. Contraindications for heat include peripheral vascular disease, bleeding diathesis, malignancy, acute trauma, sensory deficits or in patients that are unable to communicate about their sensation of pain (Basford 1998). Therapeutic heat, like other modalities, can often provide short-term relief, but there is little evidence to support long-lasting effects. Timm (1994) studied 250 subjects who had persistent low back pain following an L5 laminectomy in a randomized, controlled trial. The subjects were randomized into five groups including: (i) control; (ii) manipulation; (iii) simple home exercise programme; (iv) supervised exercise programme; and (v) physical agents, including hot packs, ultrasound and transcutaneous electrical nerve stimulation (TENS). The physical agent group did no better than the control group on the functional Oswestry scale, but was the most costly of all groups (US$1842 per subject). The exercise groups had the most improvement in the Oswestry disability scores and had fewer recurrences of low back pain; the simple home exercise programme was also the most economical (US$1392 per subject).

Superficial heat modalities

The common denominator of superficial heat modalities is direct heat penetration. Penetration is greatest within 0.5 cm from the skin surface, depending on the amount of adipose tissue (Lehmann *et al.* 1966; Michlovitz 1986). The more commonly used modes for sports rehabilitation are hydrocollator packs, whirlpools and contrast baths (see above). Other forms of superficial heat include infrared lamps, paraffin baths, fluidotherapy and moist air.

Hydrocollator packs

Hydrocollator packs serve to transfer heat via conduction. These packs come in three standard sizes and are heated in stainless steel containers containing water at temperatures between 65 and 90°C (Griffin & Karselis 1982). After appropriate heating, toweling is applied to the packs in order to minimize burning of the skin and to maintain heat insulation. The highest temperatures produced by the hydrocollator packs are at the skin surface. The pack is able to maintain heat for approximately 30 min with treatment sessions lasting 20–30 min

Other heating packs are also available and include hot water bottles, electric heating pads and chemical packs. The major disadvantage of using these devices is limited temperature control.

Hydrotherapy

EXERCISE IN WATER

Hydrotherapy is a term that can describe two distinct entities: warm water immersion or exercise performed in the water. Warm water immersion is discussed below.

A patient exercising in the water can get the therapeutic benefit of exercise while using the buoyancy principles of water to decrease the biomechanical stresses on the musculoskeletal system. The temperature of the water can be modified to fulfil individual needs. Patients with acute injuries and pregnant women are typically treated in cooler pools of 28°C whereas subacute or chronic injuries are treated in warmer temperatures of 33–34.5°C (Konlian 1999). Water exercises can also be used to cross-train patients who require weightbearing restrictions, such as those with stress fractures. Buoyancy-assisting devices can be used to allow patients to run in water (cooler temperatures of 29–29.5°C) and maintain cardiovascular fitness (Konlian 1999). Oxygen consumption of an activity performed in water has been shown to be greater than oxygen consumption of the same activity done on land (Cassidy & Nielsen 1992; Fyestone *et al.* 1993; Routi *et al.* 1994). Hall *et al.* (1996) compared water-based exercise, land-based exercise, seated water immersion and progressive relaxation in 139 chronic rheumatoid arthritis patients in a randomized trial. At 3 months, the water-based exercise group maintained the most improvement in emotional and psychological scales. Post anterior cruciate ligament repair patients obtained quicker range of motion gains with water-based exercise when compared with conventional land-based therapy (Norton *et al.* 1996). It is important to incorporate land-based as well as water-based exercises together in the rehabilitation programme. The goal is to prepare the body for function on land because most people function in life on the ground and do not live their life in the water.

Heating through the use of submersion in water is a form of convection. Whirlpools are used when a small area of the body is to be heated, such as a part of the upper or lower extremity, while Hubbard tanks are used to treat larger surface areas. The Hubbard tank, due to its larger size, also allows for range of motion manoeuvres. Since larger body areas are exposed to heat during hydrotherapy, there is an increased risk of elevation in core body temperature. Therefore, water temperature rarely exceeds 40°C for total body immersion, whereas temperatures as high as 43°C may be used for partial limb immersion.

The benefits of whirlpool treatment stem from the principle of buoyancy, in which a gravity-eliminated environment assists the patient in upward movement. An additional benefit comes from the resistance to flow, which provides low resistance for muscle strengthening and training. Agitation created by the water flow provides sensory input to the skin, assisting with pain control as well as maintaining appropriate water temperature (Hayes 1984).

As larger areas of the body are immersed in the heated water, diminished regulation of core body temperature occurs, as sweating and heat exchange can only occur in the non-immersed portions (Lehmann & de Lateur 1990). As an area with poor circulation is exposed to heat, a greater demand for blood supply is created due to increased metabolic needs. However, this demand for increased circulation may not be adequately met, leading to ischaemic results. Lowering of water temperature may limit such adverse effects. The indications and contraindications to hydrotherapy are the same as for therapeutic heat.

Paraffin baths

Paraffin baths are used in conjunction with manual joint mobilization, scar desensitization, scar mobilization and active range of motion exercises of the distal upper body or limbs of patients. This may include patients who have hand or foot contractures, healed ankle or hand fractures, postoperative Achilles tendon reconstruction and healed elbow dislocations. Paraffin baths are a mixture of paraffin and mineral oil which provide a useful means of delivering heat to the smaller joints of the body by conduction. The addition of mineral oil creates a lower melting point for the paraffin and therefore provides increased thermal energy release in comparison with water. The bath mixture is kept at a temperature of 52–58°C for upper extremity use and a somewhat lower temperature (45–52°C) for lower extremity application (Griffin & Karselis 1982). Two methods of heating are commonly employed: the dip/wrap method and the immersion method. With dipping, the extremity is immersed in the bath and then withdrawn after a few seconds, thereby allowing the wax to harden. This procedure is then repeated until a glove of wax has been created. Wrapping follows dipping whereby the extremity is enclosed within a plastic or terry towel wrap to create an insulating effect. The glove is then removed after approximately 20 min. The immersion method keeps the extremity within the paraffin bath for a period of 20–30 min. This provides for higher and more prolonged tissue temperatures than that created by the dip and wrap method. Contraindications to paraffin bath use includes patients with open wounds and severe peripheral vascular disease.

Fluidotherapy

Although infrequently used today, fluidotherapy may sometimes be used for postoperative hand and ankle rehabilitation in conjunction with manual joint mobilization, scar desensitization, scar mobilization and active range of motion exercises. Fluidotherapy involves placement of the extremity into a container through which hot air is blown within a medium of dry powder or glass beads (Borell et al. 1977). Treatment provides both therapeutic heat with its associated physiological responses, as well as mechanical stimulation that may further assist with pain control. Borell et al. (1980) found that fluidotherapy, in comparison with hydrotherapy and paraffin wax, caused the most significant temperature rise in the joint capsule and muscle.

Diathermy or deep heating modalities

Diathermy utilizes the principle of conversion to heat deeper tissues. The most commonly used deep heating agents include ultrasound and phonophoresis. Shortwave and microwave diathermy are not used much anymore. Radiant heat is not frequently used any more. The general indications and contraindications are similar to those already discussed for superficial heat. However, specific clinical uses and precautions are presented here.

Ultrasound

Ultrasound is defined as sound waves classified within the acoustic spectrum above 20 000 Hz (cycles per second). It is unique among diathermy modalities in that the production of heat is due to a high-frequency alternating electric current (0.8–1.0 MHz) which is converted via a crystal transducer to acoustic vibrations, rather than to electromagnetic energy. Energy transfer occurs due to the piezoelectric effect whereby the crystal undergoes changes in shape when the voltage is applied. By altering the crystal's configuration, vibrations are created which then pass through the tissues being treated. The heating effects depend on the absorption and reflection of ultrasonic energy based on the differences in the acoustic impedance at the tissue interface. Selective heating is greatest when acoustic impedance is high, such as at the bone–muscle interface. On the other hand, ultrasonic energy is readily conducted through homogeneous structures such as subcutaneous fat or metal implants with minimal thermal effects due to the rapid removal of heat energy. Thus, ultrasound can be safely used in the presence of metal implants. However, in the presence of methyl methacrylate and high-density polyethylene, which may be used in total joint replacements, a greater amount of ultrasound energy will be absorbed

with the potential for overheating (Lehmann & de Lateur 1982b). Significant heating can occur to depths up to 5 cm below the skin surface, thereby providing therapeutic effects to bone, joint capsule, tendons, ligaments and scar tissue (Santiesteban 1985). In summary, ultrasound provides for the deepest penetration of all heating modalities since minimal energy is converted to heat in subcutaneous fat or muscle with most of the conversion occurring at the bone interface.

In addition to the thermal effects, ultrasound also has non-thermal effects, which do not relate to tissue temperature elevation but rather to molecular vibration. Although heat can increase membrane permeability, diffusion can also occur due to the non-thermal streaming/stirring effect of fluids created by the ultrasonic field. Gaseous cavitation is also a non-thermal ultrasonic event. Gas bubbles are created as a result of acoustic rarefaction and compression causing subsequent enlargement in bubble size and pressure changes within the tissues. As the gas-filled cavity vibrates due to alternating compression and rarefaction, surrounding fluid movement occurs with the potential for cell destruction. Cavitation can be minimized by the application of external pressure and the use of a stroking, rather than a stationary, technique, which will be discussed shortly.

APPLICATION METHODS

Two primary methods of ultrasound application may be used: continuous or stationary. A coupling medium, such as mineral oil/gel or water for irregular surfaces is utilized to ensure adequate transmission of sound energy (Warren et al. 1976a; Griffin 1980; Balmaseda et al. 1986). With the continuous method, the ultrasound head is moved in a stroking fashion over the area being treated. This provides for safer, more uniform heating. The size of the applicator head should be larger than the treatment field with common sizes ranging from 5 to 10 cm². The stationary method, as the name implies, does not involve the continuous movement of the applicator head. Since a rapid rise in temperature is produced over a localized area with increased risk of burning and gaseous cavitation, this method is less commonly used. When this method is employed, intensity output is reduced.

Dosimetry is measured in watts per square centimetre ($W \cdot cm^{-2}$), which reflects the applicator output divided by the surface area of the applicator. Intensities of $1-4$ $W \cdot cm^{-2}$ are most commonly used for the continuous method. Treatment often begins at 0.5 $W \cdot cm^{-2}$ and the total output gradually increases. When using the stationary head, a safe range would be $0.1-1.0$ $W \cdot cm^{-2}$ (Lehmann & de Lateur 1982b). The duration of most treatments is 5–10 min per site based on the size of the treatment area, with 10–12 treatments per series (Hayes 1984). As with all therapeutic modalities, the patient's subjective response to heating is the best guide for proper dosing.

A variation of the primary technique includes ultrasound application under water to more effectively treat irregular surfaces. Care must be taken to minimize the development of gaseous cavitation over the body part by removing the bubbles formed. Forrest and Rosen (1989) evaluated the effectiveness of heating tendons overlying the lateral epicondyle of a pig by comparing the application of the ultrasound/coupling agent directly over the limb with limb immersion in a water bath with ultrasound application 2 cm from the skin surface. They concluded that the tendon temperature reached the therapeutic range when the ultrasound was used directly over the anatomical area rather than when given under water.

Pulsed application is a method of administering ultrasound waves whereby the energy produced is intermittent. The purpose is to produce the mechanical, non-thermal reactions of ultrasound by allowing for rest periods and subsequent cooling (Prentice 1986). However, evidence is lacking that the non-thermal effects produced by pulsing have any advantage over the similar results produced by the continuous method (Lehmann & de Lateur 1982b).

MUSCULOSKELETAL CONDITIONS

General indications and contraindications for ultrasound use in muskuloskeletal conditions are the same as for therapeutic heat. Additional precautions include ultrasound over laminectomy sites, the heart, brain, cervical ganglia, tumours, acute haemorrhage sites, pacemakers, infection sites and fluid-filled cavities such as the eyes (Basford 1998). In general, ultrasound may be effective as a therapeutic modality in subacute and chronic inflammation (Hayes 1984). Pain control may occur by both thermal and non-thermal effects. Various studies have shown alteration in nerve conduction velocity after diathermy application, with the changes appearing to be related to energy intensity of the ultrasound field (Madsen & Gersten 1961; Zankel 1966; Currier et al. 1978; Halle et al. 1981). By altering the conduction velocity, analgesic effects may occur.

Studies have also documented increased levels of cortisol following ultrasound application to peripheral nerves. This release may provide increased anti-inflammatory effects (Griffin et al. 1965). However, Gnatz (1989) found that ultrasound applied to the backs of two patients with documented lumbar disc herniation caused increased pain in a radicular pattern. Thus, any pain-relieving effects secondary to cortisol release may be overcome by the increased oedema due to the deep heating effects of ultrasound. Conflicting results have also occurred with the use of ultrasound as a diagnostic technique in the evaluation of lumbosacral nerve root irritation. Cole and Gossman (1980) concluded that ultrasound application over an irritated nerve root provoked pain radiation, providing diagnostically useful results, whereas Reid et al. (1989) concluded that due to the low sensitivity, sonation of the lumbar nerve roots in patients with sciatica was not useful as a screening test for nerve irritation secondary to disc disease.

The literature is filled with uncontrolled, non-randomized studies that show only modest benefit of ultrasound for musculoskeletal disorders

(Tiidus 1999; Baker *et al.* 2001; Robertson & Baker 2001). A closer look at just the randomized, controlled studies, however, failed to produce convincing evidence of the efficacy of ultrasound (van der Windt *et al.* 1999).

Gam *et al.* (1998) studied the effects of ultrasound, massage and exercise in 58 patients with neck and shoulder myofascial trigger points in a randomized, controlled study. The first group received all three treatments, the second group received massage, exercise and sham ultrasound, and the third group was a control group receiving no treatment. Both of the treatment groups had significantly improved numbers of myofascial trigger points compared with the non-treated control group, but there was no difference between the therapeutic ultrasound and the sham ultrasound groups.

Van der Heijden *et al.* (1999) studied 180 patients with soft tissue shoulder disorders in a randomized, blinded, controlled trial comparing bipolar interferential electrotherapy with ultrasound as adjuvants to a supervised exercise programme. All 180 subjects received exercise therapy; 73 subjects received active treatments, 72 subjects received dummy ultrasound and interferential electrotherapy, and 35 subjects received no adjuvants. At the 6-week and 12-month follow-ups, the ultrasound and electrotherapy groups had received no additional benefit above the exercise programme alone. Crawford and Snaith (1996) found no difference between ultrasound and sham ultrasound in patients with plantar heel pain. There is conflicting evidence whether ultrasound may be beneficial for delayed-onset muscle soreness (Hasson *et al.* 1990; Plaskett *et al.* 1999).

Ebenbichler *et al.* (1999) studied ultrasound therapy in 54 patients with radiographically confirmed calcific rotator cuff tendinitis in a randomized, double-blinded, sham-controlled study. Thirty-two shoulders were treated with ultrasound and 29 shoulders were treated with sham ultrasound five times a week for the first 3 weeks, then three times a week for the following 3 weeks. At 6 weeks, the treatment group reported greater improvement in pain and quality of life; however, there was no significant difference at the 9-month follow-up. Interestingly, 42% of the ultrasound-treated shoulders demonstrated resolution of calcium deposits and 23% showed improvement. In contrast, the sham group showed calcium deposit resolution in only 8% and improvement in only 12% of subjects ($P = 0.002$). Perron and Malouin (1997) did not, however, find improvement with ultrasound and acetic acid iontophoresis above the control for their smaller group of 22 patients with calcific shoulder tendinitis. Nykanen (1995) also found no benefit in using ultrasound over sham ultrasound in 72 inpatients with shoulder pain in a randomized, double-blinded, sham-controlled study. Downing and Weinstein (1986) also found no benefit from ultrasound in subacromial bursitis in a double-blinded, sham-controlled study.

Tiidus (1999) reviewed the literature and found little data to support the use of ultrasound for postexercise muscle damage.

There is some evidence to suggest that ultrasound may hasten the healing of bone and tendon. Kristiansen *et al.* (1997) studied 61 distal radius fractures in a multicentre, prospective, randomized, double-blind clinical trial comparing low intensity non-thermal pulsed ultrasound versus a placebo device. The ultrasound group experienced significantly faster radiographic fracture healing (mean of 61 days in the treatment group vs 98 days in the placebo group). Ramirez *et al.* (1997) performed work with ultrasound and Achilles tendon injuries of neonatal rats to suggest that ultrasound stimulates collagen synthesis in tendon fibroblasts and stimulates cell division during phases of rapid cell growth. Jackson *et al.* (1991) also found that ultrasound facilitated the rate of rat Achilles tendon repair by promoting synthesis of collagen which also proved to have a greater breaking strength. Enwemeka (1989) found similar increased tensile strength in the Achilles tendons of rabbits that were treated with ultrasound.

Binder *et al.* (1986) reported statistically significant results studying 38 patients having ultrasound (1 MHz, 1–2 W·cm^{-2}) versus 38 patients receiving sham ultrasound for lateral epicondylosis. Twenty-four subjects in the treatment group compared with only 11 in the sham group reported satisfactory results. Other studies evaluating ultrasound as treatment for lateral epicondylosis do not show statistically significant improvement (Halle *et al.* 1986; Lundeberg *et al.* 1988; Haker & Lundeberg 1991; Vasseljen 1992; Pienimaki *et al.* 1996).

Gam and Johannsen (1995) and van der Windt *et al.* (1999) reviewed well-designed trials evaluating ultrasound therapy and concluded that there is little evidence to show efficacy in the treatment of musculoskeletal disorders. Taking the available literature as a whole, there is evidence to support improved tendon and bone healing and only little evidence suggesting a modest benefit of ultrasound in rotator cuff calcific tendonitis and lateral epicondylosis.

Phonophoresis

Phonophoresis is sometimes used as a therapeutic modality in the rehabilitation of sports injuries. There are few good controlled studies documenting the clinical effectiveness of phonophoresis. Griffin showed that it is possible to drive a cortisol ointment onto pig skin *in situ* and to drive it into underlying muscle with ultrasonic energy using levels within the clinical range (Griffin & Touchstone 1963). Newman *et al.* (1958) reported that hypospray injection of cortisol followed by local application of ultrasonic energy showed an improvement in symptoms of shoulder bursitis compared with ultrasound used alone. Davick *et al.* (1988) demonstrated that ultrasonically treated topical application of tritiated cortisol can lead to significant increases in cortisol penetration beyond the stratum corneum and into the viable epidermis as compared with topical cortisol alone. They concluded that once beyond the stratum corneum, the cortisol may penetrate over time and be absorbed into the deep soft tissue structures.

In Kleinkort and Wood's (1975) retrospective study of 285 patients treated for a variety of common inflammatory conditions, phonophoresis using 10% hydrocortisone demonstrated better subjective and objective outcomes as compared with phonophoresis using 1% hydrocortisone.

Klaiman *et al.* (1998) studied phonophoresis versus ultrasound in 49 patients with various soft tissue injuries in a randomized, double-blinded, uncontrolled trial. Each group had treatments three times a week for 3 weeks; each group had decreased pain levels at the end of 3 weeks, but there was no significant difference between the groups.

In summary, ultrasonic energy in conjunction with topical hydrocortisone may produce some anti-inflammatory effect, possibly related to the use of ultrasound alone and in part as a result of the penetration of cortisone.

Therapeutic electricity

The use of therapeutic electricity dates back many centuries. One of the earliest accounts of the use of electricity for a musculoskeletal problem occurred in 1747 when a man with rheumatoid arthritis and involvement of the small joint in his hands received marked relief of his pain symptoms through the use of electricity (Licht 1983). Today, different forms of therapeutic electricity are used in the treatment of musculoskeletal and sports injuries. Electric currents are used to promote healing of injured tissue, to stimulate muscles, to stimulate sensory nerves in treating pain or to create an electrical field on the skin surface to drive ions beneficial to the healing process into or through the skin. This section describes different forms of therapeutic electricity, the scientific basis for their use, their indications and contraindications, briefly describes the techniques used in their applications, and elaborates on their use in sports medicine. Electrical devices can put out either alternating current (AC or faradic), which is the form usually found in household appliances, or direct current (DC or galvanic), which is found in a generator or battery. Direct current can be continuous or intermittent, and can have different waveforms, frequencies, duration and amplitudes. Adjustments in any or all of these parameters will have an effect on the quality, type and form of stimulation received by the patient. Details of these parameters can be found in the cited texts (Prentice 1986).

It is important to note that the responses muscle and nerve have to electricity vary. Nerve tissue accommodates rapidly to current. Nerve stimulation requires a current which rises rapidly to maximum intensity. High frequencies and short durations are used. Motor nerves respond to 25 cycles·s⁻¹ and 500 μs or shorter of stimulus duration. Sensory nerves respond to 100–150 cycles·s⁻¹ and 100 μs or shorter stimulus duration. Muscle tissue does not accommodate as rapidly. Muscle can be stimulated with very slowly rising currents. Lower frequency and longer duration stimuli are used in stimulating muscle as compared with nerve. The various forms of therapeutic electricity include TENS, muscle electrical stimulation, percutaneous electrical nerve stimulation, iontophoresis and interferential current.

Electrical stimulation to promote tissue healing

Medical galvanism, or the use of galvanic stimulation, uses direct current modalities that deliver a unidirectional, uninterrupted current flow within the tolerance of the patient and without the destruction of tissue. The action of direct current on the body is primarily chemical. This type of modality can be used to directly stimulate muscle following a nerve injury, to produce ionic changes within the tissues and to decrease oedema; or it can be used to introduce topically applied medications into the skin, when it is termed iontophoresis (Hillman & Delforge 1985). The purpose of this electrical stimulation is primarily for the vasomotor effects, i.e. increased circulation. These effects are most often seen in resolution of inflammation, relief of pain and reduction of interstitial oedema through electro-osmosis and the shifting of water toward the electrical cathode (Prentice 1986). Motor nerves are not stimulated by a steady flow of direct stimulation. The sensations experienced result in part

from accumulation of ions in the skin under the electrodes, which act as a physiological stimulus to the sensory nerve endings, producing reflex vasodilatation (Marino 1986).

Direct, uninterrupted electric current tends to be quite uncomfortable and may cause superficial skin burns. For this reason, a modification of the technique has been developed whereby the current is applied in an alternating or 'pulsed' manner, termed high-voltage pulsed galvanic stimulation (HVPGS). Although the main use of HVPGS in sports rehabilitation is for relief of pain, it can also be used to aid in tissue healing (Ross & Segal 1981). Electrically induced muscle contraction, such as that obtained with direct current or HVPGS, can be used to duplicate regular muscle contractions. These contractions help stimulate circulation by pumping blood through venous and lymphatic channels after acute injuries, when fluid accumulation is significant. Intermittent muscle contraction, which permits increased blood flow, may also produce relaxation of the muscles. Electrical stimulation of muscle contractions can allow resolution of inflammatory fluid, while keeping an injured joint protected. In order to be successful in reducing swelling, the current intensity must be high enough to provide a strong, comfortable muscle contraction, therefore interrupted or surge-type pulses must be used (Prentice 1986).

There are a number of contraindications to the use of electrical current in sports rehabilitation. Contraindications of electrical therapy include stimulation over cardiac pacemakers, electrical implants, carotid sinus, epiglottis, abdomen and gravid uterus (Basford 1998). Treatment should be avoided over any area that is anaesthetic to avoid local burns. Recent scars in the area to be treated should also be avoided because of the potential for wound dehiscence. Any area where metal is embedded close to the skin in the area to be treated should be avoided for fear of concentrating the heat source at the metal surface. Any form of electricity should be avoided near an area of acute injury if active bleeding is still present to prevent worsening of the haemorrhage.

Iontophoresis: driving ions with electrical stimulation

Iontophoresis uses direct current to drive medicinal ions locally into the skin and mucous membranes. Ions of the medicinal compounds are absorbed subcutaneously. This absorption occurs slowly into the local soft tissue, while some is ultimately absorbed systemically. Evidence for penetration much beyond the skin is variable and may depend on the particular substance (O'Malley & Oester 1955). James *et al.* (1986) showed that percutaneous iontophoresis of 1% prednisolone sodium phosphate through human skin and nails gives peak plasma levels of about one-third that produced by oral ingestion of 10 mg prednisolone. Similarly, Zankel *et al.* (1959) showed that the absorption of the negative ion I through unbroken skin only occurred in those conditions which included iontophoresis. Bertolucci (1982), in a double-blind study, found that patients below the age of 45 years with shoulder dysfunction related to primary tendonitis responded well to iontophoresis steroid administration, whereas the placebo group received no benefit from the iontophoretic treatment with sodium chloride. However, Chantraine *et al.* (1986), in studies done both *in vivo* and *in vitro* failed to demonstrate the transcutaneous migration of corticosteroids with iontophoresis.

Iontophoresis has been used to drive multiple substances into the skin, some of which include calcium chloride, hydrocortisone, lithium chloride, lidocaine and acetic acid. Acetic acid theoretically replaces carbonate in calcium carbonate to become calcium acetate, which is blood soluble, thereby leaching the calcium away from the site of bony spur and inflammation. Japour *et al.* (1999) reported very encouraging results using acetic acid iontophoresis in 35 patients with chronic heel pain in an uncontrolled case series. Ninety-four per cent of patients reported relief of heel pain, after an average of only 5.7 sessions, over an average 2.8-week treatment period. Pain scores decreased from 7.5 to 1.8, which continued to be low at 0.64 at the 27-month follow-up.

Without a control group, however, it is not known whether these encouraging results are from treatment effect or the natural course of heel pain.

Perron and Malouin (1997) did not, however, find improvement with ultrasound and acetic acid iontophorosis above the control in their small group of 22 patients with calcific shoulder tendinitis. Gudeman *et al.* (1997) studied 0.4% dexamethasone iontophoresis in the treatment of 40 feet with plantar fasciitis in a randomized, double-blinded, placebo-controlled trial. After six treatments over 2 weeks, the treatment group significantly improved, but were no different than placebo at the 1-month follow-up. Taniguchi *et al.* (1995) reported a significantly increased pain threshold in 30 healthy volunteers with clonidine iontophoresis, as compared with amitriptyline and imipramine iontophoresis; the clinical implications of this finding are not known. Hasson *et al.* (1992) studied 18 females with delayed-onset muscle soreness with dexamethasone iontophoresis, placebo iontophoresis and no treatment. Perceived muscle soreness was significantly less in the treatment group 48 h later, but no change in strength was noted.

The clinical effectiveness of iontophoresis is still debatable. Some of the claimed benefits for pain relief may be due to the effects of the direct current used as opposed to the medicinal compounds purportedly driven into the circulation. Few side effects have been described other than drug sensitivity and sensitive skin.

Electrical stimulation of muscle

Electrical stimulation of muscle is accomplished with either direct or alternating current, or a combination of the two. Alternating current is usually preferred to direct current because of greater patient comfort (Hillman & Delforge 1985). Muscles are stimulated for one of four reasons. The first is to aid in muscle pumping for oedema reduction and tissue healing as described in the previous section. The other reasons include re-educating muscle, retarding atrophy in immobilized or partially denervated muscle and enhancing strength.

Certain general principles need to be adhered to when performing electrical stimulation of muscle (Stillwell 1982). Good contact should be maintained between the skin and the electrodes. The active electrode should be placed over the motor point of the muscle. The two electrodes used should generally be placed on the same side of the body. Finally, since denervated muscle does not have a motor point, the active electrode may be placed at the point that gives the best motor response, or the two electrodes may be placed one at each end of the muscle so that the current will pass through the muscle and stimulate all of it.

MUSCLE RE-EDUCATION

Electrical muscle stimulation can be used for muscular re-education after sports injuries (Amrein et al. 1971). Muscular inhibition is quite common after traumatic injuries or surgery. Central nervous system inhibition is often the cause, as muscle contraction causes pain. This then causes decreased contraction and ultimate immobilization of the affected muscle. The injured patient or athlete may have a difficult time initiating contraction of an injured muscle because of the pain associated with movement and the lack of sensory input from that muscle due to disuse. Forcing the muscle to contract causes an increase in the sensory input from the muscle, allowing the patient to see the muscle contract, and then attempt to duplicate this muscular response (Prentice 1986). The focus of this type of training is on kinetic training and the sensory awareness of muscular contraction. For muscle re-education to occur, the current intensity must be adequate for a muscle contraction, but not too uncomfortable for the athlete. HVPGS or high-frequency alternating current may be most effective (Prentice 1986). Although the clinical implications are not clear, electrical muscle stimulation has been shown to selectively increase strength when applied to the abdominal muscles (Alon et al. 1987), triceps brachii (Snyder-Mackler et al. 1988) and erector spinae (Kahanovitz et al. 1987). Improved motor performance was demonstrated in the deltoid and pectoralis major

(Fleury & Lagasse 1979) and in the abductor hallicis (LeDoux & Quinones 1981).

RETARDATION OF MUSCLE ATROPHY

Electrical muscle stimulation may help prevent strength losses (Eriksson & Haggmark 1979; Godfrey et al. 1979; Gould et al. 1979; Grove-Lainey et al. 1983; Morrissey et al. 1985; Wigerstad-Lossing et al. 1988; Delitto et al. 1989; Snyder-Mackler 1990; Abdel-Moty et al. 1994), as well as prevent muscular atrophy (Eriksson & Haggmark 1979; Morrissey et al. 1985; Nitz & Dobner 1987; Wigerstad-Lossing et al. 1988), which occur when a limb is immobilized. Stanish et al. (1982) and Eriksson et al. (1981) have shown that the biomechanical changes occurring in the muscles of immobilized limbs are retarded by electrical muscle stimulation. Eriksson and Haggmark (1979) showed better muscle function in a group of patients after reconstruction of the anterior cruciate ligament when treated with electrical muscle stimulation and isometric exercise than with isometric exercise alone. However, Halbach and Straus (1980) examined isokinetic only and electrical stimulation only exercise programmes and found that the isokinetic workload was greater than the electrical stimulation workload after 3 weeks of training and stimulation.

In general, it is agreed that electrical muscle stimulation programmes are more effective than no exercise programme, but no more effective than traditional strengthening exercise programmes (Currier et al. 1979; Halbach & Straus 1980; Kramer & Mendryk 1982; Currier & Mann 1983; Kramer & Semple 1983; Laughman et al. 1983; McMiken et al. 1983; Kubiak et al. 1987; Lieber et al. 1996). Snyder-Mackler et al. (1995) showed there may be some functional benefit from using high-intensity muscle stimulation in addition to an exercise programme. They studied 110 patients following anterior cruciate ligament reconstruction and randomized them to receive high-intensity neuromuscular electrical stimulation, high-level volitional exercise, low-intensity neuromuscular electrical stimulation, or combined high- and low-intensity neuromuscular

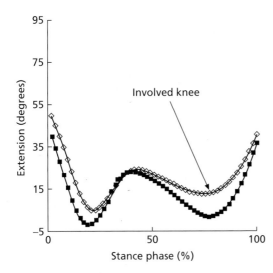

Fig. 10.2 Graph of the kinematics of the knee in the sagittal plane, showing a lack of extension of the involved knee during stance. (From Snyder-Mackler *et al.* 1995, with permission.)

stimulation in addition to a standard closed kinetic chain strengthening programme. At 4 weeks, the high-intensity stimulation group enjoyed the best quadriceps strength gains of 70% of the uninvolved side, as opposed to 57% in the high-level volitional exercise group. With knee joint kinematic analysis, the high-intensity stimulation group showed significantly more normal knee flexion–extension sagittal plane excursions during the stance phase when compared with the other groups (Fig. 10.2). However, long-term benefits and other functional outcomes were not studied.

In order to improve strength under any circumstances, either electrically stimulating muscle or through voluntary contraction, maximal or near maximal contractions must occur to the point of muscle fatigue. The discomfort of the stimulation remains a major limitation (Currier 1991). Most research to date indicates that, with few exceptions, maximal contractile forces can be produced by voluntary contractions (Singer *et al.* 1989).

Also, while electrical stimulation retards denervation atrophy, its effect depends on the pulse duration, the frequency and intensity of the current, the placement of the stimulating electrode, the duration and number of treatment sessions, the rest periods between the treatment sessions and the resting length of the muscle during stimulation. Further discussions of all these parameters are beyond the scope of this chapter, but are well described by Licht (1983). Gibson *et al.* (1988) suggest that electrical stimulation seems to prevent the fall in muscle protein synthesis that is related to immobility. Cabric *et al.* (1987) found that lower frequency electrical stimulation (50 Hz) of muscle increased muscle fibre size, which was thought to be correlated to the proliferation of muscle cell nuclei.

MUSCLE STRENGTH GAINS

Increasing the strength of a muscle can be accomplished by repeated maximal or submaximal contractions of that muscle. The rationale behind the strength enhancement is that electrical stimulation can either increase the maximum contractile force in the muscle, or that it can recruit more fibres to contract with a given stimulus, thereby enhancing the strength of contraction (Singer *et al.* 1989). When done via electrical stimulation, tetanic contractions, which are achieved at pulse rates above 20–30 per second, are required for maximum muscle contraction. Electrical stimulation is achieved by stimulating the motor nerve to a muscle by means of electrodes placed on the skin. Most of the research done with muscle stimulation for strength gains has been done with electrical stimulation in the isometric mode. Because of the many variables of stimulation of muscle—including frequency, duration, pulse shape, intensity and charge—no studies exist that compare the effectiveness of these variables in inducing effective strength-improving muscle contractions (Singer *et al.* 1989).

Significant strength gains in normal muscles have been described by Kots (1977). Kots' 'Russian' stimulation used an alternating-type current of high pulse rate and high intensity to produce strong, involuntary muscle contractions with associated stimulation of local blood flow (Hillman & Delforge 1985). The actual benefit of such a programme is questionable as similar results have not been duplicated. To date, there are no good studies to warrant electrical stimulation for gaining strength in normal muscle.

There has also been some suggestion that neuromuscular electrical stimulation can help in controlling oedema after injury (Gould *et al.* 1979; Lake 1989; Griffin *et al.* 1990). Hsueh *et al.* (1997) studied 60 patients with upper trapezius myofascial trigger points in a randomized, placebo-controlled trial. They found electrical muscle stimulation significantly improved immediate cervical range of motion over the placebo and electrical nerve stimulation groups. The electrical nerve stimulation group, however, showed significantly decreased immediate pain scores when compared with the other two groups. Pope *et al.* (1994) showed no statistical difference in physical measures in a randomized trial of 164 patients with subacute low back pain who received 3 weeks of electrical muscle stimulation, manual manipulation, massage or corset wearing.

In summary, the literature suggests that electrical muscle stimulation may be helpful in strengthening normal muscle, preventing loss of muscle bulk and strength associated with immobilization, selective strengthening, enhancing motor control and controlling oedema after injury (Lake 1992).

Electrical stimulation of nerves

The use of alternating and direct current for pain reduction via nerve stimulation is commonly used in the rehabilitation of sports injuries. The goal of nerve stimulation is to stimulate sensory nerves to change the patient's perception of a painful stimulus coming from an injured area. Nerves, being more sensitive to electric current than muscle, are usually stimulated at a high frequency and short duration. Three theories have been put forward to explain the analgesic effects of electrical stimulation—the gate-control theory, the central biasing theory and the opiate pain control theory.

Melzack and Wall (1965) proposed the gate-control theory in 1965. It postulates that when large-diameter afferent nerve fibres are electrically stimulated, painful stimuli arriving at the spinal cord through small fibres at the dorsal horn are blocked from transmission to the central nervous system where pain is perceived. By stimulating the large fibres, the 'gate' to allowing further impulses to be transmitted centrally is closed.

The central biasing theory also uses the idea of gating impulses. In this model, intense stimulation of smaller fibres (C fibres or pain fibres) at peripheral sites, for short periods, causes stimulation of the descending neurones, which then affects transmission of pain information by closing the gate at the spinal cord level (Prentice 1986).

The opiate pain control theory is premised on the fact that endogenous opiate enkephalins and β-endorphins exist in our systems. Electrical stimulation of sensory nerves may stimulate the release of these compounds from local sites throughout the central nervous system, causing pain relief.

TRANSCUTANEOUS ELECTRICAL NERVE STIMULATION (TENS)

TENS is usually defined as the application of an electric current therapy through the skin to a peripheral nerve or nerves for the control of pain (Singer *et al.* 1989). TENS units are very commonly used in sports rehabilitation (Roeser *et al.* 1976). There are a number of advantages of using TENS, including that it is comfortable, fast-acting, can be used in many types of pain problems, and can be used continuously. The disadvantages are that the carry-over is often variable and adaptations may need to be made for continued benefit, i.e. increasing the pulse width or amplitude.

There are two major forms of TENS—high frequency and low frequency. High-frequency TENS stimulates sensory nerves and causes an increase in pain threshold, although it does not stimulate the release of endorphins. Low-frequency TENS will cause pain relief, which can be blocked by administration of opiate antagonists, implicating the opiate theory of pain control. It is sometimes likened to acupuncture. Walsh *et al.* (1995) found that low-frequency TENS (4 Hz) was the best in decreasing immediate pain visual analogue scores for ischaemically induced pain in a randomized, double-blinded, controlled trial of 32 subjects comparing 4 Hz TENS, 110 Hz TENS, placebo and no treatment. When applying electrodes for either type of TENS, electrodes may be placed on or around the painful area, over specific dermatomes, myotomes or sclerotomes that correspond to the painful area, close to the spinal cord segment that innervates an area that is painful, or over trigger or acupuncture points.

The efficacy of TENS is not clear-cut (Licht 1983; Robinson 1996). Although it has been argued that blinding for TENS studies may be difficult to truly achieve (Deyo *et al.* 1990b), few studies have been done in a double-blind manner (Gersh 1978; Robinson 1996). Thorsteinsson *et al.* (1977) studied 93 patients with various disorders in a double-blind, randomized, sham-controlled, cross-over study. Forty-nine per cent of the TENS group versus 32% of the sham group reported partial or complete pain relief, but this difference was not statistically significant.

Ordog (1987) studied 100 patients with acute traumatic disorders—including sprains, fractures and contusions—in a randomized study comparing four groups: active TENS plus acetaminophen/codeine, sham TENS plus acetaminophen/codeine, active TENS and sham TENS. Pain levels in 2 days dropped 63% in the active TENS plus drug, 58% in the sham TENS plus drug, 45% in the active TENS, and 17% in the sham TENS groups. There was no statistical difference between the active TENS and the sham TENS plus drug groups suggesting that TENS may be as effective as acetaminophen/codeine for acute traumatic disorders.

Lehmann *et al.* (1986) studied 54 patients with chronic low back pain in a randomized study of active subthreshold TENS, sham TENS or electroacupuncture. They found that although all groups improved from baseline, there were no statistically significant differences between the groups at 6 months.

Deyo *et al.* (1990a) studied 145 volunteers with chronic low back pain in a randomized trial comparing four groups: active TENS, sham TENS, active TENS with exercise and sham TENS with exercise. At 8 weeks following the 4-week treatment period, there were no significant differences between the active TENS groups and the sham TENS groups.

Marchand *et al.* (1993) studied 43 patients with chronic low back pain in a randomized sham TENS (placebo) and no intervention ('nocebo') controlled study. Immediately after two treatments of 30 min each, the active TENS group showed a 43% reduction of pain intensity as compared with a 17% reduction in the sham TENS group—this finding was statistically significant. Active TENS patients maintained significantly decreased pain intensity scores at 1 week as compared with sham TENS patients. Both sham and active TENS groups' pain intensity scores were significantly better than the no treatment group at the 3- and 6-month follow-ups, but there was no statistically significant difference between the sham TENS and active TENS groups.

Herman *et al.* (1994) studied 58 work-related acute low back injuries of 3–10 weeks duration in a randomized study of active TENS versus sham TENS. Both groups received the same exercise programme. Outcome measures showed the active TENS group produced a drop in visual analogue pain scores immediately after TENS but showed no difference in disability, return to work rates or pain scores at the 4-week follow-up.

Jensen *et al.* (1985) showed that a group of patients treated with TENS following arthroscopic surgery experienced less pain, required less narcotics and regained strength more quickly than the control group. Sluka *et al.* (1998) showed that high-intensity TENS was more effective in providing immediate pain relief than low-intensity TENS for induced knee pain following injection.

Some studies have shown that TENS may provide short-term relief for delayed-onset muscle soreness (Denegar & Huff 1988; Denegar *et al.* 1989; Denegar & Perrin 1992), but others have not (Craig *et al.* 1996). TENS can also be helpful for postoperative pain (Smith *et al.* 1983; Cornell *et al.* 1984; Jensen *et al.* 1985; Arvidsson & Eriksson 1986; Carrol & Badura 2001).

Overall, clinical experiences seem to show that TENS appears to give the best benefit in the treatment of early postoperative pain or pain from acute injuries; however, the response can be variable, unpredictable and short lived. There are no good studies to prove the benefits of TENS in chronic pain problems. It appears that TENS is not harmful, may sometimes provide pain relief above the placebo response, is more effective in acute pain relief with short-term benefit, and is more effective at higher stimulation intensities (Robinson 1996).

No serious complications have been observed from the use of TENS (Licht 1983). Hypersensitivity of the skin has been observed in up to 10% of patients, either due to the electrode or the electrode jelly. Minor burns were observed when high-frequency stimulation and high-intensity stimulation were used at the same time. TENS should not be used in patients with pacemakers, stimulation should not be applied over the carotid sinus, and it should probably not be used during pregnancy, as the effects are unknown (Singer *et al.* 1989).

INTERFERENTIAL CURRENT

Interferential current is another type of electrical stimulation that is used to control pain. Electric signals from two sets of electrodes with the same waveform are applied so that they arrive at the point to be stimulated from two directions. The area where the current overlaps is called the interference pattern, and the intensity summates in a manner that can be effective in modifying pain (Singer *et al.* 1989). The frequency obtained at the interference pattern, through cancellation of some waveforms, allows stimulation of local muscle and nerve at a greater depth than if applied only from the surface at that point. Thus, interferential current uses high-frequency carrier circuits to afford deeper penetration. The main use of interferential currents in sports is for pain reduction.

PERCUTANEOUS ELECTRICAL NERVE STIMULATION (PENS)

PENS combines the therapeutic effects of TENS and electroacupuncture by placing small-gauge needles (32 gauge) 2–4 cm into soft tissues and muscles in a dermatomal distribution, with subsequent stimulation with electrical impulses (< 25 mA) at a frequency of around 4 Hz. Ghoname *et al.* (1999b) investigated the efficacy of PENS. They studied 60 patients with stable chronic non-radicular low back pain from radiographically confirmed degenerative disc disease in a randomized, single-blinded, sham-controlled, cross-over study. Each subject received all of the following four treatments in a randomized order: sham PENS, PENS, TENS and exercise. Sham PENS consisted of needle placement but no electrical stimulation. Exercise only consisted of one exercise where the patient performed spinal flexion and extension while sitting in a chair. At 24 h, the PENS group showed significant improvements on pain, activity, sleep, sense of well being and narcotic usage scores as compared with the other three groups. Ninety-one per cent identified the PENS treatment as the preferred pain therapy and 81% identified it as a treatment for which they would be willing to pay extra. Ghoname *et al.* (1999a) also found that a stimulus frequency of 15–30 Hz is more effective than 4 or 100 Hz.

There are numerous potential uses of therapeutic electricity in the rehabilitation of sports injuries. The most common indications are for stimulation of muscle to retard atrophy, to aid in tissue healing and muscle re-education, the stimulation of nerves for pain modification, and to drive ions through the skin for their medicinal effects (Table 10.2).

Traction

Traction is the technique in which a distractive force is applied to a part of the body to stretch soft tissues and to separate joint surfaces or bone fragments (Hinterbucher 1985). Cyriax popularized traction in the 1950s as a treatment for

Table 10.2 Types of therapeutic electricity and typical uses.

• Alternating current or faradic stimulation	Muscle re-education
• Direct current or galvanic stimulation	Retard muscle atrophy
• High-voltage pulsed galvanic stimulation	Improve muscle strength
• Iontophoresis	Pain control
• Transcutaneous electrical nerve stimulation	Pain control
• Percutaneous electrical nerve stimulation	Pain control
• Interferential current	Pain control

lumbar disc lesions. Prior to that, traction was mainly used in the treatment of fractures. Over the years, traction has gained some popularity in the field of sports rehabilitation, particularly with respect to cervical and lumbosacral spine injuries.

Cervical traction

Cervical traction is used for a number of types of injuries of the cervical spine including cervical herniated nucleus pulposus, radiculopathy, strains, zygapophyseal joint syndromes and myofascial pain. The main reason for its use is relief of pain. Pain relief may occur through one of several mechanisms, including rest through immobilization and support of the head, distraction of the zygapophyseal joints and associated improved nutrition to the articular cartilage, tightening of the longitudinal ligament and decreasing the intradiscal pressure. The last two both press a bulging disc more centrally, relieving nerve root pressure via increased foraminal diameter, improving head posture, and elongating muscles to improve blood flow and reduce spasm.

Determination as to whether the patient has any contraindications is the first step in administering traction of the cervical spine. Contraindications to the use of spinal traction include an unstable spine, ligamentous instability, vertebrobasilar artery insufficiency, atlantoaxial instability, rheumatoid arthritis, osteomyelitis, discitis, neoplasm, severe osteoporosis, untreated hypertension, severe anxiety, cauda equina syndrome and myelopathy (Rechtein *et al.* 1998). Clinically, the examiner can first try manual traction with

the patient for a few minutes to see what kind of therapeutic response they can expect with traction.

To achieve separation of the spinal segments, a force of significant magnitude and duration must be exerted. Traction can be delivered manually, through weights and pulleys or via a mechanical device. The direction of pull can be vertical, horizontal or at an angle. Traction can be performed while the patient is standing, sitting, lying on a horizontal or inclined plane, or in the prone or supine position. Traction can be continuous, sustained, intermittent or intermittent/pulsed. Surface resistance to traction is dependent on the weight of the body or body segment undergoing traction and the size, quality, contour and texture of the two surfaces in contact (Hinterbucher 1985).

With cervical traction, the optimal angle of pull to obtain the most distractive force with the least weight is at 20–30° of head flexion (Fig. 10.3). The supine position may be more effective than sitting, as it allows more relaxation. In the supine position the force must be sufficient enough to overcome friction and must have a pull that is at least half the weight of the head; 3.6–4.5 kg is a usual starting point. In sitting, the pull must be sufficient to support the head; usually 11–18 kg is necessary.

Cervical traction can be continuous or intermittent. Continuous traction will allow quieting of the stretch reflex and decrease muscle guarding. It will also allow separation of the posterior structures (zygapophyseal joints) if maintained for at least 7 s at a time. Intermittent traction is believed to act by cyclically causing muscle contraction and relaxation, thereby increasing blood flow in a 'massage-like' action.

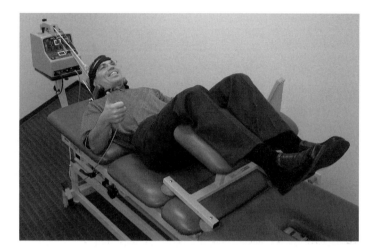

Fig. 10.3 Cervical traction mechanical unit.

Goldie and Landquist (1970) carried out a blind study of patients with cervical pain, using traction, exercise and control groups. Results showed no difference between the three groups, although there were a somewhat larger number of improved patients among those who were subjected to traction. Zylbergold and Piper (1985) studied 100 patients with disorders of the cervical spine in a randomized, controlled trial comparing static traction, intermittent traction, manual traction and no traction. At 6 weeks, all groups improved significantly compared with baseline, but the intermittent traction group scored significantly better than the no traction group in pain and cervical range of motion measures. Swezey *et al.* (1999) showed that 81% of their 58 patients with cervical spondylosis had symptomatic relief with home cervical traction in a retrospective, uncontrolled study.

Lumbar traction

The traction load necessary to produce vertebral separation in the lumbar spine is much greater than that required to produce vertebral separation in the cervical spine. De Seze and Levernieux (1951) estimated that a tractive force of 330 kg was required to obtain a separation of 1.5 mm at the L4/5 vertebral level and that 365 kg were required to obtain a separation of 2 mm at the L3/4 level. Numerous other studies discuss the

great amount of force necessary to obtain separation of even a small amount in the lumbar spine (Frazer 1954; Lawson & Godfrey 1958). Therefore, clinically, lumbar traction functions to limit the activity of the patient. It may assist to decrease muscle spasm by forcing rest. There is no evidence that lumbar traction facilitates nuclear migration of the disc.

Lumbar traction is set up in a similar manner to cervical traction except that a corset rather than a head halter is used. Various types of lumbar traction are described including gravity inversion traction, gravity lumbar reduction and autotraction. Inversion traction must be avoided in patients with hypertension or retinal problems because of the potential for increasing blood and retinal pressures. Generally, at least one-quarter of the bodyweight must be used just to overcome the friction of lumbar traction. The maximum force that a patient can tolerate is often used (Hinterbucher 1985).

Although ample experimental evidence that a traction force of sufficient magnitude and duration applied to the spine produces separation of the vertebrae and zygapophyseal joints and increases the size of the foramen, no clear scientific evidence of its therapeutic value has been reported in the few controlled studies to date (Hinterbucher 1985). Christie's (1955) controlled study of traction in the treatment of acute and chronic lumbar pain—with and without root signs—showed that traction, when effective, was most useful in patients with chronic backaches with root signs. Weber's (1973) double-blinded, controlled study of patients with sciatica from a prolapsed disc treated with traction or simulated traction failed to show any significant difference in pain, mobility of the lumbar spine or the presence of neurological signs in either group. Beurskens *et al.* (1997) studied 151 patients with non-specific low back pain in a randomized, sham-controlled trial which showed no difference between the treatment and control groups. Van der Heijden *et al.* (1995) reviewed only randomized clinical trials studying traction. Beneficial effects of lumbar traction were suggested in only three of 14 randomized studies and in only one of the 11 studies that the authors considered to be of better quality. They concluded that there was no evidence to support or refute the use of traction.

Although hard data supporting the use of traction are not available, many clinicians and patients will speak of its benefits. Some of these positive experiences may be related to enforced bed rest or the effects of some active intervention for their back complaints. Cheatle and Esterhai (1990) surveyed 369 orthopaedic surgeons and 165 physiatrists about their use of pelvic traction. Twenty-eight per cent of the responding physicians said they would prescribe traction; the chief rationale (54% of respondents) of this prescription was to ensure bed rest. Similarly, there are a lack of scientific data that traction is not physiologically sound or even harmful.

Magnetic therapy

Magnetic therapy has been used for pain relief for centuries and is replete with anecdotal successes. The strongest scientific evidence in support of the therapeutic use of magnetic fields in treating musculoskeletal disorders involves using pulsating magnetic fields of strengths over 10 G. The World Health Organization reported that there is no available evidence to show adverse effects on humans exposed to static magnetic fields up to 2 T, which is equal to 20 000 G

(United Nations Environment Programme 1987). The mechanism of action of possible therapeutic effects is unknown (Blank & Findl 1987; Ayrapetyan *et al.* 1994). Increased peripheral blood flow has been proposed as a mechanism of action by Erdman (1960), Fenn (1969) and Ross (1990). The increased blood flow may also be associated with changes in fibroblast concentration, fibrin fibres and collagen at wound sites (Goldin *et al.* 1981). Other postulates include blockage of action potentials (McLean *et al.* 1995), the role of water (Carpenter & Ayrapetyan 1994), resonance, ions, induction, subatomic magnetic field interactions, and closed electrical circuits within endothelium (Hazlewood & VanZandt 1995).

Pulsating electromagnetic field therapy has shown some promise in the treatment of osteoarthritis of the knee and spine (Miner & Markoll 1993; Trock *et al.* 1994). Trock *et al.* (1994) studied 86 subjects with knee osteoarthritis and 81 subjects with cervical spondylosis in a randomized, double-blinded, placebo-controlled trial. The group treated with pulsating electromagnetic fields (10–20 G) showed significant changes from baseline at a follow-up interval of 1 month; this change was not seen in the placebo group. Foley-Nolan *et al.* (1992) studied the use of pulsating electromagnetic therapy in acute whiplash syndrome in a double-blinded, randomized, controlled study. Twenty patients wore active pulsed electromagnetic therapy collars and 20 patients wore placebo collars for 8 h·day^{-1}. The treatment group had statistically significant improved visual analogue scales at 2 and 4 weeks compared with placebo. Pujol *et al.* (1998) randomized a small group of 30 patients to receive 40 min of real or sham current magnetic coil stimulation over localized tender body regions. Postprocedure pain scores decreased by 59% in the treatment group versus only 14% in the sham group—this finding reached statistical significance.

Non-union fracture rate healing can be improved with pulsating high magnetic fields (O'Connor *et al.* 1990; Bassett 1994). Sharrard (1990) studied electromagnetic therapy in the treatment of delayed union tibial shaft fractures using active electromagnetic stimulation units in 20 patients versus dummy control units in 25 patients. Nine subjects in the treatment group and only three subjects in the control group showed union of the fracture, which was a statistically significant finding.

There are fewer studies to support the use of static magnets placed over the skin of the affected areas. Washnis (1998) cites a multitude of studies using static magnets, but few have been randomized, double-blinded, placebo-controlled trials appearing in peer-reviewed journals (Vallbona & Richards 1999). No controlled studies have been conducted in an athletic population.

Conclusions

1 Therapeutic modalities play a small, but important, part in the rehabilitation of sports injuries. Knowledge of their indications, contraindications, methods of application and efficacy is essential if they are used.
2 Cold therapies have many applications in sports rehabilitation. Cryotherapy can be used alone in any of its application methods or in conjunction with heat in contrast baths.
3 Heat modalities work via conduction, convection or conversion. Heating can be accomplished through superficial heat modalities, such as hydrocollator packs, hydrotherapy, radiant heat, paraffin baths and fluidotherapy. Heating can also be accomplished through deeper heating modalities, such as ultrasound, phonophoresis and shortwave and microwave diathermy.
4 Therapeutic electricity can be used to promote tissue healing, to stimulate muscles, to stimulate nerves for pain reduction or to drive medicinal compounds into circulation. Stimulation of muscle fibres can be used for muscle re-education, to retard muscle atrophy or possibly to gain muscle strength. Stimulation of nerve tissue is accomplished through the use of TENS, interferential current or PENS.
5 Traction is occasionally used in sports rehabilitation, particularly with neck and low back injuries. The most useful indication for traction is with cervical injuries. The efficacy of lumbar traction is not well proven.

6 Pulsating high magnetic fields may be helpful in osteoarthritis and bone healing, but there are few data to support the use of static magnets for musculoskeletal disorders.
7 Modalities may be used as an adjunct to the rehabilitation of musculoskeletal injuries. There are no definite scientific data to strongly support their use, certainly not as a primary treatment option. They may, however, help to decrease pain and oedema to allow an exercise-based rehabilitation programme to proceed.

References

Abdel-Moty, E., Fishbain, D., Goldberg, M. *et al.* (1994) Functional electrical stimulation treatment of post-radiculopathy associated muscle weakness. *Archives of Physical Medicine and Rehabilitation* **75** (6), 680–686.

Alon, G., McCombe, S., Koutsantonis, S., Stumphauzer, L. & Burgwin, K. (1987) Comparison of the effects of electrical stimulation and exercise on abdominal musculature. *Journal of Orthopaedic and Sports Physical Therapy* **8**, 567–573.

Amrein, L., Garrett, T. & Martin, G. (1971) Use of low voltage electrotherapy and electromyography in physical therapy. *Physiotherapy Canada* **51**, 1283–1286.

Arvidsson, I. & Eriksson, E. (1986) Postoperative TENS pain relief after knee surgery: objective evaluation. *Orthopedics* **9** (10), 1346–1351.

Ayrapetyan, S., Avanesian, R. & Avetisian, T. (1994) Physiological effects of magnetic fields may be mediated through actions of the state of calcium ions in solutions. In: *Biological Effects of Electric and Magnetic Fields—Sources and Mechanisms* (Carpenter, D.O. & Ayrapetyan, S., eds). Academic Press, San Diego: 181–192.

Baker, K., Robertson, V. & Duck, F. (2001) A review of therapeutic ultrasound: biophysical effects. *Physical Therapy* **81** (7), 1351–1358.

Balmaseda, M., Fatehl, M., Koozekanani, S. & Lee, A. (1986) Ultrasound therapy: a comparative study of different coupling media. *Archives of Physical Medicine and Rehabilitation* **67**, 147–150.

Basford, J. (1998) Physical agents. In: *Rehabilitation Medicine: Principles and Practice*, 3rd edn (DeLisa, J., & Gans, B., eds). Lippencott-Raven, Philadelphia: 483–520.

Bassett, A. (1994) Therapeutic uses of electric and magnetic fields in orthopedics. In: *Geological Effect of Electric and Magnetic Fields*, Vol. 2 (Carpenter, D.O. & Ayrapetyan, S., eds). Academic Press, San Diego: 13–48.

Basur, R., Shepard, E. & Mouzas, G. (1976) A cooling method in the treatment of ankle sprains. *Practitioner* **216**, 708–711.

Bertolucci, L. (1982) Introduction of antiinflammatory drugs by iontophoresis: double blind study. *Journal of Orthopaedic and Sports Physical Therapy* **4** (2), 103–108.

Beurskens, A., de Vet, H., Koke, A. *et al.* (1997) Efficacy of traction for nonspecific low back pain. 12-week and 6-month results of a randomized clinical trial. *Spine* **22** (23), 2756–2762.

Binder, A., Hodge, G., Greenwood, A., Hazleman, B. & Page-Thomas, D. (1986) Is therapeutic ultrasound effective in treating soft tissue lesions. *British Medical Journal* **290**, 512–514.

Blank, M. & Findl, E. (1987) *Mechanistic Approaches to Interactions of Electric and Electromagnetic Fields with Living Systems*. Plenum Press, New York.

Borell, R., Henley, E., Ho, P. & Hubbell, M. (1977) Fluidotherapy: evaluation of a new heat modality. *Archives of Physical Medicine and Rehabilitation* **58**, 69–71.

Borell, R., Parker, R. & Henley, E. (1980) Comparison of *in vivo* temperatures produced by hydrotherapy, paraffin wax treatment, and fluidotherapy. *Physical Therapy* **60**, 1273–1276.

Cabric, M., Appell, H. & Resic, A. (1987) Effects of electrical stimulation of different frequencies on the myonuclei and fiber size in human muscle. *International Journal of Sports Medicine* **8** (5), 323–326.

Carpenter, D. & Ayrapetyan, S. (1994) *Biological Effects of Electric and Magnetic Fields—Sources and Mechanisms*. Academic Press, San Diego.

Carrol, E. & Badura, A. (2001) Focal intense brief transcutaneous electric nerve stimulation for treatment of radicular and postthoracotomy pain. *Archives of Physical Medicine and Rehabilitation* **82**, 262–264.

Cassidy, S. & Nielsen, D. (1992) Cardiovascular responses of healthy subjects to calisthenics performed in land versus water. *Physical Therapy* **72**, 532–538.

Chambers, R. (1969) Clinical uses of cryotherapy. *Physical Therapy* **49**, 245–249.

Chantraine, A., Ludy, J. & Berger, D. (1986) Is cortisone iontophoresis possible? *Archives of Physical Medicine and Rehabilitation* **67**, 38–41.

Cheatle, M. & Esterhai, J. (1990) Pelvic traction as treatment for acute back pain. Efficacious, benign, or deleterious? *Spine* **16** (12), 1379–1381.

Christie, B. (1955) Discussion on the treatment of backache by traction. *Proceedings of the Society of Medicine (Section of Physical Medicine)* **49**, 811.

Cole, J. & Gossman, D. (1980) Ultrasonic stimulation of low lumbar nerve roots as a diagnostic procedure: a preliminary report. *Clinical Orthopedics* **153**, 126–131.

Cornell, P., Lopez, A. & Malofsky, H. (1984) Pain reduction with transcutaneous electrical nerve stimulation after foot surgery. *Journal of Foot Surgery* **23** (4), 326–333.

Cox, J., Andrish, J., Indelicato, P. & Walsh, W. (1986) Heat modalities. In: *Therapeutic Modalities for Sports Injuries* (Drez, D., ed.). Year Book Medical Publishers, Chicago: 1–23.

Craig, J., Cunningham, M., Walsh, D., Baxter, G. & Allen, J. (1996) Lack of effect of transcutaneous electrical nerve stimulation upon experimentally induced delayed onset muscle soreness in humans. *Pain* **67** (2/3), 285–289.

Crawford, F. & Snaith, M. (1996) How effective is therapeutic ultrasound in the treatment of heel pain? *Annals of the Rheumatic Diseases* **55** (4), 265–267.

Currier, D. (1991) Neuromuscular electrical stimulation for improving strength and blood flow, and influencing changes. In: *Clinical Electrotherapy* (Nelson, R. & Currier, D., eds). Appleton & Lange, Norwalk, CT: 35–103.

Currier, D. & Mann, R. (1983) Muscular strength development by electrical stimulation in normal subjects. *Physical Therapy* **63**, 915–921.

Currier, D., Greathouse, D. & Swift, T. (1978) Sensory nerve conduction: effect of ultrasound. *Archives of Physical Medicine and Rehabilitation* **59**, 181–185.

Currier, D., Lehman, J. & Lightfoot, P. (1979) Electrical stimulation in exercise of the quadriceps femoris muscle. *Physical Therapy* **59**, 1508–1512.

Davick, J., Martin, A. & Albright, J. (1988) Distribution and deposition of tritiated cortisol using phonophoresis. *Physical Therapy* **68**, 1672–1675.

de Seze, S. & Levernieux, J. (1951) Pratique rhumatologle des tractions vertebrales. *Seminars in Hop Paris* **27**, 2085.

Delitto, A., Brown, M., Strube, M., Rose, S. & Lehman, R. (1989) Electrical stimulation of quadriceps femoris in an elite weight lifter: a single subject experiment. *International Journal of Sports Medicine* **10**, 187–191.

Denegar, C. & Huff, C. (1988) High and low frequency TENS in treatment of induced musculoskeletal pain: a comparison study. *Athletic Training* **23**, 235–237.

Denegar, C. & Perrin, D. (1992) Effect of transcutaneous electrical nerve stimulation, cold, and a combination treatment on pain, decreased range of motion, and strength loss associated with delayed onset muscle soreness. *Journal of Athletic Training* **27**, 200–206.

Denegar, C., Perrin, D., Rogoi, A. & Rutt, R. (1989) Influence of transcutaneous electrical nerve stimulation on pain, range of motion and serum cortisol concentration in females experiencing delayed onset muscle soreness. *Journal of Orthopaedic and Sports Physical Therapy* **11** (3), 100–103.

Deyo, R., Walsh, N., Martin, D., Schoenfeld, L. & Ramamurthy, S. (1990a) A controlled trial of transcutaneous electrical nerve stimulation (TENS) and exercise for chronic low back pain. *New England Journal of Medicine* **322** (23), 1627–1634.

Deyo, R., Walsh, N., Schoenfeld, L. & Rammamurthy, S. (1990b) Can trials of physical treatments be blinded? The example of transcutaneous electrical nerve stimulation for chronic pain. *American Journal of Physical Medicine and Rehabilitation* **69** (1), 6–10.

Downing, D. & Weinstein, A. (1986) Ultrasound therapy of subacromial bursitis. A double blind trial. *Physical Therapy* **66** (2), 194–199.

Drez, D., Faust, D. & Evans, J. (1981) Cryotherapy and nerve palsy. *American Journal of Sports Medicine* **9**, 256–257.

Ebenbichler, G., Erdogmus, C., Resch, K. *et al.* (1999) Ultrasound therapy for calcific tendinitis of the shoulder. *New England Journal of Medicine* **340** (20), 1533–1584.

Enwemeka, C. (1989) The effects of therapeutic ultrasound on tendon healing. *American Journal of Physical Medicine Rehabilitation* **68**, 283–287.

Erdman, W. (1960) Peripheral blood flow measurement during application of pulsed high frequency currents. *American Journal of Orthopaedics* **2**, 196–197.

Eriksson, E. & Haggmark, T. (1979) Comparison of isometric muscle training and electrical stimulation supplement isometric muscle training in the recovery after major knee ligament surgery. *American Journal of Sports Medicine* **7**, 169–171.

Eriksson, E., Haggmark, T., Keissling, K. & Karlsson, J. (1981) Effects of electrical stimulation on human skeletal muscle. *International Journal of Sports Medicine* **2** (1), 18–22.

Fenn, J. (1969) Effect of pulsed electromagnetic energy (Diapulse) on experimental hematomas. *Canadian Medical Association Journal* **100**, 251–254.

Fleury, M. & Lagasse, P. (1979) Influence of functional electrical stimulation training on pre-motor and motor reaction time. *Perceptual and Motor Skills* **48**, 387–393.

Foley-Nolan, D., Moore, K., Codd, M., Barry, C., O'Connor, P. & Coughlan, R. (1992) Low energy high frequency pulsed electromagnetic therapy for acute whiplash injuries. A double blind randomized controlled study. *Scandinavian Journal of Rehabilitation Medicine* **24** (1), 51–59.

Forrest, G. & Rosen, K. (1989) Ultrasound: effectiveness of treatments given under water. *Archives of Physical Medicine and Rehabilitation* **70**, 28–29.

Fountain, F., Gersten, J. & Sengir, O. (1960) Decrease in muscle spasm produced by ultrasound, hot packs, and infrared radiation. *Archives of Physical Medicine and Rehabilitation* **41**, 293–298.

Frazer, E. (1954) The use of traction in backache. *Medical Journal of Australia* **41**, 694.

Fu, F., Cen, H. & Eston, R. (1997) The effects of cryotherapy on muscle damage in rats subjected to endurance training. *Scandinavian Journal of Medicine and Science in Sports* **7**, 358–362.

Fyestone, E., Fellingsham, G., George, J. & Fisher, G. (1993) Effect of water running and cycling on maximum oxygen consumption and two mile run performance. *American Journal of Sports Medicine* **21** (41), 52–59.

Gam, A. & Johannsen, F. (1995) Ultrasound therapy in musculoskeletal disorders: a meta-analysis. *Pain* **63**, 85–91.

Gam, A., Warming, S., Larsen, L. *et al.* (1998) Treatment of myofascial trigger-points with ultrasound combined with massage and exercise—a randomized controlled trial. *Pain* **77** (1), 73–79.

Gersh, M. (1978) Post-operative pain and transcutaneous electrical nerve stimulation. *Physical Therapy* **58**, 1463.

Ghoname, E., Craig, W., White, P. *et al.* (1999a) The effect of stimulus frequency on the analgesic response to percutaneous electrical nerve stimulation in patients with chronic low back pain. *Anesthesia and Analgesia* **88** (4), 841–846.

Ghoname, E., Craig, W., White, P. *et al.* (1999b) Percutaneous electrical nerve stimulation for low back pain: a randomized crossover study. *Journal of the American Medical Association* **281** (9), 818–823.

Gibson, J., Smith, K. & Rennie, M. (1988) Prevention of disuse muscle atrophy by means of electrical stimulation: maintenance of protein synthesis. *Lancet* **2** (8614), 767–770.

Gnatz, S. (1989) Increased radicular pain due to therapeutic ultrasound applied to the back. *Archives of Physical Medicine and Rehabilitation* **70**, 493–494.

Godfrey, C., Jayawardena, H., Quance, T. & Welch, P. (1979) Comparison of electro-stimulation and isometric exercise in strengthening the quadriceps muscle. *Physiotherapy Canada* **31**, 265–267.

Goldie, I. & Landquist, A. (1970) Evaluation of the effects of different forms of physiotherapy in cervical pain. *Scandinavian Journal of Rehabilitation Medicine* **2–3**, 117.

Goldin, J., Broadbent, N. & Nancarrow, J. (1981) The effects of Diapulse on the healing of wounds: a double-blind randomized controlled trial in man. *British Journal of Plastic Surgery* **34**, 267–270.

Gould, N., Donnermeyer, D., Gammon, G., Pope, M. & Ashikaga, T. (1979) Transcutaneous muscle stimulation to retard disuse atrophy after open menisectomy. *Clinical Orthopaedics and Related Research* **178**, 190–197.

Grana, W., Curl, W. & Reider, B. (1986) In: *Therapeutic Modalities for Sport Injuries* (Drez, D., ed.). Year Book Medical Publishers, Chicago: 25–31.

Grant, A. (1964) Massage with ice (cryokinetics) in the treatment of painful conditions of the musculoskeletal system. *Archives of Physical Medicine and Rehabilitation* **45**, 233–238.

Griffin, J. (1980) Transmissiveness of ultrasound through tap water, glycerin, and mineral water. *Physical Therapy* **60**, 1010–1016.

Griffin, J. & Karselis, T. (1982) *Physical Agents for Physical Therapists*. Charles C. Thomas, Springfield, IL.

Griffin, J. & Touchstone, J. (1963) Ultrasonic movement of cortisol into pig tissues, I. Movement into skeletal muscle. *American Journal of Physical Medicine and Rehabilitation* **42**, 77–85.

Griffin, J., Touchstone, J. & Liu, A. (1965) Ultrasonic movement of cortisol into pig tissues, II. Movement into paravertebral nerve. *American Journal of Physical Medicine and Rehabilitation* **41**, 20–25.

Griffin, J., Newsome, L., Stralka, S. & Wright, P. (1990) Reduction of chronic posttraumatic hand edema: a comparison of high voltage pulsed current, intermittent pneumatic compression, and placebo treatments. *Physical Therapy* **70**, 279–286.

Grove-Lainey, C., Walmsley, R. & Andrew, G. (1983) Effectiveness of exercise alone versus exercise plus electrical stimulation in strengthening the quadriceps muscle. *Physiotherapy Canada* **35**, 5–11.

Gudeman, S., Eisele, S., Heidt, R., Colosimo, A. & Stroupe, A. (1997) Treatment of plantar fasciitis by iontophoresis of 0.4% dexamethasone: a randomized, double-blind, placebo-controlled study. *American Journal of Sports Medicine* **25** (3), 312–316.

Haker, E. & Lundeberg, T. (1991) Pulsed ultrasound treatment in lateral epicondylalgia. *Scandinavian Journal of Rehabilitation Medicine* **23**, 115–118.

Halbach, J. & Straus, D. (1980) Comparison of electromyo stimulation to isokinetic power of the knee extensor mechanism. *Journal of Orthopaedic and Sports Physical Therapy* **2**, 20–24.

Hall, J., Skevington, S., Maddison, P. & Chapman, K. (1996) A randomized and controlled trial of hydrotherapy in rheumatoid arthritis. *Arthritis Care and Research* **9** (3), 206–215.

Halle, J., Scouille, C. & Greathouse, D. (1981) Ultrasound effect on the conduction latency of the superficial radial nerve in man. *Physical Therapy* **61**, 345–350.

Halle, J., Franklin, R. & Karalfa, B. (1986) Comparison of four treatment approaches for lateral epicondylitis of the elbow. *Journal of Orthopaedic and Sports Physical Therapy* **8**, 62–69.

Halvorson, G. (1989) Principles of rehabilitating sports injuries. In: *Scientific Foundations of Sports Medicine* (Teitz, C., ed.). B.C. Decker, Toronto: 345–371.

Hasson, S., Mundorf, R., Barnes, W., Williams, J. & Fujii, M. (1990) Effect of pulsed ultrasound versus placebo on muscle soreness perception and muscular performance. *Scandinavian Journal of Rehabilitation Medicine* **22**, 199–205.

Hasson, S., Wible, C., Reich, M., Barnes, W. & Williams, J. (1992) Dexamethasone iontophoresis: effect on delayed muscle soreness and muscle function. *Canadian Journal of Sport Sciences* **17** (1), 8–13.

Hayes, K. (1984) Manual for physical agents. In: *Programs in Physical Therapy*. Northwestern University Medical School, Chicago.

Hazlewood, C. & VanZandt, R. (1995) A hypothesis defining an objective end point for the relief of chronic pain. *Medical Hypotheses* **44**, 63–65.

Herman, E., Williams, R., Stratford, P., Fargas-Babjak, A. & Trott, M. (1994) A randomized controlled trial of transcutaneous electrical nerve stimulation (Codetron) to determine its benefits in a rehabilitation program for acute occupational low back pain. *Spine* **19** (5), 561–568.

Hillman, S. & Delforge, G. (1985) The use of physical agents in rehabilitation of athletic injuries. *Clinics in Sports Medicine* **4**, 431–438.

Hinterbucher, C. (1985) Traction. In: *Traction and Massage*, 3rd edn (Basmajian, J., ed.). Williams & Wilkins, Baltimore: 172–200.

Ho, S., Coel, M., Kagawa, R. & Richardson, A. (1994) The effects of ice on blood flow and bone metabolism in knees. *American Journal of Sports Medicine* **22**, 537–540.

Hocutt, J. (1981) Cryotherapy. *American Family Physician* **23**, 141–144.

Hsueh, T., Cheng, P., Kuan, T. & Hong, C. (1997) The immediate effectiveness of electrical nerve stimulation and electrical muscle stimulation on myofascial trigger points. *American Journal of Physical Medicine and Rehabilitation* **76** (6), 471–476.

Jackson, B., Schwane, J. & Starcher, B. (1991) Effect of ultrasound therapy on the repair of Achilles tendon injuries in rat. *Medicine and Science in Sports and Exercise* **23**, 171–176.

James, M., Graham, R. & English, J. (1986) Percutaneous iontophoresis of prednisolone—a pharmacokinetic study. *Clinical and Experimental Dermatology* **11**, 54–61.

Japour, C., Vohra, R., Vohra, P., Garfunkel, L. & Chin, N. (1999) Management of heel pain syndrome with acetic acid iontophoresis. *Journal of the American Podiatric Medical Association* **89** (5), 251–257.

Jensen, J., Conn, R., Hazelrigg, G. & Hewitt, J. (1985) The use of transcutaneous neural stimulation and isokinetic testing in arthroscopic knee surgery. *American Journal of Sports Medicine* **13** (1), 27–33.

Kahanovitz, N., Nordin, M., Verderame, R. *et al.* (1987) Normal trunk muscle strength and endurance in women and the effect of exercises and electrical stimulation. Part 2: Comparative analysis of electrical stimulation and exercises to increase trunk muscle strength and endurance. *Spine* **12**, 112–118.

Karlsson, J., Rydgren, G., Eriksson, B., Järvholm, U., Lundin, O. & Swärd, L. (1994) Cryo-Cuff for control of post-operative pain. *Scandinavian Journal of Medicine and Science in Sports* **4**, 279.

Klaiman, M., Shrader, J., Danoff, J., Hicks, J., Pesce, W. & Ferland, J. (1998) Phonophoresis versus ultrasound in the treatment of common musculoskeletal conditions. *Medicine and Science in Sports and Exercise* **30** (9), 1349–1355.

Kleinkort, J. & Wood, F. (1975) Phonophoresis with 1 percent versus 10 percent hydrocortisone. *Physical Therapy* **55**, 1320–1324.

Konlian, C. (1999) Aquatic therapy: making a wave in the treatment of low back injuries. *Orthopaedic Nursing* **18** (1), 11–18.

Konrath, G., Lock, T., Goitz, H. & Scheidler, J. (1996) The use of cold therapy after anterior cruciate ligament reconstruction. *American Journal of Sports Medicine* **24** (5), 629–633.

Kots, Y. (1977) Electrostimulation (translated). Paper presented at the Symposium of Electrostimulation of Skeletal Muscle, Canadian Soviet Exchange Symposium, Concordia University, 6–10 December 1977.

Kramer, J. & Mendryk, S. (1982) Electrical stimulation as a strength improvement technique: a review. *Journal of Orthopaedic and Sports Physical Therapy* **4**, 91–98.

Kramer, J. & Semple, J. (1983) Comparison of selected strengthening techniques for normal quadriceps. *Physiotherapy Canada* **35**, 300–304.

Kristiansen, T., Ryaby, J., McCabe, J., Frey, J. & Roe, L. (1997) Accelerated healing of distal radial fractures with the use of specific, low-intensity ultrasound. *Journal of Bone and Joint Surgery* **79A**, 961–973.

Kubiak, R., Whitman, K. & Johnston, R. (1987) Changes in quadriceps femoris muscle strength using isometric exercise versus electrical stimulation. *Journal of Orthopaedic and Sports Physical Therapy* **8**, 537–541.

Lake, D. (1989) Increases in range of motion of the edematous hand with the use of electromesh glove. *Physical Therapy Forum* **8**, 6.

Lake, D. (1992) Neuromuscular electrical stimulation: an overview and its application in the treatment of sports injuries. *Sports Medicine* **13** (5), 320–336.

Laughman, R., Youdas, J., Garrett, T. & Chao, E. (1983) Strength changes in the normal quadriceps femoris muscle as a result of electrical stimulation. *Physical Therapy* **63**, 494–499.

Lawson, G. & Godfrey, C. (1958) A report on studies of spinal-traction. *Medical Services Journal of Canada* **14**, 762.

LeDoux, J. & Quinones, M. (1981) An investigation of the use of percutaneous electrical stimulation in muscle reeducation (abstract R183). *Physical Therapy* **61**, 737.

Lehmann, J. & de Lateur, B. (1982a) Cryotherapy. In: *Therapeutic Heat and Cold* (Lehmann, J., ed.). Williams & Wilkins, Baltimore: 563–602.

Lehmann, J. & de Lateur, B. (1982b) Diathermy and superficial heat and cold therapy. In: *Krusen's Handbook of Physical Medicine and Rehabilitation*, 3rd edn (Kottke, F., Stillwell, G. & Lehmann, J., eds). W.B. Saunders, Philadelphia: 275–350.

Lehmann, J. & de Lateur, B. (1982c) Therapeutic heat. In: *Therapeutic Heat and Cold* (Lehmann, J., ed.). Williams & Wilkins, Baltimore: 404–562.

Lehmann, J., Sliverman, D., Baum, B., Kirk, N. & Johnston, V. (1966) Temperature distributions in the human thigh produced by infrared, hot pack and microwave applications. *Archives of Physical Medicine and Rehabilitation* **47**, 291–299.

Lehmann, J., Masock, A., Warren, C. & Koblanski, J. (1970) Effect of therapeutic temperatures on tendon extensibility. *Archives of Physical Medicine and Rehabilitation* **51**, 481–486.

Lehmann, T., Russell, D., Spratt, K. *et al.* (1986) Efficacy of electroacupuncture and TENS in the rehabilitation of chronic low back pain patients. *Pain* **26**, 277–290.

Lessard, L., Scudds, R., Amendola, A. & Vaz, M. (1997) The efficacy of cryotherapy following arthroscopic knee surgery. *Journal of Orthopaedic and Sports Physical Therapy* **26** (1), 14–22.

Levy, A. & Marmar, E. (1993) The role of cold compression dressings in the postoperative treatment of total knee arthroplasty. *Clinical Orthopaedics and Related Research* **297**, 174–178.

Levy, A., Kelly, B., Lintner, S. & Speer, K. (1997) Penetration of cryotherapy in treatment after shoulder arthroscopy. *Arthroscopy* **13** (4), 461–464.

Licht, S. (1983) History of electrotherapy. In: *Therapeutic Electricity and Ultraviolet Radiation*, 3rd edn (Stillwell, G., ed.). Williams & Wilkins, Baltimore: 1–64.

Lundeberg, T., Abrahamsson, P. & Haker, E. (1988) A comparative study of continuous ultrasound, placebo ultrasound and rest in epicondylagia. *Scandinavian Journal of Rehabilitation Medicine* **20**, 99–101.

MacAuley, D. (2001) Do textbooks agree on their advice on ice? *Clinical Journal of Sports Medicine* **11**, 67–72.

Madsen, P. & Gersten, J. (1961) The effect of ultrasound on conduction velocity of peripheral nerve. *Archives of Physical Medicine and Rehabilitation* **42**, 645–649.

Marchand, S., Charest, J., Li, J., Chenard, J., Lavignolle, R. & Laurencelle, L. (1993) Is TENS purely a placebo effect? A controlled study on chronic low back pain. *Pain* **54**, 99–106.

Marino, M. (1986) Principles of therapeutic modalities: implications for sports injuries. In: *The Lower Extremity and Spine in Sports Medicine* (Nicholas, J. & Herschmena, E., eds). Mosby, St Louis: 195–244.

Martin, S., Spindler, K., Tarter, J., Detwiler, K. & Petersen, H. (2001) Cryotherapy: an effective modality for decreasing intraarticular temperature after knee arthroscopy. *American Journal of Sports Medicine* **29**, 288–291.

McLean, M., Holcomb, R. & Wamil, A. (1995) Blockage of sensory neuron action potentials by a static magnetic field in the 10mT range. *Bioelectromagnetics* **16** (1), 20–32.

McMaster, W. (1982) Cryotherapy. *Physician and Sportsmedicine* **10**, 112–119.

McMaster, W., Liddle, S. & Waugh, T. (1978) Laboratory evaluation of various cold therapy modalities. *American Journal of Sports Medicine* **6**, 291–294.

McMiken, D., Todd-Smith, M. & Thompson, C. (1983) Strengthening of human quadriceps muscles by cutaneous electrical stimulation. *Scandinavian Journal of Rehabilitation Medicine* **15**, 25–28.

Melzack, R. & Wall, P. (1965) Pain mechanisms: a new theory. *Science* **150** (699), 971–979.

Mennell, J. (1975) The therapeutic use of cold. *Journal of the American Osteopathic Association* **74**, 1146–1158.

Merrick, M., Rankin, J., Andres, F. & Hinman, C. (1999) A preliminary examination of cryotherapy and secondary injury in skeletal muscle. *Medicine and Science in Sports and Exercise* **31**, 1516–1521.

Michlovitz, S. (1986) Biophysical principles of heating and superficial heat agents. In: *Thermal Agents in Rehabilitation* (Michlovitz, S. & Wolf, S., eds). F.A. Davis, Philadelphia: 99–118..

Miner, W. & Markoll, R. (1993) A double-blind trial of the clinical effects of pulsed electromagnetic fields in osteoarthritis. *Journal of Rheumatology* **20**, 456–460.

Morrissey, M., Brewster, C., Shields, C. & Brown, M. (1985) The effects of electrical stimulation on the quadriceps during postoperative knee immobilization. *American Journal of Sport Medicine* **13**, 40–45.

Newman, M., Kill, M. & Frampton, G. (1958) Effects of ultrasound alone and combined with hydrocortisone injections by needle or hypospray. *American Journal of Physical Medicine and Rehabilitation* **37**, 206–209.

Nitz, A. & Dobner, J. (1987) High intensity electrical stimulation effect on thigh musculature during immobilization for knee sprain: a case report. *Physical Therapy* **67**, 219–222.

Norton, C., Shaha, S. & Stewart, L. (1996) *Aquatic versus Traditional Therapy: Contrasting Effectiveness of Acquisition Rates.* Orthopaedic Specialty Hospital, Salt Lake City.

Nykanen, M. (1995) Pulsed ultrasound treatment of the painful shoulder: a randomized, double-blind, placebo-controlled study. *Scandinavian Journal of Rehabilitation Medicine* **27** (2), 105–108.

O'Connor, M., Bentall, R. & Monahan, J. (1990) *Emerging Electromagnetic Medicine.* Springer Verlag, New York.

Ohkoshi, Y., Ohkoshi, M., Nagasaki, S., Ono, A., Hashimoto, T. & Yamane, S. (1999) The effect of cryotherapy on intraarticular temperature and postoperative care after anterior cruciate ligament reconstruction. *American Journal of Sports Medicine* **27** (3), 357–362.

O'Malley, E. & Oester, Y. (1955) Influence of some physical chemical factors on iontophoresis using radio isotopes. *Archives of Physical Medicine and Rehabilitation* **36**, 310–316.

Ordog, G. (1987) Transcutaneous electrical nerve stimulation versus oral analgesic: a randomized double blind controlled study in acute traumatic pain. *American Journal of Emergency Medicine* **5**, 6–10.

Ork, H. (1982) Uses of cold. In: *Physical Therapy for Sports* (Kuprian, W., ed.). W.B. Saunders, Philadelphia: 62–68.

Paddon-Jones, D. & Quigley, B. (1997) Effect of cryotherapy on muscle soreness and strength following eccentric exercise. *International Journal of Sports Medicine* **18**, 588–593.

Perron, M. & Malouin, F. (1997) Acetic acid iontophoresis and ultrasound for the treatment of calcifying tendonitis of the shoulder: a randomized control trial. *Archive of Physical Medicine and Rehabilitation* **78** (4), 379–384.

Pienimaki, T., Tarvainen, T., Siira, P. & Vanharanta, H. (1996) Progressive strengthening and stretching exercises and ultrasound for chronic lateral epicondylitis. *Physiotherapy* **82**, 522–530.

Plaskett, C., Riidus, P. & Livingston, L. (1999) Ultrasound treatment does not affect postexercise muscle strength recovery or soreness. *Journal of Sports Rehabilitation* **8**, 1–9.

Pope, M., Phillips, R., Haugh, L., Hsieh, C., MacDonald, L. & Haldeman, S. (1994) A prospective randomized three-week trial of spinal manipulation, transcutaneous muscle stimulation, massage and corset in the treatment of subacute low back pain. *Spine* **19** (22), 2571–2577.

Prentice, W. (1986) *Therapeutic Modalities in Sports Medicine.* Times Mirror/Mosby College Publishing, St Louis.

Pujol, J., Pascual-Leone, A., Dolz, C., Delgado, E., Dolz, J. & Aldoma, J. (1998) The effect of repetitive magnetic stimulators on localized musculoskeletal pain. *Neuroreport* **9** (8), 1745–1748.

Quillen, W. & Rouillier, L. (1982) Initial management of acute ankle sprains with rapid pulsed pneumatic compression and cold. *Journal of Orthopaedic and Sports Physical Therapy* **4**, 39–43.

Ramirez, A., Schwane, J., McFarland, C. & Starcher, B. (1997) The effect of ultrasound on collagen synthesis and fibroblast proliferation *in vitro. Medicine and Science in Sports and Exercise* **29**, 326–332.

Rechtein, J., Andary, M., Holmes, T. & Wieting, M. (1998) Manipulation, massage, and traction. In: *Rehabilitation Medicine: Principles and Practice*, 3rd edn (DeLisa, J. & Gans, B., eds). Lippencott-Raven, Philadelphia: 521–552.

Reid, D., De Borba, D. & Saboe, L. (1989) Sonation of lumbar nerve roots as a diagnostic procedure in patients with sciatica. *Archives of Physical Medicine and Rehabilitation* **70**, 25–27.

Robertson, V. & Baker, K. (2001) A review of therapeutic ultrasound: effectiveness studies. *Physical Therapy* **81** (7), 1339–1350.

Robinson, A. (1996) Transcutaneous electrical nerve stimulation for the control of pain in musculoskeletal disorders. *Journal of Orthopaedic and Sports Physical Therapy* **24** (4), 208–226.

Roeser, W., Meeks, L., Venis, R. & Strickland, G. (1976) The use of transcutaneous nerve stimulation for pain control in athletic medicine: a preliminary report. *American Journal of Sports Medicine* **4** (5), 210–213.

Ross, C. & Segal, D. (1981) High voltage galvanic stimulation—an aid to post operative healing. *Current Podiatry* **34**, 19.

Ross, J. (1990) Biological effects of PEMFs using Diapulse. In: *Emerging Electromagnetic Medicine* (O'Connor, M., Bentall, R. & Monahan, J., eds). Springer Verlag, New York: 269–282.

Routi, R., Toup, J. & Berger, R. (1994) The effects of non-swimming exercises on older adults. *Journal of Orthopaedic and Sports Physical Therapy* **19** (3), 140–145.

Roy, S. & Irvin, R. (1983) *Sports Medicine Prevention, Evaluation, Management, and Rehabilitation.* Prentice Hall, Englewood Cliffs, NJ.

Santiesteban, A. (1985) Physical agents and musculoskeletal pain. In: *Orthopedic and Sports Physical Therapy* (Gould, J. & Davies, G., eds). C.V. Mosby, St Louis: 199–211.

Schaubel, H. (1946) Local use of ice after orthopedic procedures. *American Journal of Surgery* **72**, 711–714.

Sharrard, W. (1990) A double-blind trial of pulsed electromagnetic fields for delayed union of tibial fractures. *Journal of Bone and Joint Surgery* **72B**, 347–355.

Simons, D., Travell, J. & Simons, L. (1990) Protecting the ozone layer. *Archives of Physical Medicine and Rehabilitation* **71**, 64.

Singer, K.D., D'Ambrosia, A. & Graf, B. (1989) In: *Therapeutic Modalities for Sports Injuries* (Drez, D., ed.). Year Book Medical Publishers, Chicago: 33–48.

Sloan, J., Giddings, P. & Hain, R. (1988) Effects of cold and compression on edema. *Physician and Sportsmedicine* **16**, 116–120.

Sluka, K., Bailey, K., Bogush, J., Olson, R. & Ricketts, A. (1998) Treatment with either high or low frequency TENS reduces the secondary hyperalgesia observed after injection of kaolin and carrageenan into the knee joint. *Pain* **77** (1), 97–102.

Smith, M., Hutchins, R. & Hehenberger, D. (1983) Transcutaneous neural stimulation in postoperative knee rehabilitation. *American Journal of Sports Medicine* **11** (2), 75–81.

Snyder-Mackler, L. (1990) *Electrically-elicited cocontraction of the quadriceps femoris and hamstring muscles: effects on gait and thigh muscle strength after anterior cruciate ligament reconstruction.* Doctoral Dissertation, Boston University, Boston.

Snyder-Mackler, L., Celluci, M., Lyons, J. et al. (1988) Effects of duty cycle of portable neuromuscular electrical stimulation on strength of the non-dominant triceps brachii. *Journal of Orthopaedic and Sports Physical Therapy* **68**, 833–839.

Snyder-Mackler, L., Delitto, A., Bailey, S. & Stralka, S. (1995) Strength of the quadriceps femoris muscle and functional recovery after reconstruction of the anterior cruciate ligament. A prospective, randomized clinical trial of electrical stimulation. *Journal of Bone and Joint Surgery* **77A** (8), 1166–1173.

Speer, K., Warren, R. & Horowitz, L. (1996) The efficacy of cryotherapy in the postoperative shoulder. *Journal of Shoulder and Elbow Surgery* **5** (1), 62–68.

Stanish, W., Valiant, G., Bonen, A. & Belcastrol, A. (1982) The effects of immobilization and of electrical stimulation on muscle glycogen and myofibrillar ATPase. *Canadian Journal of Applied Sports Sciences (Journal Candien des Sciences Appliquees au Sport)* **7** (4), 267–271.

Stillwell, G. (1982) Electrotherapy. In: *Krusen's Handbook of Physical Medicine and Rehabilitation*, 3rd edn (Kottke, F., Stillwell, G. & Lehmann, J., eds). W.B. Saunders, Philadelphia: 360–371.

Swenson, C., Swärd, L. & Karlsson, J. (1996) Cryotherapy in sports medicine. *Scandinavian Journal of Medicine and Science in Sports* **6**, 193–200.

Swezey, R., Swezey, A. & Warner, K. (1999) Efficacy of home cervical traction therapy. *American Journal of Physical Medicine and Rehabilitation* **78** (1), 30–32.

Taniguchi, K., Yoshitake, S., Iwasaka, H., Honda, N. & Oyama, T. (1995) The effects of imipramine, amitriptyline and clonidine administered by iontophoresis on the pain threshold. *Acta Anaesthesiologica Belgica* **46**, 121–125.

Taylor, B., Waring, C. & Brashear, T. (1995) The effects of therapeutic application of heat or cold followed by static stretch on hamstring muscle length. *Journal of Orthopaedic and Sports Physical Therapy* **21** (5), 283–286.

Thorsteinsson, G., Stonnington, H., Stillwell, G. & Elveback, L. (1977) Transcutaneous electrical stimulation: a double blind trial of its efficacy for pain. *Archives of Physical Medicine and Rehabilitation* **58**, 8–13.

Tiidus, P. (1999) Massage and ultrasound as therapeutic modalities in exercise-induced muscle damage. *Canadian Journal of Applied Physiology* **24**, 267–278.

Timm, K. (1994) A randomized-control study of active and passive treatments for chronic low back pain following L5 laminectomy. *Journal of Orthopaedic and Sports Physical Therapy* **20** (6), 276–286.

Travell, J. & Simons, D. (1983) *Myofascial Pain and Dysfunction: the Trigger Point Manual*. Williams & Wilkins, Baltimore.

Trock, D., Bollet, A. & Markoll, R. (1994) The effect of pulsed electromagnetic fields in the treatment of osteoarthritis of the knee and cervical spine. Report of randomized, double blind, placebo controlled trials. *Journal of Rheumatology* **21**, 1903–1911.

United Nations Environment Programme (1987) The International Labour Organization, World Health Organization, Geneva.

Vallbona, C. & Richards, T. (1999) Evolution of magnetic therapy from alternative to traditional medicine. *Physical Medicine and Rehabilitation Clinics of North America* **10** (3), 729–754.

Vallentyne, S. & Vallentyne, J. (1988) The case of the missing ozone: are physiatrists to blame? *Archives of Physical Medicine and Rehabilitation* **69**, 992–993.

van der Heijden, G., Beurskens, A., Koes, B., Assendelft, W., de Vet, H. & Bouter, L. (1995) The efficacy of traction for back and neck pain: a systematic, blinded review of randomized clinical trial methods. *Physical Therapy* **75** (2), 93–104.

van der Heijden, G., Leffers, P., Wolters, P. *et al.* (1999) No effect of bipolar interferential electrotherapy and pulsed ultrasound for soft tissue shoulder disorders: a randomized controlled trial. *Annals of the Rheumatic Diseases* **58** (9), 530–540.

van der Windt, D., van der Heijden, G., van den Berg, S., ter Riet, G., de Winter, A. & Bouter, L. (1999) Ultrasound therapy for musculoskeletal disorders: a systematic review. *Pain* **81** (3), 257–272.

Vasseljen, O. (1992) Low-level laser versus traditional physiotherapy in the treatment of tennis elbow. *Physiotherapy* **78**, 329–334.

Walsh, D., Liggett, C., Baxter, D. & Allen, J. (1995) A double-blind investigation of the hypoalgesic effects of transcutaneous electrical nerve stimulation upon experimentally induced ischaemic pain. *Pain* **61** (1), 39–45.

Warren, C., Lehmann, J. & Koblanski, J. (1971) Elongation of rat tail tendon: effect of load and temperature. *Archives of Physical Medicine and Rehabilitation* **52**, 465–474.

Warren, C., Koblanski, J. & Sigelmann, R. (1976a) Ultrasound coupling media: their relative transmissivity. *Archives of Physical Medicine and Rehabilitation* **57**, 218–222.

Warren, C., Lehmann, J. & Koblanski, J. (1976b) Heat and stretch procedures: an evaluation using rat tail tendon. *Archives of Physical Medicine and Rehabilitation* **57** (3), 122–126.

Washnis, G. (1998) *Discovery of Magnetic Health: a Health Care Alternative*. Health Research Publishers, Wheaton, MD.

Weber, H. (1973) Traction therapy in sciatica due to disc prolapse. *Journal of Oslo City Hospital* **23**, 167.

Wigerstad-Lossing, I., Grimby, G., Jonsson, T., Morelli, B., Peterson, L. & Renstrom, P. (1988) Effects of electrical stimulation combined with voluntary contractions after knee ligament surgery. *Medicine and Science in Sports and Exercise* **20** (1), 93–98.

Yackzan, L., Adams, C. & Francis, K. (1984) The effects of ice massage on delayed muscle soreness. *American Journal of Sports Medicine* **12** (2), 159–165.

Zankel, H. (1966) Effect of physical agents on motor conduction velocity of the ulnar nerve. *Archives of Physical Medicine and Rehabilitation* **47**, 787–792.

Zankel, H., Cress, R. & Kamin, H. (1959) Iontophoresis studies with radioactive tracer. *Archives of Physical Medicine and Rehabilitation* **40**, 193–196.

Zylbergold, R. & Piper, M. (1985) Cervical spine disorders. A comparison of three types of traction. *Spine* **10** (10), 867–871.

Chapter 11

Flexibility and Joint Range of Motion

MARTIN SCHWELLNUS

Introduction

Musculoskeletal injuries form a large proportion of the injuries reported by athletes (Wang *et al.* 1993). There are many potential causes for these injuries and these include muscle strength imbalances, muscle fatigue, biomechanical abnormalities, incorrect training methods and musculoskeletal inflexibility (Burkett 1970; Burry 1975; Cooper & Fair 1978; Zarins 1982; Agre 1985). A decrease in musculoskeletal flexibility has been associated with both the aetiology of these injuries, as well as a consequence of these injuries (Nicholas 1970; Glick 1980; Toft *et al.* 1989; Wang *et al.* 1993). Furthermore, it has been documented that flexibility training (stretching), using a variety of techniques, effectively increases musculotendinous unit (MTU) range of motion in human subjects (De Vries 1962; Tanigawa 1972; Medeiros *et al.* 1977; Henricson *et al.* 1984).

Because there are established guidelines as to the norms for musculotendinous unit flexibility for most joints or groups of joints (Janda 1983; Kendall & McCreary 1983; Travell & Simons 1983; Clendaniel *et al.* 1984), range of motion testing can reveal values that exceed the normal (hypermobility), or are less than the normal (hypomobility or inflexibility). Hypermobility will not be discussed in detail in this chapter. However, the causes for hypermobility are largely genetic. Also, there are instances where hypermobility is related to certain athletic activities, such as gymnastics or ballet dancing (Grahame & Jenkins 1972). In addition, in general, larger

ranges of motion are present in females compared with males, and in younger compared with older individuals (Nicholas 1970). Other causes for hypermobility are an increased musculotendinous unit temperature (Wessling *et al.* 1987; Anderson & Burke 1991) and, in some instances, after injury or surgery, significant lengthening of soft tissue structures can also result in abnormally increased joint range of motion.

The use of stretching techniques as a means of treating hypomobility is widely advocated, as a means of preventing injuries, as well as forming an important component in the design of a rehabilitation programme following injury or surgery (Cureton 1941; Weber & Kraus 1949; De Vries 1962; Nicholas 1970; Cahill & Griffith 1978; Cooper & Fair 1978; Glick 1980; Beaulieu 1981; Wiktorsson-Moller *et al.* 1983; Hardy 1985; Etnyre & Abraham 1986; Williford *et al.* 1986; Toft *et al.* 1989; Zachazewski 1990; Worrell *et al.* 1991, 1994). A number of health professionals are therefore involved in the prescription of flexibility training in the primary and secondary prevention of injuries in athletes. These professionals include sports physicians, physiatrists (rehabilitation medicine practitioners), orthopaedists, physical therapists, rehabilitation workers, physical educators, athletic trainers, coaches and athletes.

This chapter focuses on the role of flexibility training in the rehabilitation of injuries. After a brief review of definitions and terminology pertaining to flexibility training, the general benefits of flexibility training and the pathophysiology of loss of range of motion after injury will be briefly reviewed. Techniques for the measurement of flexibility, and the physiology of stretching will be discussed. A scientific basis for stretching will be presented, and practical guidelines for the implementation of a flexibility training programme during rehabilitation will be provided.

Terminology and definitions

The literature uses a variety of terms when flexibility training is discussed. It is therefore necessary to define these terms at the beginning of this chapter in order to clarify what will be referred to in the text that follows. A summary of the terminology and definitions used is depicted in Table 11.1.

The terms 'musculotendinous unit length', 'joint range of motion' and 'musculotendinous unit flexibility' are often used interchangeably. *Flexibility* can be defined as the range of motion available in a joint or in a group of joints that is influenced by muscles, tendons and bones (Anderson & Burke 1991). Flexibility has also been described as the degree to which muscle length permits movement over that which it has an influence (Toppenburg & Bullock 1986).

Measurement of joint range of motion is thereby an indirect measure of the extensibility of the tissues that have an influence over that particular joint. *Joint range of motion* is thus a functional measurement and not a measurement of the physical dimensions of the muscle or the length of the musculotendinous unit (Toppenburg & Bullock 1986). Measurements of the joint angle provide an 'index' of *musculotendinous unit length* or flexibility (Bullock-Saxton & Bullock 1994). For the purposes of this chapter, the term flexibility will be used to indicate an increase in joint range of motion.

Flexibility in the musculotendinous unit is directly related to tension in that musculotendinous unit (Starring *et al.* 1988; Taylor *et al.* 1990). Tension in the musculotendinous unit is made up of both a passive component and an active component (Taylor *et al.* 1990). The passive component lies in the connective tissue while the active component lies in the reflex activity of the muscle. The passive, connective tissue component has both viscous and elastic properties and therefore behaves in a viscoelastic fashion when subjected to a tensile force (Fung 1967; Ciullo & Zarins 1983; Herbert 1988; Taylor *et al.* 1990; Kwan *et al.* 1992).

Table 11.1 Definitions and terminology.

Term	Description
Flexibility	The range of motion in a joint or in a group of joints that is influenced by muscles, tendons and bones
Flexibility training	A training programme that is aimed at increasing the range of motion of specific joints or groups of joints (stretching programme)
Elasticity	The property in tissues that refers to the return of the tissue to its original length when the force is removed
Viscous	The property in tissues that refers to the elongation of a tissue that remains once the force applied to it is removed
Viscoelastic	A tissue that exhibits both viscous and elastic properties
Extensibility	The ability of a tissue to elongate
Stiffness	The ratio of the change in stress (force per unit area) and the change in length (strain)
Stress relaxation	The decline in tissue tension that results when a tissue is lengthened and then held at that constant length
Creep	The change in length of a tissue in response to a load that is applied and then maintained at that constant magnitude
Hysteresis	The change in length of a tissue in response to a load that is applied in a cyclic fashion

The elastic component of viscoelasticity implies that length changes in the musculotendinous unit are directly proportional to the loads imposed on the musculotendinous unit (Halbertsma & Goeken 1994). This is well described in Hooke's model of a perfect spring (Burns & MacDonald 1975; Sapega *et al.* 1981; Taylor *et al.* 1990). *Elasticity* implies the ability of a structure to stretch when a force is applied to it, and then to return to the original length when the force is removed. Extensibility and stiffness comprise elasticity (Cavagna 1970; Halbertsma & Goeken 1994). *Extensibility* refers to the ability, in this case of the musculotendinous unit, to lengthen. *Stiffness* refers to the ratio of change in muscle length to the change in muscle tension (Halbertsma & Goeken 1994). Therefore, high stiffness implies a greater resistance to stretch. Thus, flexibility is comprised of two components—tension and stiffness (Fung 1967; Stromberg & Wiederheilm 1969; Herbert 1988).

In muscles, flexibility can also be defined as the point where tension first develops in the muscle when it is stretched passively. Stiffness is the ratio between tension and the amount of lengthening. *Stiffness* can therefore also be defined as the slope of the stress–strain curve (stress = tension/cross-sectional area; strain = change in length/initial length) (Burns & MacDonald 1975). The greater the stiffness, the steeper the slope of the stress–strain curve.

The viscous component of viscoelasticity is both rate change-dependent and time-dependent (Taylor *et al.* 1990). The rate of deformation is directly proportional to the applied force. This is illustrated by Newton's hydraulic piston known as a dash pot (Burns & MacDonald 1975). The connective tissue in the musculotendinous unit responds as a viscoelastic material where the ground substances, collagen and elastin, which comprise the connective tissue, determine this response (Sapega *et al.* 1981; Starring *et al.* 1988). The relationship between length and tension, which changes with time as stretch is applied, implies viscoelasticity in the musculotendinous unit (Herbert 1988).

Stress relaxation occurs in viscoelastic substances when the tissue is stretched to a specified length and is then held at that constant length. The force or stress in the tissue, which will gradually decline over time, is known as stress relaxation (Taylor *et al.* 1990). In living soft tissue, this relationship is non-linear (Fung 1967; Herbert 1988; Taylor *et al.* 1990; Kwan *et al.* 1992). Generally, the elasticity of living tissue is characterized by a very small stress even when it is subjected to a large strain. When this stress begins to rise, however, it does so rapidly and exponentially (Fung 1967). Because the tension in the musculotendinous unit, when it is stretched, decreases over time, the tissue exhibits viscous behaviour, and because there is still a degree of tension present it also exhibits elastic behaviour (Taylor *et al.* 1990).

When the musculotendinous unit is placed under a constant force, the musculotendinous unit responds by lengthening in a viscous way. This implies an irreversible increase in musculotendinous unit length. The deformation in the musculotendinous unit occurs up to a point where the increase plateaus at a new length. This is known as 'creep' (LaBan 1962; Kottke *et al.* 1966; Fung 1967; Warren *et al.* 1976; Taylor *et al.* 1990). Prolonged, low load stretching of the musculotendinous unit results in more viscous deformation than short, high load stretching (LaBan 1962; Kottke *et al.* 1966; Fung 1967; Warren *et al.* 1976).

When a musculotendinous unit is stretched, it may not return to its original length or natural state because of its deviation from an ideal elastic substance (Starring *et al.* 1988). When the loads or stretches applied to the musculotendinous unit are cyclic, it becomes possible to predict the deformation to the musculotendinous unit. This is known as 'hysteresis' (Fung 1967). The effect of hysteresis is progressive, and further changes can be expected with repeated stretching (Starring *et al.* 1988).

Flexibility of the musculotendinous unit can, therefore, also be defined by the amount of extensibility and stiffness in that musculotendinous unit (Halbertsma & Goeken 1994). The degree to which the flexibility of the musculotendinous unit increases when a stress or stretch is applied to it, is determined by its viscoelasticity (Herbert 1988). The viscoelasticity of the musculotendinous unit allows for stress relaxation, creep and hysteresis to occur in that musculotendinous unit, when forces are applied at varying magnitudes, durations and repetitions (Kottke *et al.* 1966; Fung 1967; Warren *et al.* 1976; Starring *et al.* 1988; Taylor *et al.* 1990). Musculotendinous unit flexibility is also described as musculotendinous unit length and joint range of motion (ROM). The parameter, which is physically measurable, is joint ROM and this term will therefore be used to describe musculotendinous unit flexibility. An increase in joint ROM will indicate an increase in musculotendinous unit flexibility of the musculotendinous unit, which directly affects the joint ROM (Anderson & Burke 1991; Toppenburg & Bullock 1986).

General benefits of flexibility training

Athletes and trainers commonly perform flexibility training as part of regular training and in preparation for competition. It is also an integral part of most rehabilitation programmes following injury or surgery. The general benefits of flexibility training are usually cited as decreasing the risk of injury (primary and secondary prevention), decreasing muscle soreness and improving sports performance. Evidence that flexibility training does benefit the athlete will now be briefly reviewed.

Decreased risk of injury

Flexibility training is routinely recommended to increase ROM and thereby to reduce the risk of injury (Liemohn 1978; Glick 1980; Ekstrand & Gillquist 1982; Ciullo & Zarins 1983; Ekstrand *et al.* 1983; Zachazewski 1990; Beaulieu 1991). The rationale behind this recommendation is that musculotendinous units possessing greater flexibility are less likely to be overstretched, lessening the likelihood of injury (Bryant 1984). It has also been stated that increased flexibility decreases the risk of injury, because flexible joints can withstand a greater amount of 'stress of torque'

before injury, compared to relatively stiff joints (Klafs & Arnheim 1981). It is important to consider independently whether increased flexibility reduces the risk of new injuries (primary prevention) or reinjury (secondary prevention). The scientific evidence for each of these two possibilities will now be briefly reviewed.

DOES FLEXIBILITY TRAINING DECREASE THE RISK OF INJURIES?

A number of authors have proposed that decreased flexibility results in musculotendinous unit injuries (Liemohn 1978; Ekstrand & Gillquist 1982; Ekstrand *et al.* 1983; Worrell *et al.* 1991). It has been reported that hamstring flexibility was decreased in a group of injured athletes compared with a non-injured group participating in the same sport. Athletes with decreased ROM are more likely to suffer from musculotendinous unit tears than their flexible counterparts (Nicholas 1970; Worrell *et al.* 1991). It has also been suggested that muscle inflexibility may predispose athletes to certain injuries (Ekstrand & Gillquist 1982; Ekstrand *et al.* 1983). These investigations were conducted on soccer players, where the incidence of injuries was related to measures of flexibility. In a more recently published prospective study in military recruits, increased hamstring flexibility was related to a decrease in the overall incidence (% injuries in 13 weeks) (flexible group = 16.7%, control group = 29.1%) of injuries (Hartig & Henderson 1999).

However, there are studies that do not show that increased flexibility reduces the risk of injury. An early study on badminton players showed flexible players did not report less injuries than their inflexible team-mates (Henricson *et al.* 1983). More recently, in a well-conducted randomized prospective study, pre-exercise stretching did not reduce lower limb soft tissue, bony or all-injury risk in military recruits (Pope *et al.* 2000). However, the stretching protocol used in this study group (one static stretch of 20 s prior to training) may not have been sufficient to increase ROM.

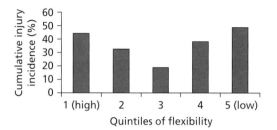

Fig. 11.1 The relationship between flexibility and the cumulative incidence of lower extremity injuries in male military recruits. The relative risk of injury for quintile 1 compared with 3 was 2.2 ($P < 0.05$).

Furthermore, a recently published comprehensive review of the literature has failed to produce strong evidence of a direct link to increased flexibility and a reduction in injuries (Shrier & Gossal 2000). Data from military populations seem to indicate that both increased flexibility as well as reduced flexibility is related to increased risk of injury (Jones & Knapik 1999). The relationship between injury risk and flexibility may well be a U-shaped curve with increased risk in both extremes (Fig. 11.1).

Despite these conflicting reports, stretching is still widely advocated and used by sportspersons and clinicians. In particular, the use of flexibility training to restore normal ROM following injury or surgery is still sound clinical practice. However, more studies are required to define the precise role of flexibility training in the prevention of injuries in sport.

Decreased muscle soreness

Muscle soreness, which follows vigorous or unaccustomed exercise, is known as delayed-onset muscle soreness (DOMS). Stretching has been advocated as a method to decrease DOMS (De Vries 1962; Liemohn 1978; Bryant 1984; Zachazewski 1990; Anderson & Burke 1991; Norris 1993). Despite the widespread belief that stretching decreases DOMS, there are few studies to verify this.

De Vries (1962) reported a chronic reduction of DOMS with repeated stretching. The total time

of stretch was 5 min during the first 22 h post-exercise. Other reports of stretching to reduce DOMS are purely anecdotal (Noakes 1992). Some authors report that musculotendinous units that are flexible before being subjected to vigorous exercise, suffer less from DOMS than musculotendinous units that are inflexible before exercise (Noakes 1992).

In a study conducted by Buroker and Schwane (1989), subjects stretched for a total time of 45 min on the first day after exercise and for 25 min on the second and third days, respectively. McGlynn *et al.* (1979) stretched their subjects for a total time of 10 min on the first day and for 20 min on the second and third days, respectively. Neither of the studies found a decrease in DOMS with the addition of stretching. Buroker and Schwane (1989) mention that this may have been due to their stretch being held for too long.

None of the above results proves that stretching is effective in alleviating DOMS. It is clear that the conditions under which DOMS is decreased by stretching need to be investigated and defined.

Improved performance

Improved athletic performance may be another potential benefit of increased musculotendinous unit flexibility (Bosco & Komi 1979; Godges *et al.* 1989; Zachazewski 1990; Noakes 1992; Wilson *et al.* 1992; Norris 1993; Worrell *et al.* 1994). Indeed, in Borms (1984) it has been suggested that a limited ROM can reduce work efficiency. Two possible explanations are given for the positive association between increased flexibility and enhanced performance.

The first explanation is that musculotendinous unit flexibility is necessary in order for a limb to move through its full ROM. This is a given prerequisite for optimal performance (Ciullo & Zarins 1983; Borms 1984; Shellock & Prentice 1985). The second explanation is that flexibility training could reduce musculotendinous stiffness and enhance rebound performance (Wilson *et al.* 1992). Mechanical work is absorbed by the series elastic component of the musculotendinous unit during eccentric contraction and is stored as potential energy. This energy is then available for use during the subsequent concentric contraction (Cavagna 1970; Bosco & Komi 1979).

Two studies have been conducted which investigate the effect of stretching on musculotendinous unit performance (Wilson *et al.* 1992; Worrell *et al.* 1994). Wilson *et al.* (1992) implemented a static stretching programme twice weekly for 8 weeks in the pectoral musculotendinous unit complex. At the end of this time, the bench press performance of the subjects had improved significantly. Worrell *et al.* (1994) determined the effect of hamstring stretching on hamstring musculotendinous unit performance. The subjects stretched 5 days a week for 3 weeks. Static stretching and proprioceptive neuromuscular facilitation (PNF) stretching were included as stretching methods. The results showed that both methods of stretching increased musculotendinous unit flexibility. Selective torque measurements were significantly improved for eccentric and concentric contractions of the hamstring musculotendinous unit in both groups.

It can be concluded that there is some scientific evidence that increased flexibility enhances musculotendinous unit performance. This is most probably because of the attainment of optimal ROM and the reduction of musculotendinous unit stiffness. Stored elastic strain energy is thereby utilized well during musculotendinous unit contractions.

Other benefits of stretching

Other reported benefits resulting from increased musculotendinous unit ROM are numerous. They include muscle relaxation (De Vries 1962), avoidance of skeletal dysfunction (Starring *et al.* 1988; Bullock-Saxton & Bullock 1994), prevention of scar tissue formation in the musculotendinous unit's shortened position (Reilly 1992) and prevention of imbalance at the joints (Herbert 1988; Bullock-Saxton & Bullock 1994). Skeletal dysfunction can be defined as the syndrome that is a result of prolonged incorrect biomechanical usage of the joints that comprise the skeletal system

(McKenzie 1985). Imbalance at the joints is the result of one musculotendinous unit at a joint being either significantly weaker or significantly less flexible than the other musculotendinous units at that joint (Kendall & McCreary 1983).

Summary

Numerous authors, trainers and athletes advocate the use of stretching to increase musculotendinous unit ROM. The benefits of an increase in musculotendinous unit ROM are commonly reported. These include decreased risk of musculotendinous unit injury, decreased DOMS, enhanced performance, avoidance of joint dysfunction, joint imbalance and scar tissue formation, and increased general relaxation and well being. There is, however, a paucity of scientific research data to substantiate these postulated positive effects of flexibility training.

There is some evidence that indicates that athletic performance may be enhanced by increased musculotendinous unit ROM. There is also an association between decreased injury prevalence and increased musculotendinous unit ROM. By all accounts, there are few, if any, negative side effects if stretching is implemented correctly. Therefore, the use of stretching to increase musculotendinous unit ROM is likely to continue to be supported by therapists, coaches and athletes.

Pathophysiology of soft tissue contracture following injury

The biology of soft tissue repair following injury or surgery has been discussed in detail in Chapters 3–5. However, in the context of flexibility training as part of normal rehabilitation following injury or surgery, a brief review of the mechanisms associated with soft tissue contracture is appropriate. A decrease in range of motion following injury and repair can be the result of a number of mechanisms (Table 11.2).

The healing process in soft tissues follows a continuous process consisting of four interwoven phases: immediate reaction to trauma (0–60 min), acute inflammatory phase (0–72 h), repair phase

Table 11.2 Mechanisms responsible for decreased range of motion in soft tissues following injury or surgery.

Increased fibrosis within the scar
Wound contraction
Immobilization
Nerve root tension
Decreased tissue temperature
Increased age

(2–42 days) and the remodelling phase (21 days to 1 year). During the late part of the inflammatory and early part of the repair phase, fibroblast accumulation is evident in the wound (Wahl & Renström 1990). The repair process follows and is characterized by recruitment of fibroblasts, proliferation of fibroblasts, collagen and matrix synthesis, and later, tissue remodelling.

Increased fibrosis within the scar

In normal tissue repair, matrix generation is self-limiting and minimal scar tissue formation occurs. However, in some wounds, scar tissue formation may become excessive. This process of increased fibrosis may result from: (i) increased numbers (proliferation and recruitment) of collagen-synthesizing cells; (ii) increased matrix synthesis by existing cells; (iii) deficient collagen degradation; and (iv) continued collagen synthesis (Wahl & Renström 1990). In addition to a larger volume of fibrous tissue, the fibrous tissue can also form adhesions and interfere with the normal function of adjacent tissue.

Wound contraction

Wound contraction refers to the inward movement of the wound edges by the action of cells known as myofibroblasts (Martinez-Hernandez & Amenta 1990). It is postulated that myofibroblasts are derived from mesenchymal stem cells or from perivascular cells. They appear at the wound site 3–4 days after the injury and become prominent 6–7 days after the injury. Their contraction can reduce wound size by up to 70%.

Excessive wound contraction can lead to contractures, which can result in decreased soft tissue flexibility. A detailed discussion on the control of wound contraction is beyond the scope of this chapter but has recently been reviewed (Nedelec *et al.* 2000).

Other factors

Following an injury, a decrease in musculotendinous unit flexibility may also be associated with other factors. These include: (i) increased nerve root tension (Gadjosik 1991); (ii) increased age (Norris 1993; Booth *et al.* 1994) and obesity (Norris 1993); (iii) decreased musculotendinous unit temperature (Rigby 1964; Sapega *et al.* 1981; Norris 1993); and (iv) immobilization or prolonged usage in a limited ROM (Herbert 1988; Starring *et al.* 1988).

Measurement of flexibility

The measurement of musculotendinous unit flexibility is of importance in both the laboratory and in the clinical examination room. A brief discussion on the basic method that is used to measure musculotendinous unit flexibility is therefore needed. Musculotendinous unit flexibility refers to its functional length (Toppenburg & Bullock 1986), and represents the degree to which it permits a movement over which it has an influence (Bullock-Saxton & Bullock 1994). In clinical practice, the ROM of a joint or a group of joints is usually measured and then compared with the normal values expected for a specific population. It is also useful to measure the ROM prior to starting flexibility training, in order to assess changes objectively. Practically, a clinical test of flexibility will be done by a clinician who will position a limb or a body segment, and then gradually move the segment to an end point.

For example, a number of anatomical positions have been used to assess hamstring musculotendinous flexibility. These include: (i) flexion at the hips in standing (Gadjosik *et al.* 1993); (ii) extension of the knee with the hip flexed to 90° while lying in the supine position (Gadjosik &

Lusin 1983; Gadjosik *et al.* 1993); and (iii) the straight leg raise (SLR) method (Fahrni 1966; Breig & Troup 1979; Goeken 1991, 1993; Gadjosik *et al.* 1993; Cameron *et al.* 1994). The SLR method is commonly used because it is relatively easy to measure (Janda 1983; Kendall & McCreary 1983) and evidence indicates that it is a clinically acceptable form of measurement (Gadjosik 1991; Gadjosik *et al.* 1993). The SLR method has been proven as a reliable, albeit indirect, measure of hamstring musculotendinous unit flexibility (Gadjosik 1991; Gadjosik *et al.* 1993).

A number of methods have been used to determine the end-point for a clinical range of motion measurement. These include: (i) patient sensation of the end of range (as a tolerable, uncomfortable, but not painful sensation) (Goeken 1991); (ii) subjective tester determination of end-feel (Cyriax & Cyriax 1983; Maitland 1991); (iii) the start of joint movement as felt by the tester (Bullock-Saxton & Bullock 1994; Hanten & Chandler 1994); (iv) measurement of resistance to movement through objective force measures (Gadjosik 1991); (v) the objective use of cinematography to measure a limb angle (Bohannon 1982); and (vi) the use of the electromyogram (EMG) to objectively detect a sudden spike in neuromuscular activity (Moore & Hutton 1980; Bohannon 1984; Condon & Hutton 1987; Kirsch *et al.* 1993; Chequer *et al.* 1994). The repeatability of the various measures of end-point in testing hamstring flexibility was evaluated recently in a controlled laboratory-based study. The repeatability of the four common tests is depicted in Table 11.3.

Table 11.3 The intratester repeatability of four common methods of assessing the end-point in hamstring range of motion testing (Hughes 1996).

Test of end-point	Correlation coefficient
Subject (patient sensation)	0.86
Tester end-feel	0.95
Knee bend	0.73
EMG spike	0.99

The EMG detection of the end-point is the most repeatable measurement of the end-point of the flexibility test (intratester correlation coefficient = 0.99) (Hughes 1996), and is recommended for research studies. The most repeatable clinical method of assessing end-point is the end-feel by the tester (intratester correlation coefficient = 0.95). This method is recommended for testing end-range in a clinical setting.

Physiology of stretching

Stretching implies that a force applied to the tissue elongates the tissue. The physiological effects that stretching has on the musculotendinous unit include neural effects (Beaulieu 1981; Reilly 1992; Norris 1993; Vujnovich & Dawson 1994), plastic (viscous) effects (Sapega *et al.* 1981; Starring *et al.* 1988) and elastic effects (Starring *et al.* 1988; Taylor *et al.* 1990). The physiology of each of these effects is discussed briefly.

Neural effects of stretching

There are three reflexes that primarily control the neural effects of stretching. These are the stretch reflex, inverse stretch reflex, and perception and control of pain by the Pacinian corpuscles.

When a stretch is applied to the musculotendinous unit, the first reflex evoked is the stretch reflex. The origin of this reflex is situated in the intrafusal and extrafusal fibres of the muscle spindle (Beaulieu 1981; Etnyre & Abraham 1986; Reilly 1992; Norris 1993; Vujnovich & Dawson 1994). The stretch reflex serves as a protective measure by causing a reflex contraction of the muscle to prevent overstretching of the musculotendinous unit. The magnitude and rate of contraction elicited by the stretch reflex in a musculotendinous unit are proportional to the magnitude and rate of the stretch that is applied to that musculotendinous unit (Beaulieu 1981; Matthews 1993). Both static and ballistic stretching evoke a response in the stretch reflex when the end-point of ROM is reached (Beaulieu 1981). One method of observing the stretch reflex is through the EMG device (Moore & Hutton 1980;

Condon & Hutton 1987). In this method, the stretch reflex causes a spiking of the neural activity, which is reflected by measuring EMG activity.

The inverse stretch reflex applies both to prolonged contraction and stretching of the musculotendinous unit (Beaulieu 1981; Anderson & Burke 1991). This reflex is responsible for preventing prolonged increased strain of the musculotendinous unit, caused either by powerful active contraction or by overstretching of the musculotendinous unit (Beaulieu 1981; Etnyre & Abraham 1986; Anderson & Burke 1991). The origin of the inverse stretch reflex is located in the Golgi tendon organ (GTO), which is comprised of receptors situated in the musculotendinous junction of the musculotendinous unit. The GTO causes a dampening effect on the motor neuronal discharges, thereby causing relaxation of the musculotendinous unit by resetting its resting length (Beaulieu 1981; Reilly 1992; Norris 1993; Vujnovich & Dawson 1994). This usually occurs 6–20 s after commencement of the stretch (Norris 1993).

The third reflex of the musculotendinous unit originates in the Pacinian corpuscles that are located throughout the musculotendinous unit. The Pacinian corpuscles serve as pressure sensors, and assist with the regulation of pain tolerance in the musculotendinous unit (Beaulieu 1981; Reilly 1992; Vujnovich & Dawson 1994).

The three reflexes together are responsible for the neural effects that regulate musculotendinous unit flexibility, and are active during the stretching of the musculotendinous unit. The normal sequence of activation in a vigorous stretching movement would therefore be stretch reflex activation, causing reflex contraction of the musculotendinous unit, and Pacinian corpuscle activation, leading to a perception of pain. This would be followed in a prolonged stretch by GTO inhibitory effects and Pacinian corpuscle modification. The latter two reflexes will allow relaxation in musculotendinous unit tension and decreased pain perception (Beaulieu 1981; Reilly 1992; Vujnovich & Dawson 1994).

It has also been suggested that prolonged exposure to significantly large and unusual afferent inputs can cause long-term changes in levels of neuronal excitability and thereby, indirectly, on flexibility (Vujnovich & Dawson 1994). Therefore, musculotendinous units that are exposed to repetitive stretching demonstrate increased tolerance to the manoeuvre, resulting in an apparent increased ROM.

Plastic and elastic effects of stretching

Plastic deformation within the musculotendinous unit has largely been ascribed to changes which occur in the non-contractile elements within the musculotendinous unit (Cavagna 1970; Sapega et al. 1981; Vujnovich & Dawson 1994). The non-contractile elements (ligaments, tendons, capsules, aponeuroses and fascial sheaths) are predominantly comprised of connective tissue. Connective tissue is made up of collagen fibres which vary in spatial arrangements and are of varying densities and strengths (Sapega et al. 1981). The non-contractile element of the muscle tissue is also comprised of a connective tissue framework, which is responsible for its resistance to stretch (Sapega et al. 1981). Scar tissue and adhesions are also comprised of connective tissue (Sapega et al. 1981). Prolonged stretching results in plastic elongation of the connective tissue (Sapega et al. 1981; Starring et al. 1988). The mechanisms of both increased plastic and elastic deformation have already been defined and described above.

Methods of stretching

Several stretching techniques have been developed to increase joint ROM. These include PNF, ballistic stretching and static stretching. Combinations of these techniques have also been advocated. All these techniques rely on the neural, plastic and elastic effects of deformation as previously described for their effectiveness.

Proprioceptive neuromuscular facilitation

Proprioceptive neuromuscular facilitation is based on the theory that maximal contraction of

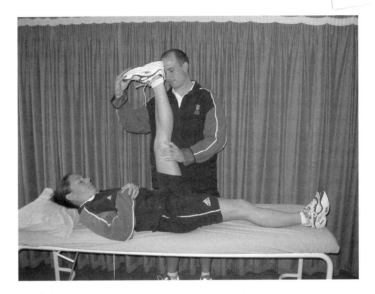

Fig. 11.2 A typical position for performing an assisted proprioceptive neuromuscular facilitation stretch technique.

the musculotendinous unit results in maximum relaxation after active contraction of that musculotendinous unit (Knott & Voss 1956; Sady *et al.* 1982; Voss 1985; Osternig *et al.* 1987; Anderson & Burke 1991). The PNF stretches that are used in sports have been adapted from neurological physical therapy treatments. The two techniques that are commonly used are contract–relax (CR) and contract–relax agonist–contract (CRAC).

1 *Contract–relax.* In CR, a therapist stretches a limb to the point where limitation of ROM is felt. The therapist then holds this stretched position while the patient actively contracts the musculotendinous unit against the resistance of the therapist (Fig. 11.2).

The muscle is then relaxed and moved passively to the new lengthened position, until a stretch is felt in the new position (Hanten & Chandler 1994; Voss 1967, 1985; Norris 1993). A rotational component which entails a movement in the horizontal plane may be added to the resistance which is in the sagittal or longitudinal plane (Hanten & Chandler 1994; Voss 1967, 1985). Modifications to this method include contraction of the musculotendinous unit before stretching and contracting as described above (Beaulieu 1981; Taylor *et al.* 1990; Noakes 1992; Bandy & Irion 1994). The rationale behind the CR

method is that increased stress through contraction of the musculotendinous unit will result in autogenic inhibition in the musculotendinous unit. The GTO activity will decrease tension and cause relaxation by resetting the musculotendinous unit length. This will facilitate the passive stretch procedure applied by the clinician (Norris 1993).

2 *Contract–relax agonist–contract.* In CRAC, the musculotendinous unit is stretched as described above in the CR procedure. In addition to this, the opposing musculotendinous unit (antagonist) of the musculotendinous unit being stretched (agonist) is contracted isometrically while the stretch is applied. The stretch procedure applied by the clinician is then aided by contraction of the opposing musculotendinous unit (antagonist). This results in reciprocal inhibition of the musculotendinous unit being stretched, in order to reduce its tension (Voss 1985; Norris 1993).

In one of the first studies on the role of PNF in flexibility training, PNF was compared with static stretching of the hamstring musculotendinous unit (Tanigawa 1972). In this study, subjects were divided into two treatment groups, and stretches were applied twice weekly for 4 consecutive weeks. The PNF stretch procedure involved taking the leg into SLR until the subject detected a stretch sensation. In this position, an isometric contraction was held for 7 s and then allowed to rest in the neutral position for 5 s. This was then repeated three more times. The static stretch procedure to the hamstring musculotendinous unit was applied to group 2 in the SLR position for 7 s and allowed to rest in the neutral position for 5 s. This static stretch was repeated three more times. The control group rested in the neutral position for 45 s. The results indicated that PNF was more effective than static stretching for increasing hamstring musculotendinous unit ROM. Static stretching was also more effective than the control group. Measurements were taken after each stretching session and these indicate that PNF resulted in greater increases in ROM at each of the individual stretching sessions and over the 4-week period.

In another study the effects of PNF, ballistic and static stretching were compared (Sady et al. 1982). Subjects were divided into four groups: PNF, ballistic stretch, static stretch and controls. Measurements of musculotendinous unit ROM were taken of the shoulder, hamstrings and trunk. These measurements were repeated at the end of the 6-week programme. Stretch procedures were performed three times weekly. The PNF procedure consisted of a stretch of the musculotendinous unit to end of range, an isometric contraction for 6 s, an unspecified relaxation period and a further unspecified stretch. This was repeated two more times. The ballistic stretch involved repeating the full ROM, rapidly, 20 times. The static stretch involved reaching the musculotendinous unit end of range, holding for 6 s, relaxing for an unspecified time and repeating the procedure twice more. The control group's procedure was not specified. Results indicate that only PNF stretching increased musculotendinous unit ROM over the 6-week period, compared with the control group. This study was limited because there was no reported detail in terms of the control group's procedure and individual measurements of musculotendinous unit ROM during the 6-week period.

Other authors also reported that PNF stretching techniques are effective in increasing muscu-

lotendinous unit ROM (Holt et al. 1970; Tanigawa 1972; Sady et al. 1982; Wallin et al. 1985; Etnyre & Abraham 1986; Osternig et al. 1987; Cobbing et al. 2001). However, if PNF is to be performed effectively, it requires expertise in all the stretching techniques, as well as an experienced clinician. These techniques, therefore, although effective, are seldom prescribed to or administered by individual athletes (Bandy & Irion 1994).

Ballistic stretching

During ballistic stretching, the limb is moved to the end of its ROM where the stretch sensation is felt, either passively by the clinician or actively by the subjects themselves (Fig. 11.3).

Once this stretched position is achieved, repetitive bouncing or jerking movements are added (Schultz 1979; Sady et al. 1982; Hardy & Jones 1986; Anderson & Burke 1991). This jerking motion during ballistic stretching could theoretically exceed the limit of available range and thereby cause a strain injury or tear in the musculotendinous unit (De Vries 1962; Anderson & Burke 1991; Noakes 1992). In addition, this rapid jerking movement also elicits the stretch reflex, which then causes a reflex contraction against the direction of stretch in the musculotendinous unit. The resulting increase in tension can therefore increase the risk of injury (Beaulieu 1981; Anderson & Burke 1991; Norris 1993). Theoretically, this technique may not be as beneficial for increasing ROM as the musculotendinous unit would undergo a reflex contraction at each bounce or jerk due to the stretch reflex. Relaxation, or lengthening, of the musculotendinous unit can therefore not be achieved (Beaulieu 1981; Voss 1985; Noakes 1992; Matthews 1993).

In one study, the effects of a combination of ballistic and static stretching with static stretching alone on the ankle dorsiflexion musculotendinous unit were compared (Vujnovich & Dawson 1994). Subjects were divided into a static (stretch applied to the musculotendinous unit for 160 s) and a static–ballistic stretch group (static stretch applied to the musculotendinous unit for 160 s followed by 160 s of ballistic stretch). The

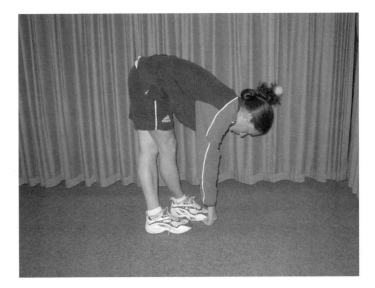

Fig. 11.3 A typical position for ballistic stretching of the hamstring muscles. The athlete performs small oscillating movements in this position.

control group was rested for an unspecified time period. The results of this study showed that a static stretch followed by ballistic stretching increased musculotendinous unit ROM more than static stretching alone. Given that all the stretching techniques are reported to increase musculotendinous unit ROM (Tanigawa 1972; Sapega *et al.* 1981; Taylor *et al.* 1990; Vujnovich & Dawson 1994), it is not surprising that the addition of one technique to the other, thereby doubling the total stretching time, will result in greater increases in musculotendinous unit ROM than with one technique alone. In this study, the one group was stretched for 160 s in total, whereas the other group was stretched for a total of 320 s. The greater increases in ROM in the static–ballistic group could not therefore be explained by the stretch type only, but also by total duration of stretch.

The use of ballistic stretching would appear to increase the risk of injury due to the increases in musculotendinous unit tension. Furthermore, due to the stretch reflex mechanism, it, indeed, may not be effective in increasing musculotendinous unit ROM. Its use is therefore not widely advocated as the technique of choice to improve musculotendinous unit ROM.

Static stretching

The most common method of stretching that is used by athletes, coaches and therapists, is the static stretch (Zachazewski 1990; Anderson & Burke 1991; Beaulieu 1991; Norris 1993). Static stretching is characterized by the limb being moved slowly and gently to the end of its available ROM, in order to obtain a stretch sensation in the tissues (Fig. 11.4).

This controlled stretch is maintained in this position for an extended period (Beaulieu 1991; Norris 1993). The end of the available range is determined by maximum tolerance of the subject to the stretch sensation just short of pain (Norris 1993; Bandy & Irion 1994).

Static stretching is sometimes referred to as passive stretching. Where this occurs, the distinction referred to is the mode of application. If the stretch is applied and held by the subject, it is referred to as static stretching. If the static stretch procedure is applied by a therapist or another person to the subject, it is sometimes referred to as passive stretching (Beaulieu 1981; Noakes 1992). The danger of the passive stretch is that when executed incorrectly by a team-mate or partner, it has the potential to overstretch the

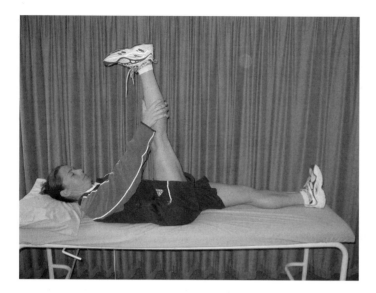

Fig. 11.4 A typical position for an athlete to perform a static stretch of the hamstring musculotendinous unit.

musculotendinous unit. When administered by an experienced clinician, though, passive stretching can be very useful and as effective as the standard static stretch (Beaulieu 1981; Noakes 1992).

When the static stretch position is obtained slowly and gently, the stretch reflex response is dampened and occurs late in the movement. As the tension in the musculotendinous unit from the stretch and from the reflex contraction increases, the inverse stretch reflex initiated by the GTO is induced (Beaulieu 1981; Voss 1985). This causes autogenic inhibition in the musculotendinous unit and allows a greater ROM to be achieved in the musculotendinous unit (Voss 1985). The GTO, therefore, overrides the stretch reflex. In this way, both neural effects and plastic deformation are utilized to increase musculotendinous unit ROM.

In one study, variations of the static stretching procedures were examined. The effect of cyclic stretch with static stretch on hamstring musculotendinous unit ROM was studied (Starring *et al.* 1988). Subjects were divided into two groups and the hamstring musculotendinous unit length was measured using the knee extension test with the hip in 90° flexion. The cyclic stretch entailed the hamstring being stretched to the end of range

and held for 10 s. The limb was then moved into a greater ROM for a further 10 s. This procedure was repeated for 15 min. Because the stretch was held statically for a period of time, this cyclic method of stretching is referred to as a repeated static stretch. The static stretch group had a constant force applied to the hamstrings for 15 min. Hamstring musculotendinous unit ROM was measured at the end of each treatment session. The procedures were repeated daily for 5 consecutive days. Another measurement was taken 5 days after the last stretching session.

Results showed that hamstring musculotendinous unit ROM increased more in the cyclic stretch group compared to the static stretch group. Increases in musculotendinous unit ROM were recorded on day 5 compared with day 1, for both groups. In both groups, there were still increases in musculotendinous unit ROM at 5 days after the last stretch session, compared with the measurements taken on day 1. These increases were, however, less on day 5 compared with those reported on day 1. The cyclic group maintained a significantly larger increase in ROM than the static group. These results show that static stretching which is held, and then repeated in the increased ROM, produces greater increases in musculotendinous unit ROM than static stretching sustained for long periods in one position.

Compared with other methods of stretching, static stretching produces the least amount of tension (Moore & Hutton 1980). Theoretically, it therefore has the lowest risk of injury, and is easy and safe to implement. The static stretching method is consequently the one most commonly advocated for use in a flexibility training programme (Bass 1965; Burry 1975; Glick 1980; Beaulieu 1981; Leach 1982; Zarins 1982; Voss 1985; Noakes 1992).

Scientific basis of a stretching session

A number of factors are important in the successful implementation of a stretching session or flexibility training programme, irrespective of the type of technique. These include: (i) the duration for which a stretch is held; (ii) the number of times the stretch is repeated in one session; (iii) the number of times the session is repeated per day or week; (iv) the effect of warm-up on the effect of stretching; and (v) the most effective anatomical position in which to stretch a particular musculotendinous unit. Despite the fact that there are guidelines in most sports medicine textbooks on the method of static and PNF stretching (Zachazewski 1990; Noakes 1992; Norris 1993), there are very few clinical research data available to support the currently advocated methods of static and PNF stretching. This section will focus on the recently acquired data from research studies that identified the scientific basis for optimum static and PNF stretching.

Optimum duration of a stretch at one stretching session

STATIC STRETCHING

The duration of the force applied in static stretching can be defined as the time for which a stretch is applied at a single stretching session. Investigators have studied the effects of various durations of passive stretch in animal models. One study compared the effects of high load, short duration (5 min) stretch with low load (25% of high load), long duration (50 min) stretch (Warren et al. 1976). This study was conducted on rat tail tendon. The high load, short duration protocol resulted in almost twice the elongation compared to the low load, long duration group. However, in the high load, short duration group, elongation was retained for only half as long as in the low load, long duration group.

Lehmann et al. (1970) compared short-term stretch (time not reported) with long-term stretch (20 min) on rat tail tendon. This study found that long duration stretches were more effective in increasing tendon length. Both Lehmann et al. (1970) and Warren et al.'s (1976) studies did not investigate some of the commonly used stretching durations and therefore offer limited information on the optimum duration of static stretching. In addition, both these studies were conducted on animal tail tendon and therefore cannot be extrapolated to human musculotendinous units.

In one animal study, performed on rabbit musculotendinous units, stress relaxation was used to determine the effects of static stretch duration on musculotendinous unit ROM (Taylor et al. 1990). In this study, the musculotendinous unit was taken to a predetermined tension of 78.4 N (this magnitude of force was selected on the basis that it did not cause any irreversible damage but resulted in significant elastic deformation of the musculotendinous unit) and held at that length for 30 s. The stress relaxation was then measured by recording the change in tension in the musculotendinous unit over that time period. It was documented that significant relaxation in the musculotendinous unit occurred after 12–18 s, although relaxation continued over the entire 30 s period. Because the measurements were only taken over 30 s, it is impossible to state whether the same overall stress relaxation would have occurred if held for a period of 48–72 s (i.e. $4 \times$ 12–18 s).

The optimum duration of a static stretch that is to be used in the normal population, and in athletes in particular, has also been investigated in human studies. The optimum duration of static stretching has been reported on numerous

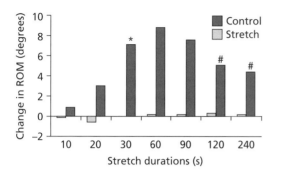

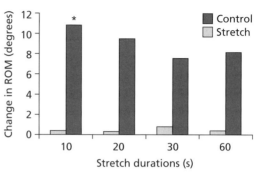

Fig. 11.5 The effect of different static stretch durations on changes in hamstring ROM. All stretch durations (except the 10 s duration) were significantly different from controls. *, significant difference from change in ROM after 20 s; #, significant difference from change in ROM after 60 s. (From Hughes *et al.* 2001.)

Fig. 11.6 The effect of different PNF stretch durations on changes in hamstring ROM. All stretch durations were significantly different from controls. *, significant difference from change in ROM between 10 and 30 s. (From Cobbing *et al.* 2001.)

occasions and varies from 6 s to 20 min (De Vries 1962; Tanigawa 1972; Medeiros *et al.* 1977; Moore & Hutton 1980; Beaulieu 1981; Klafs & Arnheim 1981; Sady *et al.* 1982; Bohannon 1984; Henricson *et al.* 1984; Madding *et al.* 1987; Zachazewski 1990; Bandy & Irion 1994).

Until recently, only three studies have been reported in humans where different durations of static stretch were compared with another. Bohannon (1984) measured increases in musculotendinous unit length at 15 s and then at 30 s intervals thereafter, for 8 min. Madding *et al.* (1987) measured only at 15, 45 and 120 s. Bandy and Irion (1994) measured at 12, 30 and 60 s over a 6-week period.

A definitive study described by Hughes *et al.* (2001) examined the effects of different durations of static stretching on hamstring musculotendinous unit ROM. In this study, 10 normal subjects underwent static stretching durations of 10, 20, 30, 60, 90, 120 and 240 s. ROM was measured using EMG activity as the end-point. Three stretches were applied with a 1 min rest in between. The results of this study are depicted in Fig. 11.5.

The results of this study clearly show that a static stretch duration of 30–60 s is optimal to increase ROM in static stretching.

PNF STRETCHING

The precise duration of a PNF stretch on increases in hamstring ROM has only recently been reported. In this study, human subjects (experimental and a control group) were subjected to durations of PNF stretch of 10, 20, 30 and 60 s. The increases in hamstring ROM following different durations of PNF stretches are depicted in Fig. 11.6.

The results of this study show that a 10 s PNF stretch is as effective in increasing ROM as longer durations, i.e. up to 60 s.

Number of repetitions (frequency) of stretches at one stretching session

STATIC STRETCHING

The optimum number of repetitions that should be performed at a single static stretching session has not been investigated until recently. In the past, between one and 20 repetitions have been advocated to increase ROM (Beaulieu 1991; Norris 1993). However, this advice has not been based on scientific data from human studies.

In one animal study on rabbit musculotendinous units, this parameter was investigated (Taylor *et al.* 1990). In this study, the stress–relaxation procedure was used. This involved taking the musculotendinous unit to a predetermined 78.4 N point of tension. This point was determined as the point where no irreparable damage was done to the musculotendinous unit, but where lengthening occurred. The length of the musculotendinous unit where this point of tension occurred was maintained for 30 s. During the 30 s period, the tension in the musculotendinous unit and its length was measured. The tension decreased during the 30 s period. After 30 s, the musculotendinous unit was returned to the initial resting tension of the musculotendinous unit of 1.96 N. This cycle of stretching was repeated 10 consecutive times for each musculotendinous unit. Results showed significant increases in musculotendinous unit length during the first four cycles, with cycles 1 and 2 showing the largest increments in increased musculotendinous unit length. Cycles 5–10 also showed increases in musculotendinous unit length, but these were not as significant as those occurring during cycles 1–4.

This study indicates that the optimal number of repetitions in a single stretching session is four. However, because all the stretches were only held for 30 s, it was not possible to determine whether the same increases in ROM would have been attained had the stretch been held for a total of 48–72 s (i.e. 4×12–18 s) in one session. Although this was a very thorough and useful study, it required validation in the human model.

It was therefore necessary to investigate the number of repetitions in a static stretch session that are required to gain optimum increases in ROM in the human musculotendinous unit. Recently this study was undertaken, using normal subjects that were subjected to stretches of 30 s duration (Hughes 1996). The frequency of stretches varied from one to 10 stretches. The results of this study are depicted in Fig. 11.7.

The results of this study indicate that three stretches are optimum in increasing ROM and that additional stretches do not add any further advantage to increasing the ROM.

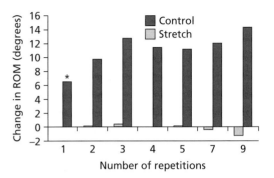

Fig. 11.7 The effect of different static stretch repetitions on changes in hamstring ROM. All stretch repetitions were significantly different from controls. *, significant difference from change in ROM from after repetitions. (From Hughes *et al.* 2001.)

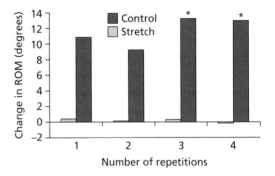

Fig. 11.8 The effect of different PNF stretch repetitions on changes in hamstring ROM. All stretch repetitions were significantly different from controls. *, significant difference from change in ROM from after two repetitions. (From Cobbing *et al.* 2001.)

PNF STRETCHING

The optimum frequency of PNF stretches to increase hamstring ROM has only very recently been reported. Healthy subjects underwent 10 s repeated PNF stretches of different frequencies. Hamstring ROM was assessed in a stretch and control group using EMG spikes as the end-point to determine ROM. The results of this study are depicted in Fig. 11.8.

The results of this study show that three PNF stretches result in the largest increase in ROM, but that this was not significantly more than performing a single stretch.

Retention of increased ROM after one stretching session

STATIC STRETCHING

Until recently, it had not been well documented how long the retention in increased ROM following a static stretch session would last. A number of authors have suggested time periods for the retention of ROM, but none of these have been tested in a well-conducted clinical trial. Suggested time periods for retention of ROM ranged from 3 h (Beaulieu 1981) to days (Atha & Wheatley 1976). Data on the retention of ROM after a static stretching session are vitally important in order to implement a scientifically based stretching programme.

In a study on rat tail tendon by Warren *et al.* (1976), it was demonstrated that the application of low load forces (25% of high load) for 50 min resulted in the retention of more than twice the elongation compared with the high load, short duration applied for 5 min. The retention of elongation was measured 10 min poststretch. This study was conducted on animal tendon and is therefore not representative of the complete musculotendinous unit and may also not be applicable to human subjects.

In a recent study (Hughes 1996), the retention in ROM achieved by a static stretch session (3 × 30 s stretches) was evaluated. Normal subjects underwent a static stretch session, and ROM was then measured over a 24 h period to determine residual increases in ROM at periodic intervals. The results of this study are depicted in Fig. 11.9.

The results of this study indicate that following a stretch session that is conducted optimally, based on recent scientific evidence, ROM is only retained for 4–6 h. The practical implication is that the frequency with which stretch sessions should be conducted during a day to achieve maximal benefit, is approximately every 6 h (during awake hours).

PNF STRETCHING

The retention in ROM following a PNF stretch session has not been well investigated. In one study by Toft *et al.* (1989), it was documented that there was a residual effect of increased musculotendinous unit ROM for at least 90 min after a PNF stretching bout. In this study, measurements of ankle dorsiflexion were taken. PNF stretching was obtained by maximal contraction of the plantar flexors for 8 s in the stretched position, followed by 2 s of relaxation and finally 8 s of slow static stretching. This procedure was repeated five times, and 90 min later ankle dorsiflexion was remeasured. It was found that the increases in musculotendinous unit ROM were maintained over this 90 min period. Here the static stretching procedure was administered for 40 s only in total (15 × 8 s) and was preceded by an isometric contraction before each stretch. The duration of retention of ROM following PNF stretching requires further investigation.

Cumulative effect of repeated static stretching sessions

STATIC STRETCHING

Until recently, there had been no studies that documented the cumulative effect, if any, of

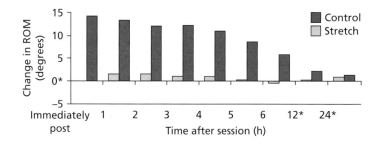

Fig. 11.9 The retention in hamstring ROM after a static stretch session (3 × 30 s stretches). *, significant difference from change in ROM from value immediately poststretch. (From Hughes *et al.* 2001.)

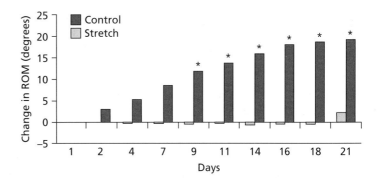

Fig. 11.10 The cumulative effects of daily static stretching (3 × 30 s every 6 h) on hamstring ROM. *, significant difference from change in ROM from day 1. (From Hughes *et al.* 2001.)

repeated bouts of static stretching on joint ROM. In one study by Bandy and Irion (1994), subjects were placed on a stretching programme for 3 weeks. Measurements of hamstring musculotendinous unit ROM were made before and after the study. Subjects in the three experimental groups performed one 15 s, one 30 s or one 60 s static stretch. This static stretch was performed daily, 5 days a week, for 3 weeks. At the end of this period, hamstring musculotendinous unit had increased significantly in the groups stretching for 30 and 60 s, but not in the group stretching for 15 s. However, because measurements were only taken prior to the onset of the study and after 3 weeks, it was not possible to determine when the changes in ROM occurred.

More recently, the cumulative effects of static stretching were investigated. In this study healthy subjects underwent daily stretching every six hours (3 × 30 s static stretches). ROM measurements of the hamstring musculotendinous unit were conducted over a 22-day period. The results of this study are depicted in Fig. 11.10.

The results of this study indicate that daily static stretching (every 6 h) can result in retention of ROM after as short a period as 7 days. There is also a progressive increase in ROM (approximately 1% per degree, in general). From Fig. 11.10 it can be seen that the increase in ROM achieved using this stretching programme is approximately 15–20%, and that a plateau effect had not yet been achieved after 3 weeks.

PNF STRETCHING

Retention in ROM following PNF stretching has not been well investigated either. In one study, a PNF stretching programme was implemented where subjects stretched twice daily for 3 weeks (Toft *et al.* 1989). Ankle dorsiflexion ROM was measured before implementing the stretch procedure and after 3 weeks of stretching. The stretch procedure consisted of a maximal isometric contraction of the plantar flexors for 8 s in the stretched position, followed by a 2 s rest period and finally an 8 s slow static stretch of the plantar flexors. This was repeated five times. The whole procedure was carried out twice daily for 3 weeks. No measurements of ankle ROM were taken during the 3-week period. Ankle ROM was remeasured at the end of the 3-week period. At the final measurement, no stretching procedures were carried out for at least 20 h prior to measurement. There were still large residual increases in ankle musculotendinous unit ROM.

Role of warm-up prior to static stretching on musculotendinous unit ROM

The inclusion of warm-up prior to stretching is widely advocated (Dominguez 1982; Wathen 1987; Zachazewski 1990). However, its role in altering the effectiveness of the stretching procedure is not clear. It has been suggested that increases in flexibility occur as a result of increases in tissue temperatures (Cureton 1941; De Vries 1962; Lehmann *et al.* 1970; Nicholas 1970; Warren *et al.* 1976). Other authors suggest that increased tissue temperatures do not result in increases in musculotendinous unit flexibility (Halkovich *et al.* 1981; Wiktorsson-Moller *et al.* 1983; Williford *et al.* 1986; Cornelius *et al.* 1988).

It is also important to determine whether the warm-up is passive or active. Passive warm-up occurs when the muscles are warmed by means of external heating such as direct heat application (heat packs) or in the form of therapeutic ultrasound. Active warm-up refers to a warm-up of the muscles by active contraction. This would be in the form of a jog or any other exercise where the muscles to be stretched are repeatedly contracted prior to stretching.

PASSIVE WARM-UP

It has been postulated that in passive warm-up, the increases in tissue temperatures increase the extensibility to the musculotendinous unit. This increased extensibility is due to the effects of heat on the intermolecular bonding of collagenous tissue. It is probable that heating of the musculotendinous unit results in the collagen being partially destabilized and consequently more pliable and extensible (Rigby 1964; Lehmann *et al.* 1970; Warren *et al.* 1976; Sapega *et al.* 1981; Ciullo & Zarins 1983).

In an animal study, Warren *et al.* (1976), showed that rat tail tendon extensibility was increased with the addition of heat prior to the static stretch procedure. The tendons were either exposed to temperatures of 25, 39 or 45°C. A load of 100 g was applied to all the tendons and increases in length were measured. The groups exposed to higher temperatures experienced significantly greater increases in extensibility compared with the 25°C group at the load of 100 g. There was also less resultant tissue damage in these two groups than in the 25°C group.

Studies on the effects of passive warm-up on static stretching have also been performed on human subjects. In 1984, Henricson *et al.* conducted a trial on the effects of heat and stretching

on musculotendinous unit ROM. Measurements of hip flexion, abduction and external rotation were taken. Subjects were divided into three groups. The first group had an electric heat pad applied for 20 min at 43°C. A second group had the electric heat pad applied as above and this was then followed by a modified PNF technique consisting of 7 s isometric contraction of the musculotendinous unit, followed by 7 s relaxation, followed by 7 s static stretching. The third group performed only the PNF technique of stretching. Results show that no increases in ROM occurred in the first (heating only) group. The other two groups showed significant increases in ROM, with the combined heat and PNF group showing the greatest increases in ROM. This study indicates that passive heating alone is not effective in increasing musculotendinous unit ROM. However, when combined with stretching, passive heating is more effective in increasing musculotendinous unit ROM than stretching alone. The PNF stretching technique is notable in that it includes a muscle contraction as well as a static stretch. Therefore, PNF techniques employ an element of active warm-up as well.

In another human study, the effect of passive heating on the stretching procedure was studied (Wessling *et al.* 1987). In this study, the triceps surae musculotendinous unit either had static stretching applied to it for 1 min, or 1 min of static stretching applied after 7 min of continuous ultrasound. Ultrasound causes a deep heating effect in tissues (Gerston 1955; Low & Reed 1990). This study showed that the addition of deep heating to static stretching of the musculotendinous unit resulted in greater increases in ROM than static stretching alone. The difference between this study and the one conducted by Henricson *et al.* (1984) may lie in the deep heating effect of ultrasound compared with the more superficial heating of the heat pad.

ACTIVE WARM-UP

Although knowledge of the effects of the addition of passive heat to the effectiveness of stretching in increasing musculotendinous unit ROM is valuable to the clinician, active warm-up is more practical and of more value to the sportsperson. As muscles contract repeatedly, heat is produced and the intramuscular temperature increases (Zachazewski 1990). This process is known as active warm-up or physiological preconditioning (Safran *et al.* 1988; Zachazewski 1990). There have been a number of studies conducted to determine the effect of active warm-up on musculotendinous unit ROM.

In an animal study conducted by Safran *et al.* (1988), the effect of active warm-up on the ROM of the musculotendinous unit was investigated in rabbits. In one group, musculotendinous unit length was measured and then this musculotendinous unit was electrically stimulated to its maximum wave summated tension for 15 s. This was classified as the active warm-up period. The electrode was then removed and the musculotendinous unit was statically stretched to failure. In the second group the musculotendinous unit length was measured and then statically stretched to failure without active warm-up. An average of 7% more force was needed to reach failure in the active warm-up group. The actively warmed-up musculotendinous units could also be stretched to a significantly greater length before reaching failure. Intramuscular temperatures were recorded to increase by 1°C in the actively warmed-up musculotendinous units. The results of this study are valuable because they indicate that actively warmed-up musculotendinous units obtain significant increases in musculotendinous unit ROM and can absorb significantly higher forces before failure. This would indicate that actively warmed-up musculotendinous units would significantly increase their musculotendinous unit ROM when statically stretched and also have a lower risk of injury.

In another study, the effects of active warm-up, massage and stretching on ROM and muscle strength were conducted (Wiktorsson-Moller *et al.* 1983). In this study, hip flexion, hip extension, hip abduction, knee flexion and ankle dorsiflexion ROM, and hamstring and quadriceps strength were measured. There were four groups that were compared. The first group received an active warm-up consisting of 15 min of stationary cycling. The second group received 15 min of warm-up as above and 12 min of massage. The third group received 12 min of massage only. The fourth group received warm-up as above and PNF stretching. The PNF stretch consisted of a maximal isometric contraction for 4–6 s, followed by relaxation for 2 s and finally by a static stretch for 8 s. Results showed that other than for ankle dorsiflexion, warm-up alone, massage alone and warm-up plus massage have no effect on musculotendinous unit ROM. Warm-up combined with stretching showed significant increases in ROM for all joints. None of the groups showed any changes in muscle strength with the intervention. No measurements were done on the effects of stretching alone, and therefore the effect of the addition of warm-up to stretching could not be determined.

In 1986, Williford *et al.* conducted a study on the effects of active warm-up on musculotendinous unit flexibility over a period of 9 weeks. The flexibility of the shoulder, hamstrings, trunk and ankle were measured. The subjects were divided into two groups. The first group performed only static stretching that entailed a static stretch, which was held for 30 s and then repeated once more, totalling 60 s of static stretching. The second group actively warmed-up by jogging lightly but progressively for 5 min, prior to performing the same static stretching as in group 1. The subjects performed their respective stretching routines twice per week for 9 weeks. Results indicated that the active warm-up group gained significantly greater increases (approximately 14%) in ROM than the stretching only group. Gains (approximately 11%) in ROM were also documented in the stretching-only group.

In another study, the effects of the placement of a stretching session in a work-out in increasing ROM was determined (Cornelius *et al.* 1988). Subjects were divided into three groups. The first group performed static stretching for 10 s before the exercise session, which consisted of 20–30 min of jogging. The second group performed static stretching after the exercise session described. The third group performed the

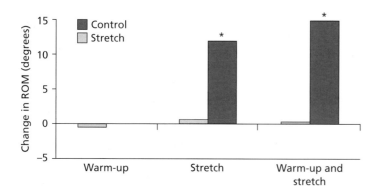

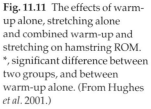

Fig. 11.11 The effects of warm-up alone, stretching alone and combined warm-up and stretching on hamstring ROM. *, significant difference between two groups, and between warm-up alone. (From Hughes *et al.* 2001.)

stretching both before and after the exercise session. The stretching and exercise sessions were performed 3–5 times per week, for 6 weeks. Results showed increases in musculotendinous unit ROM in all the groups, but no significant differences between the groups. This study is limited in its value because the stretching procedure was not well defined, and the subjects in the groups were not well matched. There was a wide variation in the amount of stretching and exercise that was performed by the subjects.

From the above studies, it is difficult to determine the effects of active warm-up on musculotendinous unit ROM. Passive warm-up appears to have little effect on musculotendinous unit ROM (Henricson *et al.* 1984). When passive warm-up is combined with stretching it appears to be more effective than stretching alone for increasing musculotendinous unit ROM (Henricson *et al.* 1984; Wessling *et al.* 1987). Active warm-up before static stretching in human subjects appears more beneficial in increasing musculotendinous unit ROM than static stretching alone, over a period of 9 weeks (Williford *et al.* 1986). The most valuable study on the effect of active warm-up was conducted on rabbit musculotendinous units (Safran *et al.* 1988). However, the results of this study cannot be directly extrapolated to humans. In this study, active warm-up increased musculotendinous unit ROM, musculotendinous unit length to failure, and the force necessary to reach failure.

In a recent study, the effects of active warm-up alone, static stretching alone and active warm-up combined with static stretching on musculotendinous unit ROM were determined. Normal subjects underwent either active warm-up only (running until 70% maximum heart rate was achieved), static stretching (3×30 s) only, or combined active warm-up and then static stretching. Hamstring ROM measurements were conducted in all groups after the interventions, and in a control group. The results of this study are depicted in Fig. 11.11. The results of this study indicate that active warm-up alone is not effective in increasing ROM, but that it may have an additive effect if it is performed prior to static stretching.

There have been no studies that compare active versus passive warm-up, with and without stretching.

Effect of stretch position during the stretching session on musculotendinous unit ROM

It is a widely held belief that stretch position alters the efficacy of the stretching procedure (Voss 1985). For example, it is generally believed that increased ROM in a musculotendinous unit cannot be achieved when the musculotendinous unit is contracting. In a recent study, the effect of limb position on hamstring ROM has been evaluated. Normal subjects underwent three types of stretching procedures: (i) standing and stretching a weightbearing (contracting) hamstring muscle; (ii) standing but stretching a non-weightbearing hamstring muscle; and (iii) lying supine and stretching a non-weightbearing

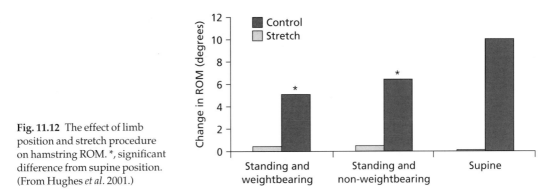

Fig. 11.12 The effect of limb position and stretch procedure on hamstring ROM. *, significant difference from supine position. (From Hughes *et al.* 2001.)

hamstring muscle. The ROM immediately after the stretches (3×30 s static stretches) was measured. The results are depicted in Fig. 11.12.

The results of this study show that limb position is important when performing static stretch procedures. It is advised that static stretching should take place in the relaxed, non-weightbearing position.

Conclusions and practical guidelines for stretching

- Musculoskeletal injuries are common in athletes and require rehabilitation following injury or surgery.
- Injury or surgery can result in decreased joint ROM mainly due to fibrosis and wound contraction.
- Flexibility training is an important component of rehabilitation in order to minimize the decrease in joint ROM.
- Flexibility training should begin in the first week following injury or surgery to prevent decrease in ROM due to wound contraction and fibrosis.
- The main postulated benefits of flexibility training for the non-injured athlete are injury prevention (weak scientific evidence), increased athletic performance (good scientific evidence) and the prevention of muscle soreness (some scientific evidence).
- A variety of stretching techniques can be used in improving range of motion, including PNF, ballistic stretching and static stretching.

- Static stretching is most commonly used, is safe and effective.
- PNF is more effective than static stretching but it requires some training to master the technique and requires an assistant in some instances.
- Ballistic stretching may be effective but it has been postulated to increase the risk of injury while performing the stretch.
- An optimum static stretch session should consist of three stretches lasting 30 s each.
- Two to three static stretch sessions should be performed daily for maximum benefit.
- Static stretch sessions performed two or three times per day will result in a permanent increase in joint range of motion after 7 days.
- A cumulated benefit to daily static stretches (every 6 h) for up to 21 days has been demonstrated.
- A warm-up alone will not increase ROM but has an additive effect if it precedes a static stretch session.
- A static stretch should be performed in the non-weightbearing position with the muscle relaxed for maximum gain in ROM.

References

Agre, J.C. (1985) Hamstring injuries: proposed etiological factors, prevention and treatment. *Sports Medicine* **2**, 21–23.

Anderson, B. & Burke, E.R. (1991) Scientific, medical, and practical aspects of stretching. *Clinical Sports Medicine* **10**, 63–86.

Atha, J. & Wheatley, D.W. (1976) The mobilising effect of repeated measurement on hip flexion. *British Journal of Sports Medicine* **10** (1), 22–25.

Bandy, W.D. & Irion, J.M. (1994) The effect of time on static stretch on the flexibility of the hamstring muscles. *Physical Therapy* **74** (9), 845–852.

Bass, A.L. (1965) Athletic and soft tissue injuries. *Physical Therapy* **51**, 112–114.

Beaulieu, J.E. (1981) Developing a stretching program. *Physical Sportsmedicine* **9** (11), 59–69.

Bohannon, R.W. (1982) Cinematographic analysis of the passive straight-leg-raising test for hamstring muscle length. *Physical Therapy* **62** (9), 1269–1274.

Bohannon, R.W. (1984) Effect of repeated eight-minute muscle loading on the angle of straight-leg-raising. *Physical Therapy* **64** (4), 491–497.

Booth, F.W., Weeden, S.H. & Tseng, B.S. (1994) Effect of aging on human skeletal muscle and motor-function. *Medicine and Science in Sports and Exercise* **26** (5), 556–560.

Borms, J. (1984) Importance of flexibility in overall physical fitness. *International Journal of Physical Education* **11**, 2.

Bosco, C. & Komi, P.V. (1979) Potentiation of the mechanical behaviour of the human skeletal muscle through prestretching. *Acta Physiologica Scandinavica* **106**, 467–472.

Breig, A. & Troup, J.D.G. (1979) Biomechanical considerations in the straight-leg-raising test. *Journal of Orthopaedic and Sports Physical Therapy* **4** (3), 242–250.

Bryant, S. (1984) Flexibility and stretching. *Physical Sportsmedicine* **12** (2), 171.

Bullock-Saxton, J.E. & Bullock, M.I. (1994) Repeatability of muscle length measures around the hip. *Physiotherapy Canada* **46** (2), 105–109.

Burkett, L.N. (1970) Causative factors in hamstring strains. *Medical Science Sports* **2** (1), 39–42.

Burns, D.M. & MacDonald, S.G.G. (1975) *Physics for Biology and Pre Medical Students*, 2nd edn. Addison–Wesley, London.

Buroker, K.C. & Schwane, J.A. (1989) Does postexercise static stretching alleviate delayed muscle soreness? *Physical Sportsmedicine* **17** (6), 65–83.

Burry, H.C. (1975) Soft tissue injury in sport. *Exercise and Sport Sciences Reviews* **3**, 275–301.

Cahill, B.R. & Griffith, E.H. (1978) Effect of preseason conditioning on the incidence and severity of high school football knee injuries. *American Journal of Sports Medicine* **6** (4), 180–184.

Cameron, D.M., Bohannon, R.W. & Owen, S.V. (1994) Influence of hip position on measurements of the straight-leg-raise test. *Journal of Orthopaedic and Sports Physical Therapy* **19** (3), 168–172.

Cavagna, G.A. (1970) Elastic bounce of the body. *Journal of Applied Physiology* **29** (3), 279–282.

Chequer, R.S., Goodin, D.S. & Aminoff, M.J. (1994) Late electromyographic activity following stretch in human forearm muscles: physiological role. *Brain Research* **641**, 273–278.

Ciullo, J.V. & Zarins, B. (1983) Biomechanics of the musculotendinous unit: relation to athletic performance and injury. *Clinical Sports Medicine* **2** (1), 71–86.

Clendaniel, R.A., Gossman, M.R., Katholi, C.R. *et al.* (1984) Hamstring muscle length in men and women: normative data. *Physical Therapy* **64** (5), 716–717.

Cobbing, S.E., Schwellnus, M.P. & Noakes, T.D. (2002) Scientific basis for stretching III: duration, frequency and type of proprioceptive neuromuscular facilitation (PNF) stretching. (In review.)

Condon, S.M. & Hutton, R.S. (1987) Soleus muscle electromyographic activity and ankle dorsiflexion range of motion during four stretching procedures. *Physical Therapy* **67** (1), 24–30.

Cooper, D.L. & Fair, J. (1978) Hamstring strains. *Physical Sportsmedicine* **6**, 104.

Cornelius, W.L., Hagemann, R.W. & Jackson, A.W. (1988) A study on placement of stretching within a workout. *Journal of Sports Medicine and Physical Fitness* **28** (3), 234–236.

Cureton, T.K. (1941) Flexibility as an aspect of physical fitness. *Research Quarterly for Exercise and Sport* **12**, 390.

Cyriax, J.H. & Cyriax, P.J. (1983) *Illustrated Manual of Orthopaedic Medicine*, 1st edn. Butterworths, London.

De Vries, H.A. (1962) Evaluation of static stretching procedures for improvement of flexibility. *Research Quarterly* **33** (2), 222–229.

Dominguez, R.H. (1982) To stretch or not to stretch? *Physical Sportsmedicine* **10** (9), 137–140.

Ekstrand, J. & Gillquist, J. (1982) The frequency of muscle tightness and injuries in soccer players. *American Journal of Sports Medicine* **10** (2), 75–78.

Ekstrand, J., Gillquist, J., Moller, M. *et al.* (1983) Incidence of soccer injuries and their relation to team training and team success. *American Journal of Sports Medicine* **11**, 63–67.

Etnyre, B.R. & Abraham, L.D. (1986) H-reflex changes during static stretching and two variations of proprioceptive neuromuscular facilitation techniques. *Electroencephalography and Clinical Neurophysiology* **63**, 174–179.

Fahrni, W. (1966) Observations on straight-leg-raising with special reference to nerve root adhesions. *Canadian Journal of Surgery* **9**, 44–48.

Fung, Y.C.B. (1967) Elasticity of soft tissues in simple elongation. *Journal of Physiology* **213** (6), 1532–1544.

Gadjosik, R.L. (1991) Effects of static stretching on the maximal length and resistance to passive stretch of short hamstring muscles. *Journal of Orthopaedic and Sports Physical Therapy* **14** (6), 250–255.

Gadjosik, R. & Lusin, G. (1983) Reliability of an active knee extension test. *Physical Therapy* **63** (7), 1085–1090.

Gadjosik, R.L., Rieck, M.A., Sullivan, D.K. *et al.* (1993) Comparison of four clinical tests for assessing hamstring muscle length. *Journal of Orthopaedic and Sports Physical Therapy* **18** (5), 614–618.

Gersten, J.W. (1955) Effect of ultrasound on tendon extensibility. *American Journal of Physical Medicine* **34**, 359–368.

Glick, J.M. (1980) Muscle strains: prevention and treatment. *Physical Sportsmedicine* **8** (11), 73–77.

Godges, J.J., Holden, McR., Langdon, C. *et al.* (1989) The effects of two stretching procedures on hip range of motion and gait economy. *Journal of Orthopaedic and Sports Physical Therapy* **10**, 350–357.

Goeken, L.N. (1991) Instrumental straight-leg-raising: a new approach to Lasegue's test. *Archives of Physical Medical Rehabilitation* **72**, 959–966.

Goeken, L.N. (1993) Instrumental straight-leg-raising: results in healthy subjects. *Archives of Physical Medical Rehabilitation* **74**, 194–203.

Grahame, R. & Jenkins, J.M. (1972) Joint hypermobility—asset or liability. *Annals of the Rheumatic Diseases* **31**, 109–111.

Halbertsma, J.P.K. & Goeken, L.N.H. (1994) Stretching exercises: effects on passive extensibility and stiffness in short hamstrings of healthy subjects. *Archives of Physical Medicine and Rehabilitation* **75**, 976–981.

Halkovich, L.R., Personius, W.J., Clamann, H.P. *et al.* (1981) Effect of fluori-methane spray on passive hip flexion. *Physical Therapy* **61** (2), 185–189.

Hanten, W.P. & Chandler, S.D. (1994) Effects of myofascial release leg pull and sagittal plane isometric contract-relax techniques on passive straight-leg raise angle. *Journal of Orthopaedic and Sports Physical Therapy* **20** (3), 138–144.

Hardy, L. (1985) Improving active range of hip flexion. *Research Quarterly for Exercise and Sport* **56** (2), 111–114.

Hardy, L. & Jones, D. (1986) Dynamic flexibility and proprioceptive neuromuscular facilitation. *Research Quarterly for Exercise and Sport* **57** (2), 150–153.

Hartig, D.E. & Henderson, J.M. (1999) Increasing hamstring flexibility decreases lower extremity overuse injuries in military basic trainees. *American Journal of Sports Medicine* **27** (2), 173–176.

Henricson, A., Larsson, A., Olsson, E. *et al.* (1983) The effect of stretching on the range of motion of the ankle joint in badminton players. *Journal of Orthopaedic and Sports Physical Therapy* **5** (2), 74–77.

Henricson, A.S., Fredriksson, K., Persson, I. *et al.* (1984) The effect of heat and stretching on the range of hip motion. *Journal of Orthopaedic and Sports Physical Therapy* **6** (2), 110–115.

Herbert, R. (1988) The passive mechanical properties of muscle and their adaptations to altered patterns of use. *Australian Journal of Physical Therapy* **34** (3), 141–149.

Holt, L.E., Travis, T.M. & Okha, T. (1970) Comparative study of three stretching techniques. *Perceptual and Motor Skills* **31**, 611–616.

Hughes, H.G. (1996) *The effects of static stretching on the hamstring musculotendinous unit.* MSc Thesis, University of Cape Town, Cape Town.

Hughes, H.G., Schwellnus, M.P. & Noakes, T.D. (2002) Scientific basis for stretching II: retention of range of motion after 24 hours, and regular static stretching over 3 weeks. (In review.)

Janda, V. (1983) *Muscle Function Testing.* Butterworths, Sydney.

Jones, B.H. & Knapik, J.J. (1999) Physical training and exercise-related injuries. Surveillance, research and injury prevention in military populations. *Sports Medicine* **27** (2), 111–125.

Kendall, F.P. & McCreary, E.K. (1983) *Muscle Testing and Function,* 3rd edn. Williams & Wilkins, Baltimore.

Kirsch, R.F., Kearney, R.E. & MacNeil, J.B. (1993) Identification of time-varying dynamics of the human triceps surae stretch reflex. *Experimental Brain Research* **97**, 115–127.

Klafs, C.E. & Arnheim, D.D. (1981) *The Science of Sports Injury Prevention and Management: Modern Principles of Athletic Training,* 5th edn. CV Mosby, St Louis.

Knott, M. & Voss, D.E. (1956) *Proprioceptive Neuromuscular Facilitation.* Harper & Row, New York.

Kottke, F.J., Pauley, D.L. & Ptak, R.A. (1966) The rationale for prolonged stretching for correction of shortening of connective tissue. *Archives of Physical Medicine and Rehabilitation* **47**, 345–352.

Kwan, M.K., Wall, E.J., Massie, J. *et al.* (1992) Strain, stress and stretch of peripheral nerve. *Acta Orthopaedica Scandinavica* **63** (3), 267–272.

LaBan, M.M. (1962) Collagen tissue: implications of its response to stress *in vitro. Archives of Physical Medicine and Rehabilitation* **43**, 461–466.

Leach, R.E. (1982) The prevention and rehabilitation of soft tissue injuries. *International Journal of Sports Medicine* **3**, 18–20.

Lehmann, J.F., Masock, A.J., Warren, C.G. *et al.* (1970) Effect of therapeutic temperatures on tendon extensibility. *Archives of Physical Medicine and Rehabilitation* **51**, 481–487.

Liemohn, W. (1978) Factors relating to hamstring strains. *Journal of Sports Medicine* **18**, 71–76, 168–171.

Low, J. & Reed, A. (1990) *Electrotherapy Explained: Principles and Practice,* 1st edn. Butterworth–Heinemann, Oxford.

Madding, S.W., Wong, J.G., Hallum, A. *et al.* (1987) Effect of duration of passive stretch on hip abduction range of motion. *Journal of Orthopaedic and Sports Physical Therapy* **8** (8), 409–416.

Maitland, G.D. (1991) *Peripheral Manipulation*, 3rd edn. Butterworth–Heinemann, Oxford.

Martinez-Hernandez, A. & Amenta, P.S. (1990) Basic concepts in wound healing. In: *Sports-Induced Inflammation* (Leadbetter W.B., Buckwalter, J.A. & Gordon, S.L., eds). American Academy of Orthopaedic Surgeons, Park Ridge, IL: 55–101.

Matthews, P.B.C. (1993) Interaction between short and long latency components of the human stretch reflex during sinusoidal stretching. *Journal of Physiology* **426**, 503–527.

McGlynn, G.H., Laughlin, N.T. & Rave, V. (1979) Effect of electromyographic feedback and static stretching on artifically induced muscle soreness. *American Journal of Physical Medicine* **58** (3), 139–148.

McKenzie, R. (1985) *Treat Your Own Back*, 3rd edn. Sygma Books, Kloof.

Medeiros, J.M., Smidt, G.L., Burmeister, L.F. *et al.* (1977) The influence of isometric exercise and passive stretch on hip joint motion. *Physical Therapy* **57** (5), 518–523.

Moore, M.A. & Hutton, E.S. (1980) Electromyographic investigation of muscle stretching techniques. *Medicine and Science in Sports and Exercise* **12**, 322–329.

Nedelec, B., Ghahary, A., Scott, P.G. *et al.* (2000) Control of wound contraction: basic and clinical features. *Hand Clinics* **16** (2), 289–302.

Nicholas, J.A. (1970) Injuries to knee ligaments. *Journal of the American Medical Association* **212** (13), 2236–2239.

Noakes, T.D. (1992) *Lore of Running*, 3rd edn. Oxford University Press, Cape Town.

Norris, C.M. (1993) *Sports Injuries and Management for Physiotherapists*. Butterworth–Heinemann, Oxford.

Osternig, L.R., Robertson, R., Troxel, R. *et al.* (1987) Muscle activation during proprioceptive neuro-muscular facilitation (PNF) stretching techniques. *American Journal of Physical Medicine* **66** (5), 298–307.

Pope, R.P., Herbert, R.D., Kirwan, J.D. *et al.* (2000) A randomized trial of preexercise stretching for prevention of lower-limb injury. *Medicine and Science in Sports and Exercise* **32** (2), 271–277.

Reilly, T.I. (1992) *Sports Fitness and Sports Injuries*. Wolfe Publishing, London.

Rigby, B.J. (1964) The effect of mechanical extension upon the thermal stability of collagen. *Biochemica et Biophysica Acta* **79**, 634–636.

Sady, S.P., Wortmann, M. & Blanke, D. (1982) Flexibility training: ballistic, static or proprioceptive neuro-muscular facilitation? *Archives of Physical Medicine and Rehabilitation* **63**, 261–263.

Safran, M.R., Garrett, W.E., Seaber, A.V. *et al.* (1988) The role of warmup in muscular injury prevention. *American Journal of Sports Medicine* **16** (2), 123–129.

Sapega, A.A., Quendenfeld, T.C., Moyer, R.A. *et al.* (1981) Biophysical factors in range-of-motion exercise. *Physical Sportsmedicine* **9** (12), 57–65.

Schultz, P. (1979) Flexibility: day of the static stretch. *Physical Sportsmedicine* **7**, 109–117.

Shellock, F.G. & Prentice, W.E. (1985) Warming up and stretching for improved physical performance and prevention of sports-related injuries. *Sports Medicine* **2**, 267–278.

Shrier, I. & Gossal, K. (2000) Myths and truths of stretching. *Physical Sportsmedicine* **28** (2), 57–63.

Starring, D.T., Gossman, M.R., Nicholson, G.G. *et al.* (1988) Comparison of cyclic and sustained passive stretching using a mechanical device to increase resting length of hamstring muscles. *Physical Therapy* **68** (3), 314–320.

Stromberg, D.D. & Wiederheilm, C.A. (1969) Viscoelastic description of a collagenous tissue in simple elongation. *Journal of Applied Physiology* **26** (6), 857–862.

Tanigawa, M.C. (1972) Comparison of the hold-relax procedure and passive mobilization on increasing muscle length. *Physical Therapy* **52** (7), 725–735.

Taylor, D.C., Dalton, J.D., Seaber, A.V. *et al.* (1990) Viscoelastic properties of muscle tendon units. *American Journal of Sports Medicine* **18** (3), 300–309.

Toft, E., Espersen, G.T., Kalund, S. *et al.* (1989) Passive tension of the ankle before and after stretching. *American Journal of Sports Medicine* **17** (4), 489–494.

Toppenburg, R. & Bullock, M. (1986) The interrelation of spinal curves, pelvic tilt and muscle lengths in adolescent females. *Australian Journal of Physiotherapy* **36** (2), 6–12.

Travell, J.G. & Simons, D.G. (1983) *Myofascial Pain and Dysfunction—the Trigger Point Manual*, 1st edn. Williams & Wilkins, Baltimore.

Voss, D.E. (1967) Proprioceptive neuromuscular facilitation. *American Journal of Physical Medicine* **46**, 838–898.

Voss, D.E. (1985) *Proprioceptive Neuromuscular Facilitation*, 3rd edn. Harper & Row, Philadelphia.

Vujnovich, A.L. & Dawson, N.J. (1994) The effect of therapeutic muscle stretch on neural processing. *Journal of Orthopaedic and Sports Physical Therapy* **20** (3), 145–153.

Wahl, S. & Renström, P. (1990) Fibrosis in soft-tissue injuries. In: *Sports-Induced Inflammation* (Leadbetter W.B., Buckwalter, J.A. & Gordon, S.L., eds). American Academy of Orthopaedic Surgeons, Park Ridge, IL: 637–647.

Wallin, D., Ekbom, V., Grahn, R. *et al.* (1985) Improvement of muscle flexibility: a comparison between two techniques. *American Journal of Sports Medicine* **13**, 263–268.

Wang, S.S., Whitney, S.L., Burdett, R.G. *et al.* (1993) Lower extremity muscular flexibility in long distance runners. *Journal of Orthopaedic and Sports Physical Therapy* **17** (2), 102–107.

Warren, C.G., Lehmann, J.F. & Koblanski, J.N. (1976) Heat and stretch procedures: an evaluation using rat tail tendon. *Archives of Physical Medicine and Rehabilitation* **57**, 122–126.

Wathen, D. (1987) Flexibility: its place in warmup activities. *National Strength and Conditioning Association Journal* **9** (5), 26–27.

Weber, S. & Kraus, H. (1949) Passive and active stretching of muscles. *Physical Therapy Review* **29** (9), 407–411.

Wessling, K.C., DeVane, D.A. & Hylton, C.R. (1987) Effects of static stretch versus static stretch and ultrasound combined on triceps surae muscle extensibility in healthy women. *Physical Therapy* **67** (5), 647–679.

Wiktorsson-Moller, M., Oberg, B., Ekstrand, J. *et al.* (1983) Effects of warming up, massage, and stretching on range of motion and muscle strength in the lower extremity. *American Journal of Sports Medicine* **11** (4), 249–252.

Williford, H.N., East, J.B., Smith, F.H. *et al.* (1986) Evaluation of warm-up for improvement in flexibility. *American Journal of Sports Medicine* **14** (4), 316–319.

Wilson, G.J., Elliott, B.C. & Wood, G.A. (1992) Stretch shorten cycle performance enhancement through flexibility training. *American Journal of Sports Medicine* **24** (1), 116–123.

Worrell, T.W., Perrin, D.H., Gansneder, B.M. *et al.* (1991) Comparison of isokinetic strength and flexibility measures between hamstring injured and non-injured athletes. *Journal of Orthopaedic and Sports Physical Therapy* **13** (3), 118–125.

Worrell, T.W., Smith, T.L. & Winegardener, J. (1994) Effect of hamstring stretching on hamstring muscle performance. *Journal of Orthopaedic and Sports Physical Therapy* **20** (3), 154–159.

Zachazewski, J.L. (1990) Flexibility in sports injuries. In: *Sports Physical Therapy*. Appleton & Lange, East Norwalk, CT: 229–230.

Zarins, B. (1982) Soft tissue injury and repair—biomechanical aspects. *International Journal of Sports Medicine* **3**, 9–11.

Chapter 12

Strength and Endurance

GUNNAR GRIMBY AND ROLAND THOMEÉ

Introduction

Injuries to the musculoskeletal system could result in skeletal muscle hypotrophy and weakness, loss of aerobic capacity and fatigability. Often there is a combination of these negative effects of injuries and immobilization with usually one or the other dominating, depending on the type of injury. This chapter will discuss the time sequence and extent of these changes in the perspective of rehabilitation measures. Rehabilitation techniques and exercise prescription will especially be described for resistance training and cardiovascular (aerobic) conditioning training during the second phase (after the acute phase with immobilization).

Reduction in skeletal muscle strength

Reduction in skeletal muscle strength and increased fatigue after injury and/or immobilization with disuse depend on several factors (Kannus et al. 1992b,c; Behm & St Pierre 1998). The specific effects of immobilization have been described in detail in Chapter 6 and the physiological and functional implications of injury in Chapter 7. In the clinical management nowadays, immobilization is avoided, if possible. The reduction in muscle strength can in principle depend on impaired neuromuscular activation and/or reduced muscle volume, as it can be assumed that the number of muscle fibers are protected.

Impaired muscular activation

An impaired muscular activation can depend on factors such as: (i) inhibition due to pain or other afferent nerve influence; or (ii) reduced muscle activity at immobilization and/or injury.

Pain, joint effusion and knee angle are factors influencing the degree of inhibition. Pain from a joint may result in involuntary inhibition of activity in muscles acting across that joint, and a considerable lack of ability for muscle activation has been seen after knee pathologies and surgery (Hurley et al. 1994). However, the presence of pain is not necessary for inhibition to occur (Stokes & Young 1984; Shakespeare et al. 1985). There is not a direct relationship between the degree of pain and the amount of muscle inhibition. Inhibition may be as severe in a later postoperative period as at the first postoperative day, even in a virtually pain-free state. The activity in other receptors from the joint and adjacent structures may have similar effects as seen in animal experiments and human studies. It has been demonstrated that a very small amount of joint effusion will result in reflex inhibition of the musculature. The amount of quadriceps inhibition after knee injury may partly be dependent on the knee angle, with less inhibition in a flexed than in a fully extended position (Shakespeare et al. 1985). There might be selective inhibitions of motor units, which could explain part of the dominant hypotrophy of a specific fibre type (see below), seen after joint damage. Selective

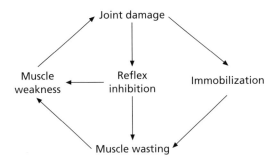

Fig. 12.1 Schematic presentation of different mechanisms leading to muscle wasting and muscle weakness. (Redrawn from Stokes & Young 1984.)

inhibition of part of the quadriceps muscle has also been noted among patients with patellofemoral pain syndrome (Thomée *et al.* 1996).

There is a vicious cycle causing muscle weakness. Figure 12.1 illustrates the relationship between joint damage, immobilization, reflex inhibition and muscle wasting. The reflex inhibition can therefore result in an immediate reduction of voluntary muscle activation causing muscle weakness, early after an injury or surgery. In a longer perspective it will also cause muscle wasting resulting in further muscle weakness.

Reduced muscle volume

The other factor causing decreased muscular strength, besides inhibition, is the reduction in muscle volume that follows an injury. In rehabilitation, aspects to consider are the importance of the different patterns of muscle hypotrophy, the difficulty in assessing the degree of muscle wasting, the difference in strength between extremities, and the strength relation between the agonist and the antagonist muscles (agonist–antagonist ratios).

Patterns of muscle hypotrophy

Different patterns of muscle hypotrophy may be seen depending on the type of immobilization and disuse (Appell 1990; Kannus *et al.* 1992b,c). Patients with longstanding pain may show

hypotrophy of slow-twitch type I fibres, as also seen after immobilization with a short muscle length. After general disuse, a reduction, especially of fast-twitch type II fibres, predominates. A reduction of the muscle size of the quadriceps equivalent to up to 30–40% may be seen after knee injury. The wasting of quadriceps usually dominates over the loss of hamstrings muscle volume.

Assessing the degree of muscle wasting

The degree of muscle wasting can not be accurately diagnosed by measurements of circumference using a standard tapemeasure device and can in fact be grossly underestimated. The reason for this is that the fat and bones structures are practically constant. With a reduction of the circumference of the muscle tissue, there will be an increase in the width of the subcutaneous fat layer masking part of the effect of muscle wasting on the total circumference. Thus, it is difficult and often misleading to use changes in circumferences as indicators of gains in muscle tissue during rehabilitation after injury or immobilization. Other more exact means have to be used including computed tomography (CT), magnetic resonance imaging (MRI) or ultrasound. In clinical practice one has often to rely on the indirect measurement of muscle strength and the interpretation of changes in muscle strength with respect to muscle volume.

Difference in strength between extremities

An important aspect when evaluating reduction in strength at follow-up, is that there may be a lack of perception of a moderate difference in strength between the two extremities. Thus, a 20% reduction, or even more, of quadriceps muscle strength has been recorded in the previously injured side compared with the non-injured side in persons who have returned to normal activity and considered themselves fully recovered (Grimby *et al.* 1980; Arvidsson *et al.* 1981). If such differences are seen in athletes, objective evaluation and further rehabilitation are needed.

Agonist–antagonist ratios

Assessment of the ratio of the agonist–antagonist strength, as the quadriceps–hamstrings ratio, may also result in recommendations for further training, but a comparison between injured and non-injured sides is of more importance in clinical practice. The knowledge of the prevalence of muscular imbalance and its functional significance is, however, rather poor.

Reduction in muscle endurance

Parallel with the reduction in muscle strength there will usually be a reduction in muscle endurance. A given level of force production will now be closer to the maximal force output of the muscle, and therefore will need a relatively higher proportion of the muscle strength. There are a number of factors which may reduce muscle endurance following disuse (Kannus *et al.* 1992b,c; Behm & St Pierre 1998), including a reduction in mitochondrial enzymes necessary for the oxidative process in the muscle and a reduction in capillarization with less ability to transport oxygen and energy supply to the muscle cell. On the other hand, a reduction in muscle fibre cross-sectional area with disuse will reduce the diffusion distances. With training these factors will be reversed. An increase in mitochondrial enzymes will be seen quite quickly during adequate training emphasizing the endurance adaptation.

Background for resistance training

There are different aspects of resistance training depending upon whether an improved neuromuscular activation or increase in muscle volume are given priority.

Neuromuscular activation

Important points to consider are time, assessment of the degree of neuromuscular activation, contralateral effects of resistance training, and speed of force development. The specific nature of the neural adaptation is relatively unknown and different aspects may be of importance, depending on the type of training, the muscles involved, and the pretraining status.

The mechanisms of adaptation may include increased activity of the prime movers for a specific movement and changes in the activation of synergists and antagonists (Sale 1988). There may be an increased activation of the number of motor units at maximal effort and/or an increased firing rate. The relative importance of these factors may vary between muscles and type of muscle activation. Motor units may be better synchronized. There may be facilitation of reflexes as well as reduction of inhibitory influence. Parallel to the activation of the prime mover, activation of the antagonist may also occur, having a functional positive or negative effect. A reduction in the activation of the antagonist during training may lead to greater activation of the prime mover, reducing any reciprocal inhibition, and also—through less force produced by the antagonists—an increased net output of force in the direction of the movement.

TIME ASPECTS

Early after an injury and/or immobilization there is most likely to be reduced neuromuscular activation (Sale 1988; Häkkinen 1994). Strength training effects will then mainly depend on neural factors and may be limited to the type of training exercise, both with respect to speed during dynamic exercise and joint angle during static exercises (Kraemer *et al.* 1996). The length of this initial period may vary depending on the type and degree of injury and disuse. For training from an initial moderately untrained state, it has been estimated to be in the order of 6–10 weeks. The initial training effect may be quite large, providing that there are no major inhibitory factors, as discussed earlier.

ASSESSMENT OF NEUROMUSCULAR ACTIVATION

One way in the laboratory setting to identify lack of neuromuscular activation is the use of single superimposed twitch electrical stimulation (Behm *et al.* 1996; Thomée *et al.* 1996). After identifying the maximal intensity of the stimulus for a single twitch by successively increasing the signal during resting conditions to get a plateau, one or several single-twitch stimuli are given during muscle actions with maximal voluntary effort. Electrical stimulation has mainly been used during static muscle activity, whereas our knowledge is more limited concerning optimal neuromuscular activation during dynamic muscle actions. During these conditions, electrical stimulation with tetanic trains has been used; however, this requires considerably cooperation from the subject due to the discomfort involved. It has been used to demonstrate the lack of maximal activation at eccentric muscle actions (Westing *et al.* 1990).

CONTRALATERAL EFFECTS OF RESISTANCE TRAINING

It has been reported that by training one leg, the other leg also may improve and show strength gains. Improvements can be in the order of 35–60% of that attained in the trained limb (Kannus *et al.* 1992a). Such a possible effect of contralateral training should be recognized and possibly be used during rehabilitation after injury and immobilization of one extremity.

SPEED OF FORCE DEVELOPMENT

Another aspect of muscle force development is a shortening of the time for tension development after activation (electromechanical delay). Speed of force development may decrease after immobilization or surgery (Komi 1984) and can increase with specific training. The force–time relationship may change using power training with high-velocity contractions or explosive training models, so that there will be a relatively faster force rise early in the muscle activation (Häkkinen 1994).

Muscle volume

As mentioned earlier, in the initial stages of weight training for sports or rehabilitation purposes, increases in strength occur mainly because of

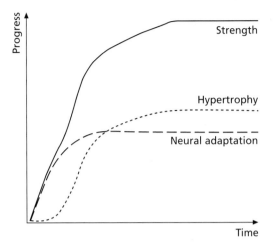

Fig. 12.2 Schematic illustration of the contribution to increased strength from neural adaptation and muscular hypertrophy. (Redrawn from Sale 1988.)

neural adaptation. In contrast, in the later stages of resistance training increases in muscle strength occur mainly by increases in muscle volume (Fig. 12.2) (Sale 1988). There is an increase in the size (cross-section) of the individual muscle fibres leading to an increase in the total muscle cross-sectional area. Whether there will also be hyperplasia (an increase in the number of muscle fibres) is more questionable, unless there is an injury of the muscle tissue. Besides an increase in cross-sectional area, there may be other structural changes of importance for force development such as increases in: (i) the length of muscle fibres due to an increase in the number of sarcomeres; (ii) the density of contractile proteins; and (iii) the intra- and extracellular connective tissue matrix, enhancing the proportion of the sarcomere force that can be transmitted to the skeletal system (Enoka 1988).

Muscle training methods

In principle, resistance exercise can be performed with static (isometric) or dynamic muscle actions. Dynamic exercise can be performed at a constant velocity throughout the range of motion, isokinetic action, or with a constant or variable load, but without control of movement velocity. The activity can be concentric or eccentric. In addition, electrical muscle stimulation can be used. The advantages of static exercise are that it can be used in the presence of limited joint mobility and also that a pain-free joint angle can be chosen. However, there will be no training through the full range of motion and static exercises are often considered 'non-functional'.

Dynamic exercise with a constant weight can be easy to arrange, but will not match the pattern of maximal torque through the range of motion and may not accommodate resistance to pain. Eccentric exercise, if not wanted, cannot easily be avoided. During dynamic exercise with variable resistance, the load and muscle torque can be matched and it may, thus, be very efficient. However, special considerations may be needed to accommodate the resistance to pain as, for example, only using part of the range of motion.

Isokinetic exercise—concentric or eccentric—is sometimes considered non-functional, but is a well-controlled method of activating the muscle through the full range of motion, reducing the risk for overload. However, at the end of the movement there will no load and thus no training effect, for example, for end of knee extension.

Eccentric muscle action results in higher maximal torque than concentric muscle action (Westing et al. 1988). Neural activation is, however, not larger with eccentric muscle action as indicated by maximal electromyographic (EMG) activity, which may be lower than in concentric actions. Eccentric muscle actions increase the risk for muscle soreness, as demonstrated in a number of studies (Fridén et al. 1983). However, by producing greater muscle tension, eccentric muscle actions may enhance protein synthesis in muscles and contractile tissues. The soreness after eccentric exercise will lessen over the first week of continuous training (Fridén et al. 1983). As eccentric muscle action is part of many natural movement patterns, especially when the stretch–shortening cycle is used, as in running, jumping or throwing, they should be included in training programmes at some point.

It has been demonstrated that a short training period before immobilization may help to prevent muscle hypotrophy and loss of strength (Appell 1990). This might be explained by a maintained effect on the adaptation of the muscle and may have clinical implications for elective surgical procedures. However, the clinical relevance and usefulness has to be studied further.

Electrical stimulation

Electrical muscle stimulation in the early phase of strength training or during immobilization may promote neural activation by the afferent signals, reducing any pain and preventing or overriding reflex inhibition. However, in order to enhance the central neural drive to the muscle, electrical muscle stimulation has to be combined with voluntary muscle activation. At voluntary activation the low-threshold motor units innervating slow-twitch type I muscle fibres will be activated first, followed by the high-threshold fast-twitch type II fibres at a higher stimulus intensity (Gollnick et al. 1974). During direct nerve stimulation, however, larger axons belonging to the fast-twitch type II fibres will be activated first, as they have the lowest excitability. Combining electrical nerve stimulation and voluntary muscle activation may have a synergistic effect. However, no convincing evidence is available of the recruitment order of motor units, and in fact during surface stimulation no difference from pure voluntary activation has been seen (Knaflitz et al. 1990).

The order of motor unit activation with electrical muscle stimulation depends on at least three factors: (i) the diameter of the motor axon; (ii) the distance between the axon and the active electrode; and (iii) the effect of input to motor neurones from cutaneous afferents by the electrical muscle stimulation. It has been demonstrated in a number of studies that a combination of electrical muscle stimulation and voluntary muscle activation may limit strength reduction during immobilization and in the early postoperative phase (Arvidsson et al. 1986; DeLitto et al. 1988; Wigerstad-Lossing et al. 1988). It will also act to maintain muscle oxidative enzymatic capacity (Wigerstad-Lossing et al. 1988).

Gender differences

There are indications that the effect of neural adaptation in strength training would plateau somewhat earlier in women than in men (Häkkinen 1994). The effect on muscle volume is, however, more dominant in men than in women reflecting different hormonal influences. In women there may still be rather large interindividual differences in training-induced muscle hypertrophy, depending on the actual serum testosterone level (Häkkinen 1994). Even if certain specific aspects may be taken into consideration when training men and women, the general principles and the phases during rehabilitation are the same, with similar recommendations.

Strength training for children and adolescents

No convincing scientific evidence supports beneficial effects of using strength training for prepubescent children. Until more convincing studies are presented strength training should be avoided in this age group or used with low intensity. Reasons for this are the imbalances between the maturation of the muscle, tendon and skeletal tissues. Using too heavy loads often results in frustrating set-backs due to overuse or overload pain symptoms. To this can be added the absence of strength gains compared with non-strength-training peers. Strength training can slowly be added to postpubescent children but the training should be carefully monitored to avoid excessive overload or overuse.

Cardiovascular endurance

This section deals with endurance for more prolonged exercise, which is dependent on the function of the cardiovascular and respiratory systems. The overall capacity of the system can be defined as the aerobic capacity (maximal oxygen uptake). Endurance is defined as the ability to sustain prolonged aerobic exercise with an acceptable level of homeostasis, expressed, for example, as a percentage of maximal oxygen uptake or absolute power output or distance with a specific speed. Another aspect is the economy for body movement, as for running, with less energy consumption at a more economic movement pattern.

There are many factors contributing to endurance for whole body exercise, including the capacity of the heart with respect to maximal cardiac output and stroke volume, the distribution of blood flow to active muscles and the ventilatory function and blood–gas exchange in the lung. Coupled to these is the metabolic capacity for aerobic metabolism in the muscles. It is now well established that the maximal perfusion capacity of particular skeletal muscles is well above that which can be used for exercise with larger muscle groups (whole body exercise) (Andersen & Saltin 1985) and that the regulation of the peripheral blood flow in relation to the pumping capacity of the heart is essential (Saltin et al. 1998). Capillary density, leg blood flow and maximal oxygen uptake all increase in similar proportion after physical conditioning (Saltin & Rowell 1980).

With immobilization there will be a rather rapid reduction in the activity of the mitochondrial enzymes in the muscles (Appell 1990), which would also have an impact on the regulation of the central circulation contributing to the increased heart rate at a certain submaximal exercise level. There will successively be a reduction in the circulatory capacity towards the untrained state. Studies of immobilization and training of one leg have demonstrated the interaction between peripheral and central adaptation to exercise at immobilization and training (Saltin 1986).

Training of cardiovascular endurance after sports injury

Endurance training should include activities that are easy to perform despite the presence of any local body restrictions, such as remaining pain, limited joint motion, reduced muscle strength and local muscular fatigability. By tradition, exercises where the effect of bodyweight is reduced, such as swimming, pool exercises, bicycling and rowing machines, are used.

An important consideration is the possible interaction of concurrent strength and endurance training (Leveritt *et al.* 1999). During such a training regime the increase in strength may be reduced or limited compared with pure strength training, but the understanding of such an inhibition is limited at present. Various combinations of resistance and endurance training have to be studied to further understand the interactions. Whether, and to what extent, this also applies to training starting from an immobilized state, as after an injury or surgery, is not well known. Hypotheses based on acute (caused by residual fatigue after endurance training) and chronic (lack of possibility to adapt metabolically and morphologically to both strength and endurance training simultaneously) effects have been suggested. Endurance training even with resistance training superimposed may tend to reduce or limit the increase in muscle fibre size seen after resistance training alone. These aspects have to be taken into consideration when designing training programmes, especially in the later stages after immobilization and sports injuries in athletes participating in sports that require both strength and endurance.

Principal rehabilitation techniques

A gradually increasing training programme, with appropriate and continuously adjusted exercises, is probably the most important tool during rehabilitation after a sports injury. The rehabilitation programme can be divided into three different phases, not rigidly separated from each other, but with a more or less obvious overlap of different treatment approaches between the different phases.

First phase (acute phase)

REHABILITATION GOALS DURING
THE FIRST PHASE

• Minimize the magnitude of the injury by correct acute management.
• Reduce or minimize loading of the injured tissue.

• Increase the circulation of blood and joint fluid with low loading exercises performed several times daily to aid in the healing process, to preserve range of motion and to accustom the tissues to an increasing load.
• Maintain strength, endurance, range of motion and function for the rest of the body.

REHABILITATION TECHNIQUES

During the first phase emphasis should be on the reduction or elimination of any reflex inhibition. Pain, joint effusion and inflammation should be addressed with proper clinical management. Therefore local anaesthesia, analgesics, transcutaneous electrical nerve stimulation (TENS) and acupuncture may serve an important role during this phase.

The last decade has also shown that physical exercises can be used with good results during the acute phase (Kannus *et al.* 1992b, 1998). Thus immobilization can be replaced with specific range of motion exercises and active muscle activation exercises. Three to five specific exercises with a low load (0–30% of 1 RM) and with many repetitions (20–50) could be recommended. These exercises should be performed several times per day.

There are several factors that can explain the beneficial effects of an early active mobilization after injury. With exercise there is an increase in blood flow, increasing the exchange of nutrients and removing waste products from the injury site. The tension created in the injured tissue serves as a positive stimulation for tissue repair. The neuromuscular activation from exercises used in early mobilization preserves coordination. Tension, compression, torsion, distraction and angular displacements at various speeds are necessary to maintain proprioceptive functions. The triggering of endorphin release achieved with active muscle activation can be beneficial, resulting in pain reduction and subsequent improved neuromuscular activation (Thorén *et al.* 1990). With early mobilization, range of motion can be preserved and, for example, joint fibrosis can be avoided or minimized.

To achieve a more than voluntary activated muscle force, superimposed electrical stimulation can be used during early immobilization. For optimal muscle effect the electrical stimulation should be given simultaneously with maximal voluntary activation, as discussed above. No randomized and double-blind studies are found in the literature studying the effects of electrical muscle stimulation during sports injury rehabilitation. However, superimposed electrical stimulation has been suggested for the recovery of quadriceps and hamstring muscle strength during rehabilitation after reconstruction of the anterior cruciate ligament (Arvidsson *et al.* 1986; Wigerstad-Lossing *et al.* 1988; Snyder-Mackler *et al.* 1995). It should be recognized that the placebo effect may have contributed to these effects. Also, the positive effect of increased motivation, with increased training effort and compliance, may have contributed to the results.

Second phase (training phase)

REHABILITATION GOALS DURING THE SECOND PHASE

• Increase load tolerance of injured tissues.
• Improve balance and coordination.
• Improve muscle strength and power and muscular endurance by gradually increasing loads and degree of difficulty regarding balance and coordination, using more demanding sport-specific exercises.
• A gradual change from one to two training sessions per day at the beginning of this phase to three or four highly demanding sessions per week at the end of the phase.

REHABILITATION TECHNIQUES

In the second phase the injured tissue and surrounding muscles can withstand higher loads and thus be more actively mobilized. The treatment programme should be concentrated on the recovery of muscle mass. The number of repetitions used in the various exercises during the first phase is therefore gradually lowered to 8–12. Two to three sets per exercise and three

training sessions per week are recommended. At the same time the load is gradually increased with a goal to reach 70–80% of maximal. At this level an optimal muscle hypertrophy can be anticipated. No major inhibitory influences should be present and an adequate motor recruitment is necessary. Therefore, at this stage, the training can be non-specific and various weight-training equipment can be used, such as leg-extension, leg-curl and leg-press weight machines. The use of repetition maximum (RM, the maximal load that can be lifted a given number of repetitions within one set) is a common method of determining the load used in resistance training. For increased maximal strength 1–5 RM are used, whereas 8–12 RM results in muscle hypertrophy.

During the late phases of anterior cruciate ligament (ACL) rehabilitation, slow and moderate improvements of quadriceps muscle strength and size have been reported (Risberg *et al.* 1999). This may indicate that rehabilitation programmes should have a greater emphasis on training for muscle volume and strength (i.e. high-intensity weight training using heavy loads which activate both high- and low-threshold motor units). Restoring muscle volume and strength is a cornerstone in rehabilitation, therefore weight training, with the optimal amount of resistance required for a maximal muscle growth process to occur, must be considered an essential training programme variable.

Interestingly, in sports training, as opposed to the rehabilitation field, a number of empirically based strategies have been developed through the years to maintain a positive response to long-term weight training (Fleck & Kraemer 1997). Thus, in advanced weight training various systems (e.g. periodization or organization of training into distinct periods) and methods (e.g. supersets, forced repetitions, power factor training and pre-exhaustion) are used to avoid performance to plateau, and for bringing about optimal gains of strength and muscle hypertrophy (Sisco & Little 1997; Bompa & Cornacchia 1998). However, current scientific knowledge of these practical strength- and power-training principles is poor.

Isokinetic training and testing equipment has been recommended for many years. However, the validity, reliability and sensitivity has been strongly questioned during recent years (Gleeson & Mercer 1996; Stone *et al.* 2000). In well-controlled studies, isokinetic training, previously thought to be superior, has been found to be inferior to other training modes (Stone *et al.* 2000). Isokinetic testing is still the most commonly used strength testing procedure, but it is suggested that greater familiarization with the technique is needed, and several pre- and postevaluations, in order to improve testing reliability and sensitivity (Gleeson & Mercer 1996; Stone *et al.* 2000).

Closed and open kinetic chain exercises

There is a debate concerning the use of closed versus open kinetic chain lower limb exercises during rehabilitation. Studies have compared the effect of closed versus open kinetic chain lower limb exercises on knee ligament strain (Henning *et al.* 1985; Yack *et al.* 1993), anteroposterior tibiofemoral translation (Panariello *et al.* 1994) and patellofemoral compression forces (Gooch *et al.* 1993; Steinkamp *et al.* 1993). The importance of using closed kinetic chain rehabilitation (De Carlo *et al.* 1992; Shelbourne *et al.* 1995) and evaluation (Wilk *et al.* 1994; Greenberger & Paterno 1995) has been stressed. However, few studies have investigated whether the effect of closed versus open kinetic chain weight training on strength and performance differs.

Despite several studies (Yack *et al.* 1993; Beynnon *et al.* 1997) concerning safety issues of closed and open kinetic chain exercises in ACL rehabilitation, and although some authors have advocated the sole use of closed kinetic chain exercises (Shelbourne & Nitz 1992; Bynum *et al.* 1995), it is concluded that both types of exercises can be performed in ways that do not place excessive strain on the ACL (Fitzgerald 1997).

Escamilla *et al.* (1998), comparing knee joint biomechanics while performing closed and open kinetic chain weight training at a 12 RM load, reported that peak ACL tension forces in open kinetic chain exercise were only 0.2 times bodyweight, and non-existent in closed kinetic chain exercise. Factors such as joint compressive forces

(e.g. axial loading) and joint geometry probably play integral roles in knee joint stability during closed kinetic chain exercise (Isear *et al.* 1997). Significant coactivation of the antagonists during maximal knee flexion/extension, indicating an inhibitory mechanism which prevents overloading of the joint and contributes to joint stabilization (Kellis & Baltzopoulos 1998), would explain the low ACL tension forces during open kinetic chain exercise.

Free weights and weight machines

Most athletes use resistance training, involving both free weights and weight machines, to improve strength and power. The pros and cons of training with free weights versus weight machines are, as closed and open kinetic chain training, widely discussed among athletes and coaches, among physical therapists, as well as in sports science. Differences of opinion exist as to which method results in optimal performance gains. Proponents of free weights emphasize functionality and a direct application to sporting activities (Panariello *et al.* 1994). Conversely, the advocators of weight machines stress safety and less requirements of coordination as compared with free weight training (Kraemer & Fleck 1993).

In studies comparing free weights versus weight machines or closed versus open kinetic chain weight training, a dilemma exists in creating matching training conditions, e.g. equating total volume of training, total work and total training time. Moreover, as the weight does not vary in free weight exercise, the resultant torque, and therefore the required muscular contraction, does vary according to the mechanics of the specific exercise. Weight machines, on the other hand, operating through, for example, a cam, enable variable resistance throughout the range of motion of an exercise. This is an attempt to approximate the strength curve of the exercise, thus forcing the muscle to contract maximally throughout the range of movement.

A barbell squat is a free weight, closed kinetic chain exercise, involving muscles working across

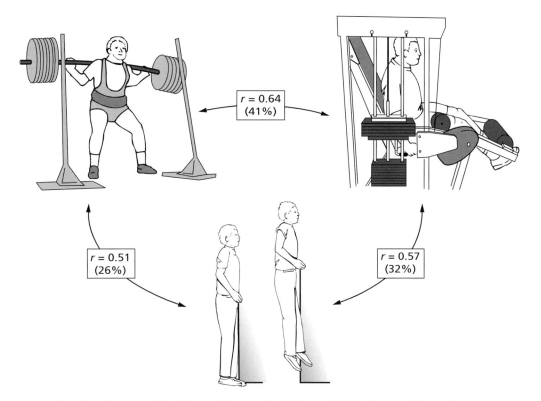

Fig. 12.3 Correlation between a closed kinetic chain test (barbell squat 3 RM) and an open kinetic chain test (concentric isokinetic knee extension), respectively, and the test of functional performance (vertical jump) in healthy male subjects. (From Augustsson & Thomeé 2000.)

multiple joints. Athletes using resistance training often include a barbell squat programme to improve lower extremity strength. Several studies have shown positive effects from a barbell squat exercise programme on strength and athletic performance (Thorstensson *et al.* 1976; Fry *et al.* 1991; Hickson *et al.* 1994).

Weight machine exercises, using muscles working across only single joints in an open kinetic chain, are also commonly used to improve lower extremity strength. The specificity of free weight and weight machine training is a critical issue, demanding accurate and sensitive tests to prove the superiority of one method over another. Dynamic (isotonic) testing such as a barbell squat or a vertical jump, activating the stretch–shortening cycle (Komi 1987), could be argued to be more valid than isokinetic testing when assessing

sporting activities. However, the isokinetic knee extension exercise, though not activating the stretch–shortening cycle, has advantages such as greater control over velocity of motion, technique and extraneous movement, which facilitates measurement reliability and objectivity (Abernethy *et al.* 1995). Augustsson and Thomeé (2000) showed that a similar correlation existed for both closed ($r = 0.51$) and open ($r = 0.57$) chain testing with a vertical jump. However only 26–32% of jumping ability was explained by the strength in the closed ($r^2 = 0.26$) and open ($r^2 = 0.32$) chain tests (Fig. 12.3).

Much time and effort is initially spent learning proper technique when training with free weights. Conversely, weight machines are probably less difficult to master as they allow movement in only one plane and direction. Therefore, it is theorized that weight machines cause greater gains of training load in short-term weight-training programmes. According to Sale (1988), increased performance as a result of weight training that lasts less than 20 weeks is associated mainly with neural adaptation, such as increased motor unit activity of prime mover muscles, and improved coordination, i.e. appropriate changes in the activation of synergists and antagonists.

Single-joint weight machine exercises allow a superior function of synergists and antagonists, enabling a high activation of motor units in prime mover muscles, as opposed to complex, multi-joint free weight exercises where full motor activation is probably more difficult to achieve due to greater demands of coordination. This theory is supported by recent studies in which open kinetic chain training resulted in larger increases of training load (Augustsson *et al.* 1998) and muscle hypertrophy (Chilibeck *et al.* 1998) than closed kinetic chain training in short-term weight training.

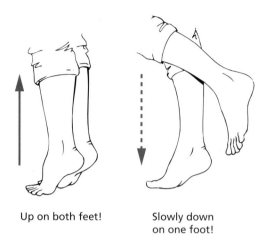

Up on both feet!   Slowly down on one foot!

Fig. 12.4 Eccentric strength training for the ankle plantor flexors.

Eccentric training

Eccentric training is different from traditional concentric/eccentric training in that a higher load is possible during eccentric training. However, the same types of exercises, with the same number of repetitions, sets and frequency of training, can be used. The higher load can be accomplished in different ways. For example, in the sitting knee extension exercise the weight can be lifted concentrically with both legs and lowered eccentrically with one leg. The same principle applies to exercise in the standing position (Fig. 12.4). Another way is to have a training partner help during the concentric phase. Current isokinetic dynamometers allow specific heavy eccentric loading.

During normal concentric/eccentric weight training higher improvements have been noticed both in concentric and eccentric strength gains compared with concentric-only weight training (Dudley *et al.* 1991). Further, Higbie *et al.* (1996) reported higher eccentric strength gains using

eccentric training and higher concentric strength gains using concentric training. A more interesting issue is, however, if eccentric strength training results in higher or faster strength gains, eccentrically or concentrically, than traditional concentric/eccentric training. No definite answer can be found in the literature, thus more research is needed. However, some studies, randomized and controlled, show better results with eccentric training programmes compared with concentric/eccentric training programmes for patients with chronic pain from the Achilles tendon (Mafi *et al.* 2000; Grävare Silbernagel *et al.* 2001).

Muscle power training

As muscle strength and load tolerance increases, the total load on the musculoskeletal system can be further increased. When close to normal strength is achieved, muscle power training and plyometrics (mainly reactive throwing and jumping exercises) can gradually be added to the rehabilitation programme, stressing time to peak muscular tension as well as stressing the stretch–shortening cycle. It is recommended that maximal or close to maximal muscle power training and plyometrics (Fig. 12.5) are added to the training programme once or twice per week.

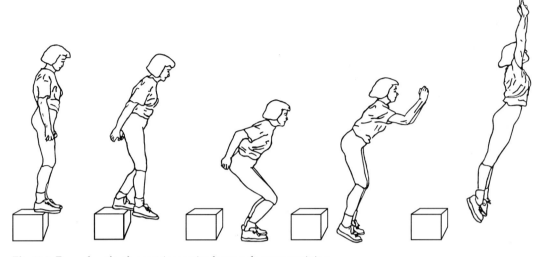

Fig. 12.5 Examples of a plyometric exercise for muscle power training.

Three to five exercises with two to three sets of 10–15 repetitions and with a total training time of 10–15 min is sufficient. Thus the rehabilitation programme should use free weights (barbells and dumbbells), medicine balls, throwing implements and various jumping exercises. Häkkinen (1994) showed that explosive-type training (i.e. power training and plyometrics) had a positive effect on the maximal average integrated electromyography (IEMG)–time curve of the leg extensor muscles. Also, positive effects were shown with explosive-type training on the average isometric force–time curve with a higher speed of force development, compared with heavy resistance training.

Muscular endurance

If the general overall goal during the second phase is to also improve muscular endurance, many repetitions should be used with very short rest pauses of only a few seconds in between sets. This type of muscular endurance training can be performed daily with close to maximal intensity. Such a programme may increase endurance as well as strength and aerobic capacity of the muscle (Grimby *et al.* 1973).

Third phase (return to sports phase)

REHABILITATION GOALS DURING THE THIRD PHASE

• Regain maximal balance and coordination during maximally loading exercises as well as maximal endurance exercises.
• Regain maximal running, jumping and throwing capacity.
• Resume sports activity by implementing sport-specific exercises with maximal loading and maximal demand on range of motion, strength, endurance and coordination.

REHABILITATION TECHNIQUES

The third phase can be arbitrarily defined to start when the muscle has regained sufficient volume, strength and endurance to approach a minimal level needed for various functional activities. Individuals have different functional needs, and the limitations will therefore vary according to the sport. A common feature, however, is the need for further improvement in muscle structure and activation, as well as improved motor control and coordination.

It has been noticed that despite 'aggressive' rehabilitation with early mobilization, full strength and muscle mass is not achieved 1 year after ACL surgery (Arangio *et al.* 1997; Pfeifer & Banzer 1999). Pfeifer and Banzer (1999) concluded, in their study of 39 patients with arthroscopically assisted ACL reconstruction, that insufficient rehabilitation schemes and not inhibition explained the large strength deficits seen 10–16 months after surgery. Despite this, many athletes resume their sports at 6 months and sometimes earlier after ACL reconstruction. It is thus not surprising that reinjury is common or that a new injury occurs. In many sports the musculoskeletal system is exposed to extreme loads. For example, during jumping the Achilles tendon is loaded with 5–10 times the bodyweight and the patellofemoral joint with up to 25 times the bodyweight.

There is, thus, a definite need for objective measurements of muscle function before full athletic activity is allowed. It is a future sports medicine challenge to develop a test battery of various strength tests, jumping, throwing and running tests, and agility and sport-specific tests. Tests need to be valid for the specific sport involved and tested for reproducibility.

During the third phase, training programmes to achieve and maintain gross motor functions must continue. More and more emphasis should be placed on specific training exercises for the specific sport that the athlete is to resume. Aspects of proprioceptive function, coordination and mechanical efficiency are discussed further in Chapter 13.

Special aspects of cardiovascular endurance training programmes

During rehabilitation after a sports injury it is important to try to maintain cardiovascular endurance. Thus regular bicycling, one-legged bicycling or arm cycling, an exercise programme in a pool using a wet vest or general major muscle exercise programmes with relatively high intensity and short rest periods (circuit weight training) can be of major importance. Increased maximal oxygen uptake has been shown to be maintained with a circuit weight programme (Gettman *et al.* 1979, 1982; Haennel *et al.* 1989). In these studies the participants trained 8–12 weeks, three times a week, using three circuits, with 8–10 exercises and with 20–30 s work and rest periods. Thus, an athlete sustaining an injury can maintain certain aspects of cardiovascular endurance by replacing, for example, running with an alternative form of cardiovascular endurance training. However, the peripheral muscular endurance close to the injury is more difficult to maintain and is limited to the recovery of the injury.

References

Abernethy, P., Wilson, G. & Logan, P. (1995) Strength and power assessment. *Sports Medicine* **19**, 401–417.

Andersen, P. & Saltin, B. (1985) Maximal perfusion of skeletal muscle in man. *Journal of Physiology (London)* **366**, 233–249.

Appell, H.-J. (1990) Muscular atrophy following immobilisation. A review. *Sports Medicine* **10**, 42–58.

Arangio, G., Chen, C., Kalady, M. & Reed, J. (1997) Thigh muscle size and strength after anterior cruciate ligament reconstruction and rehabilitation. *Journal of Orthopaedic and Sports Physical Therapy* **26**, 238–243.

Arvidsson, I., Eriksson, E., Häggmark, T. & Johnson, R.J. (1981) Isokinetic thigh muscle strength after ligament reconstruction in the knee joint. Result from a 5–10 year follow-up after reconstruction of the anterior cruciate ligament in the knee joint. *International Journal of Sports Medicine* **2**, 7–11.

Arvidsson, I., Arvidsson, H., Eriksson, E. & Jansson, E. (1986) Prevention of quadriceps wasting after immobilization—an evaluation of the effect of electrical stimulation. *Orthopaedics* **9**, 1519–1528.

Augustsson, J. & Thomeé, R. (2000) Ability of closed and open kinetic chain tests of muscular strength to assess functional performance. *Scandinavian Journal of Medicine and Science in Sports* **10**, 164–168.

Augustsson, J., Esko, A., Thomeé, R. & Svantesson, U. (1998) Weight training of the thigh muscles using closed vs. open kinetic chain exercises: a comparison of performance enhancement. *Journal of Orthopaedic and Sports Physical Therapy* **27**, 3–8.

Behm, D.G. & St Pierre, D.M.M. (1998) The effects of strength training and disuse on mechanisms of fatigue. *Sports Medicine* **25**, 173–189.

Behm, D., St Pierre, D. & Perez, D. (1996) Muscle inactivation; assessment of interpolated twitch technique. *Journal of Applied Physiology* **81**, 2267–2273.

Beynnon, B., Johnson, R., Fleming, B., Stankewich, C., Renström, P. & Nichols, C. (1997) The strain behavior of the anterior cruciate ligament during squatting and active flexion-extension. *American Journal of Sports Medicine* **25**, 823–829.

Bompa, T. & Cornacchia, L. (1998) *Serious Strength Training*. Human Kinetics, Champaign, IL.

Bynum, B.E., Barrack, R.L. & Alexander, A.H. (1995) Open versus closed chain kinetic exercises after anterior cruciate ligament reconstruction. *American Journal of Sports Medicine* **23**, 401–406.

Chilibeck, P.D., Calder, A.W., Sale, D.G. & Webber, C.E. (1998) A comparison of strength and muscle mass increases during resistance training in young women. *European Journal of Applied Physiology* **77**, 170–175.

‣ De Carlo, M., Shelbourne, D., McCarroll, J. & Rettig, A. (1992) Traditional versus accelerated rehabilitation following ACL reconstruction: a one-year follow-up. *Journal of Orthopaedic and Sports Physical Therapy* **6**, 309–316.

DeLitto, A., Rose, S., McKoven, J.M., Lehman, R.C., Thomas, J.A. & Shively, R.A. (1988) Electrical stimulation versus voluntary exercise in strengthening thigh musculature after anterior cruciate ligament surgery. *Physical Therapy* **68**, 660–663.

Dudley, G.A., Tesch, P.A., Miller, B.J. & Buchanan, P. (1991) Importance of eccentric actions in performance adaptations to resistance training. *Aviation, Space and Environmental Medicine* **62**, 543–550.

Enoka, M. (1988) Muscle strength and its development. New perspectives. *Sports Medicine* **6**, 146–168.

Escamilla, R., Fleisig, G., Zheng, N., Barrentine, S., Wilk, K. & Andrews, J. (1998) Biomechanics of the knee during closed kinetic chain and open kinetic chain exercises. *Medicine and Science in Sports and Exercise* **4**, 556–569.

Fitzgerald, G.K. (1997) Open versus closed kinetic chain exercise. Issues in rehabilitation after anterior cruciate ligament reconstructive surgery. *Physical Therapy* **77**, 1747–1754.

Fleck, S.J. & Kraemer, W.J. (1997) *Designing Resistance Training Programs*, 2nd edn. Human Kinetics, Champaign, IL.

Fridén, J., Seger, J., Sjöström, M. & Ekblom, B. (1983) Adaptive responses in human skeletal muscle subjected to prolonged exercise training. *International Journal of Sports Medicine* **4**, 177–183.

Fry, A.C., Kraemer, W.J. & Weseman, C.A. (1991) The effect of an off-season strength and conditioning program on starters and non-starters in women's intercollegiate volleyball. *Journal of Applied Sports Science Research* **5**, 174–181.

Gettman, L.R., Ayres, J.J., Pollock, M.L., Durstine, J.L. & Grantham, W. (1979) Physiological effects on adult men of circuit strength training and jogging. *Archives of Physical Medicine and Rehabilitation* **60**, 115–120.

Gettman, L.R., Ward, P. & Hagan, R.D. (1982) A comparison of combined running and weight training with circuit weight training. *Medicine and Science in Sports and Exercise* **14**, 229–234.

Gleeson, N.P. & Mercer, T.H. (1996) The utility of isokinetic dynamometry in the assessment of human muscle function. *Sports Medicine* **21**, 18–34.

Gollnick, P.D., Karlsson, J., Piehl, K. & Saltin, B. (1974) Selective glycogen depletion in skeletal muscle fibers of man following sustained contraction. *Journal of Physiology (London)* **241**, 59–67.

Gooch, J., Geiringer, S. & Akau, C. (1993) Sports medicine III. Lower extremities injuries. *Archives of Physical Medicine and Rehabilitation* **74**, 438–442.

Grävare Silbernagel, K., Thomeé, R., Thomeé, P. & Karlsson, J. (2001) Eccentric overload training for patients with chronic Achilles tendon pain—a randomised controlled study with reliability testing of the evaluation methods. *Scandinavian Journal of Medicine and Science in Sports* **11**, 197–206.

Greenberger, H. & Paterno, M. (1995) Relationship of knee extensor strength and hopping test performance in the assessment of lower extremity function. *Journal of Orthopaedic and Sports Physical Therapy* **5**, 202–206.

Grimby, G., Björntorp, P., Fahlén, M. *et al.* (1973) Metabolic effects of isometric training. *Scandinavian Journal of Clinical Laboratory Investigations* **31**, 301.

Grimby, G., Gustafson, E., Peterson, L. & Renström, P. (1980) Quadriceps function and training after knee ligament surgery. *Medicine and Science in Sports and Exercise* **21**, 19–26.

Haennel, R., Teo, K.K., Quinney, A. & Kappagoda, T. (1989) Effects of hydraulic circuit training on cardiovascular function. *Medical Science Sports Medicine* **21**, 605–612.

Häkkinen, K. (1994) Neuromuscular adaptation during strength training, ageing, detraining and immobilization. *Critical Reviews in Physical Medicine and Rehabilitation* **6**, 161–198.

Henning, C.E., Lynch, M.A. & Glick, K.R. (1985) An *in vivo* strain gage study of elongation of the anterior cruciate ligament. *American Journal of Sports Medicine* **13**, 22–26.

Hickson, R., Hidaka, K. & Foster, C. (1994) Skeletal muscle fibertype, resistance training, and strength-related performance. *Medicine and Science in Sports and Exercise* **5**, 593–598.

Higbie, E.J., Cureton, K.J., Warren III, G.L. & Prior, B.M. (1996) Effects of concentric and eccentric training on muscle strength, cross-sectional area, and neural activation. *Journal of Applied Physiology* **81**, 2173–2181.

Hurley, M.V., Jones, D.W. & Newham, D.J. (1994) Artrogenic quadriceps inhibition and rehabilitation of patients with extensive traumatic knee injuries. *Clinical Science* **86**, 305–310.

Isear Jr, J., Erickson, J. & Worrell, T. (1997) EMG analysis of lower extremity muscle recruitment patterns during an unloaded squat. *Medicine and Science in Sports and Exercise* **29**, 532–539.

Kannus, P., Alosa, D., Cook, L. *et al.* (1992a) Effect of one-legged exercise on the strength, power and endurance of the contralateral leg. *European Journal of Applied Physiology* **64**, 117–126.

Kannus, P., Jozsa, L., Renström, P. *et al.* (1992b) The effects of training, immobilization and remobilization on musculoskeletal tissue. 1. Training and immobilization. *Scandinavian Journal of Medicine and Science in Sports* **2**, 100–118.

Kannus, P., Jozsa, L., Renström, P. *et al.* (1992c) The effects of training, immobilization and remobilization on musculoskeletal tissue. 2. Remobilization and prevention of immobilization atrophy. *Scandinavian Journal of Medicine and Science in Sports* **2**, 164–176.

Kannus, P., Jozsa, L., Kvist, M., Jarvinen, T. & Jarvinen, M. (1998) Effects of immobilization and subsequent low- and high-intensity exercise on morphology of rat calf muscles. *Scandinavian Journal of Medicine and Science in Sports* **8**, 160–171.

Kellis, E. & Baltzopoulos, V. (1998) Muscle activation differences between eccentric and concentric isokinetic exercise. *Medicine and Science in Sports and Exercise* **30**, 1616–1623.

Knaflitz, M., Merlitto, R. & DeLuca, C.J. (1990) Inference of motor unit recruitment order of voluntary and electrical elicited contractions. *Journal of Applied Physiology* **68**, 1657–1667.

Komi, P. (1984) Physiological and biomechanical correlates of muscle function. Effects of muscle structure and stretch-shortening cycle on force and speed. *Exercise and Sport Sciences Reviews* **12**, 81–121.

Komi, P. (1987) Neuromuscular factors related to physical performance. *Medicine and Sport Science* **26**, 48–66.

Kraemer, W.J. & Fleck, S.J. (1993) *Strength Training for Young Athletes.* Human Kinetics, Champaign, IL.

Kraemer, W.J., Fleck, S.J. & Evans, W.J. (1996) Strength and power training: physiological mechanisms of adaptation. *Exercise and Sport Sciences Reviews* **14**, 363–397.

Leveritt, M., Abernethy, P.J., Barry, B.K. & Logan, P.A. (1999) Concurrent strength and endurance training. A review. *Sports Medicine* **28**, 413–427.

Mafi, N., Lorentzon, R. & Alfredson, H. (2001) Superior short-term results with eccentric calf muscle training compared to concentric training in a randomized prospective multicenter study on patients with chronic Achilles tendinosis. *Knee Surgery, Sports Traumatology, Arthroscopy* **99**, 42–47.

Panariello, R., Backus, S. & Parker, J. (1994) The effect of the squat exercise on anterior-posterior knee translation in professional football players. *American Journal of Sports Medicine* **6**, 768–773.

Pfeifer, K. & Banzer, W. (1999) Motor performance in different dynamic tests in knee rehabilitation. *Scandinavian Journal of Medicine and Science in Sports* **9**, 19–27.

Risberg, M.A., Holm, I., Tjomsland, O., Ljunggren, E. & Ekeland, A. (1999) Prospective study of changes in impairments and disabilities after anterior cruciate ligament reconstruction. *Journal of Orthopaedic and Sports Physical Therapy* **29**, 400–412.

Sale, D.G. (1988) Neural adaptation to resistance training. *Medicine and Science in Sports and Exercise* **20**, S135–S145.

Saltin, B. (1986) Physiological adaptation to physical conditioning. *Acta Medica Scandinavica* **711** (Suppl.), 11–24.

Saltin, B. & Rowell, L.B. (1980) Functional adaptations to physical activity and inactivity. *Federation Proceedings* **39**, 1506–1513.

Saltin, B., Rådegran, G., Koskolou, M.D. & Roach, R.C. (1998) Skeletal muscle blood flow in humans and its regulation during exercise. *Acta Physiologica Scandinavica* **162**, 421–436.

Shakespeare, D.T., Stokes, M., Sherman, K.P. & Young, A. (1985) Reflex inhibition of the quadriceps after meniscectomy. Lack of association with pain. *Clinical Physiology* **5**, 137–144.

Shelbourne, K., Klootwyk, T., Wilckens, J. & De Carlo, M. (1995) Ligament stability two to six years after anterior cruciate ligament reconstruction with autogenous patellar tendon graft and participation in accelerated rehabilitation program. *American Journal of Sports Medicine* **5**, 575–579.

Shelbourne, K.D. & Nitz, P. (1992) Accelerated rehabilitation after anterior cruciate ligament reconstruction. *Journal of Orthopaedic and Sports Physical Therapy* **15**, 256–264.

Sisco, P. & Little, J. (1997) *Power Factor Training: a Scientific Approach to Building Lean Muscle Mass.* Contemporary Books, Lincolnwood, IL.

Snyder-Mackler, L., Delitto, A., Bailey, S.L. & Stralka, S.W. (1995) Strength of the quadriceps femoris muscle and functional recovery after reconstruction of the anterior cruciate ligament. A prospective, randomized clinical trial of electrical stimulation. *Journal of Bone and Joint Surgery (American)* **77**, 1166–1173.

Steinkamp, L.A., Dillingham, M.F., Markel, M.D., Hill, J.A. & Kaufman, K.R. (1993) Biomechanical considerations in patellofemoral joint rehabilitation. *American Journal of Sports Medicine* **21**, 438–444.

Stokes, M. & Young, A. (1984) The contribution of reflex inhibition to arthrogenous muscle weakness. *Clinical Science* **67**, 7–14.

Stone, M.H., Collins, D., Plisk, S., Haff, E. & Stone, M.E. (2000) Training principles: evaluation of modes and methods of resistance training. *Strength and Conditioning Journal* **22**, 65–76.

Thomeé, R., Grimby, G., Svantesson, U. & Österberg, U. (1996) Quadriceps muscle performance at sitting and standing in young women with patellofemoral pain syndrome and healthy controls. *Scandinavian Journal of Medicine and Science in Sports* **6**, 233–241.

Thorén, P., Floras, J.S., Hoffmann, P. & Seals, D.R. (1990) Endorphins and exercise. Physiological mechanisms and clinical implications. *Medicine and Science in Sports and Exercise* **4**, 417–428.

Thorstensson, A., Karlsson, J., Viitasalo, J.H.T., Luhtanen, P. & Komi, P.V. (1976) Effect of strength training on EMG of human skeletal muscle. *Acta Physiologica Scandinavica* **98**, 232–236.

Westing, S.H., Seger, J.Y., Karlsson, E. & Ekblom, B. (1988) Eccentric and concentric torque-velocity characteristics of the quadriceps femoris in man. *European Journal of Applied Physiology* **58**, 100–104.

Westing, S.H., Seger, J.Y. & Thorstensson, A. (1990) Effects of electrical stimulation on eccentric and concentric torque-velocity relationships during knee extension in man. *Acta Physiologica Scandinavica* **140**, 17–22.

Wigerstad-Lossing, I., Grimby, G., Jonsson, T., Morelli, B., Peterson, L. & Renström, P. (1988) Effects of electrical muscle stimulation combined with voluntary contractions after knee ligament surgery. *Medicine and Science in Sports and Exercise* **20**, 93–98.

Wilk, K., Romaniello, W., Soscia, S., Arrigo, C. & Andrews, J. (1994) The relationship between subjective knee scores, isokinetic testing, and functional testing in the ACL-reconstructed knee. *Journal of Orthopaedic and Sports Physical Therapy* **2**, 60–72.

Yack, J., Collins, C. & Whieldon, T. (1993) Comparison of closed and open kinetic chain exercise in the anterior cruciate ligament-deficient knee. *American Journal of Sports Medicine* **21**, 49–54.

Chapter 13

Proprioception and Coordination

JUAN JOSÉ GONZÁLEZ ITURRI

Introduction

Proprioception can be defined as 'a special type of sensitivity that informs about the sensations of the deep organs and of the relationship between muscles and joints'. Coordination can be defined as 'the capacity to perform movements in a smooth, precise and controlled manner'.

Rehabilitation techniques increasingly refer to neuromuscular re-education. These methods have provided evidence of their efficacy and reliability in athletes, where just recovering the function of an injured joint is not sufficient, and perfect rehabilitation is required. Muscle-strengthening techniques are not sufficient since the neuromuscular and neuroarticular functions need to be re-educated. It is therefore time for rehabilitation to have a proprioceptive objective.

Ligaments, tendons and joint capsules do not just perform mechanical support functions or induce movement. They are also the bearers of deep sensitivity mechanoreceptors that gather information on the position of the joints, or how tendons and ligaments are stretched, and this information is sent to the base of the encephalon through the upper cord, initiating an effective response, resulting in dynamic stabilization and therefore a balanced reaction.

Neurological proprioception mechanisms

With regard to proprioception, as in many other fields associated with the nervous system,

Sherrington's contributions are fundamental due to his classification of sensitivity (Asirón Yribarren 1991):

1 *Exteroceptive sensation.* This is external surface sensation. It includes touch, pressure, pain, and hot and cold temperatures, which are globally known as general exteroceptive sensations; it also includes other more specialized sensations such as sight, hearing and smell, which together form special exteroceptive sensation.

2 *Proprioceptive sensation.* This covers a series of impressions on the functional state of the joints and muscles. If the individual is aware of these impressions, this is conscious proprioceptive sensation (awareness of passive and active movements, and the attitude or position of a somatic part of the body, kinaesthesia); if he or she is unaware of them, this is called unconscious proprioceptive sensation (relating to balance, tone and muscular coordination). There is also a special proprioceptive sensation, called labyrinthine.

3 *Interoceptive sensation.* This is found in the viscera and vessels (pain, oppression, etc.) and is of a general nature; it can be divided in areas such as gustatory and olfactory.

There are three types of sensation:

1 *Deep sensation.* This is the source of profound sensations, from pain to pressure, or sensations of movement.

2 *Epicritical superficial sensation.* This corresponds to fine contacts, the special difference between sensations, the perception of temperature and the location of painful and temperature-related sensations.

3 *Protopathic superficial sensation.* This produces sensations of extreme pain and temperatures.

However, it is preferable to use less topographic and more functional classifications and descriptions. Gley (1914) talks of the sensation of attitudes and movements as a synonym for muscular sensations—awareness of the position of muscles in space and the sensation of passive movements, together with active movements and resistance. He establishes a series of divisions:

• Kinetic impressions, sensations of attitude, continuous, articular and muscular sensations.

• Kinetic impressions, sensation of passive movement. The perception of passive movements depends on articular sensitivity. Nevertheless, according to Gley, it is very difficult for joint sensations alone to determine the perception of passive movements.

• Kinetic impressions, sensation of active movements. Perception is a complex phenomenon combining tactile, joint and muscular impressions.

The afferent nerves responsible for kinetic impressions are cutaneous, articular and muscular:

• Cutaneous: these nerves are found in the fold and tension of the skin, and vary with the speed, energy and length of the contraction.

• Articular: articular anaesthesia reduces the perception of active and passive movements.

• Muscular: these nerves arise in the Golgi tendon organs and in the bones. The latter sense movement and the former sense tension (Grigg *et al.* 1982).

• Feelings of central enervation, an efferent nerve, which comes from the brain and precedes the contraction. This is the sensation that an effort has to be made, of force released in the brain to provoke a movement.

Thounnard *et al.* (1986), in a critical study of the pathogenesis of a sprained ankle, reported that the passive structures are incapable of absorbing the energy produced when jumping on to an unstable surface. The time required to reach the calcaneotibial varus angle that causes the capsuloligamentous rupture is less than the reflex latencies observed in the muscles that stabilize the ankle, so it is assumed that only active

muscular rigidity beforehand could protect this joint against a ligament injury.

For Strumpell (1924) the nerve endings in the skin are sensitive to stimulant disorders: mechanical, temperature-related and pain. He claims that the deep parts of the muscles, fasciae, periosteum and joints can only feel mechanical pressure and distension stimuli, in particular tactile sensation referring to heat and cold, pain, pressure, mechanical distension, electrocutaneous sensation or sense of vibrations, and stereognostic sensation, which recognizes objects from their size, shape, hardness, etc.

For Sonjen (1986) the term exteroceptive is obsolete, whereas proprioceptive is used extensively. He points out the utility of classifying somatic sensation as superficial or deep, corresponding to the excitation of cutaneous sense organs and proprioceptors.

Sensitive receptor organs

Superficial somatic sensation is caused by exteroceptors, including: Pacinian corpuscles, mechanoreceptors for rapid, tactile and vibratory adaptations; Merkel's disks, mechanoreceptors for slow adaptations, tactile and pressure sensitivity; Meissner corpuscles, also for rapid adaptations and tactile sensation; Krause bulbs or heat receptors; Ruffini corpuscles, slow adaptation mechanoreceptors for sustained pressure; and free endings for nociception and intense tactile and temperature stimuli (Burgess & Clark 1969; Burgess & Wei 1982).

Deep somatic sensation is due to proprioceptors, found in articular receptors like the Golgi organs, Ruffini corpuscles, Pacinian corpuscles, free endings and Krause's end bulbs; and in muscular receptors like the laminated Pacinian corpuscles, Kühne's neuromuscular spindles, Golgi–Mazzoni tendinous organs and free endings (Table 13.1).

Spinal level

As afferent elements in the spine, we have those already described, and as efferent elements, the

Table 13.1 Sensory receptor organs.

Receptors	Location	Function
Superficial somatic sensation (exteroceptive)	Pacinian corpuscles	Rapid adaptations, touch, vibration
	Merkel's disks	Slow adaptations, tactile sensation, pressure
	Meissner corpuscles	Rapid adaptations, tactile sensation
	Krause bulbs	Temperature receptors
	Ruffini corpuscles	Rapid adaptations, sustained pressure
	Free nerve endings	Nociception, tactile stimuli, endings
Profound somatic sensation (proprioceptors)		
Articular receptors	Golgi receptors	
	Ruffini corpuscles	
	Pacinian corpuscles	
	Krause's free endings	Deep sensation
Muscular receptors	Pacinian corpuscles	
	Kühne's spindles	
	Golgi organs	
	Free nerve endings	

final common pathway and as a response to the segmental and suprasegmental reflexes and voluntary impulses, the motoneuron axonal process located in the anterior horn of the spine contributing muscle fibres and provoking contraction.

Reflexes

In humans, the medullar reflex circuits play a decisive role in the control of movement. Some of them are monosynaptic, including the stretching reflex and passive muscular stretching, which excite the annulospiral endings.

When walking, monosynaptic stretching reflexes are inhibited. This has been verified by examining the behaviour of the potentials evoked when walking or standing; when walking, the group I afferent signals are blocked, both on the segmentary and supraspinal levels.

On the other hand, and unlike what happens when walking, segmentary stretching reflex activity helps to activate the muscles that stretch the legs during rapid movements such as running or jumping.

Polysynaptic reflexes are mutually inhibitory, since the same afferent nerves that determine the myotatic reflex provoke antagonist inhibition by

means of an interneurone. Sherrington's law of successive induction, a sequence of reciprocal inhibition, expresses the ease of contraction of a muscular group when antagonist contraction ceases.

The flexor withdrawal, or proprioceptive reflex, response to the nociceptive afferences on any structure, activating the flexor muscles and inhibiting the extensors, which provokes bending of the stimulated limb and the extension of the contralateral muscle.

Cerebral cortex

At the head of the hierarchy is the cerebral cortex, with two relief stations: the somatosensory area and the motor areas, through which a transcortical loop of variable gain and relatively slow execution is established, unlike the segmentary loops of less improvement but much faster execution.

For afferent nerves, there are two ways in which sensations reach the cerebral cortex to become conscious—they are the lemniscal system that carries precise time and space information, and the indirect extralemniscal system, with imprecise space and time characteristics.

For efferent nerves, there is the pyramidal path, a prolongation of the pyramidal neurones of the motor cortex that is directly and indirectly projected onto the motor neurones of the anterior horn of the medulla, to which the voluntary motorial function is attributed (Dietz 1987).

Finally, we have the extrapyramidal pathways that are projected on to the thalamus, nucleus basalis, red nucleus and pontine nuclei; they are involved in muscular tone, the regulation of movement and the regulation of posture.

Conclusions

Proprioception can be considered as the individual's capacity to be aware of and recognize the instantaneous, static or dynamic situation of his/her body. According to classic proprioception classifications, it is responsible for capturing tension, force, spatial position, passive and active movements with speed, acceleration and amplitude, and the sensation of the structures, their situation and body limits (body schema).

All nerve endings, both superficial—general exteroceptive and special (sight and hearing) —and deep—general proprioceptive (articular and muscular), visceral, general interoceptive and special (taste and smell)—are involved in proprioception.

The nervous levels used include: the medullar segmentary level; the suprasegmentary level with the brainstem; and the cortical level, the activity of which is conditioned by specific and non-specific sensory afferent nerves, as well as the reticular thalamic system, or humoral regulation, cortical regulation or feedback.

Cutaneous, articular, tendinous and muscular afferent nerves follow the lemniscal path to the somatognosic areas, alert the cerebral cortex and produce proprioceptive sensation.

The use of proprioceptive mechanisms helps to correct or perfect motorial abilities (proprioceptive facilitation) and conscious proprioceptive perception provides awareness of posture and recognition of the body schema, allowing for their eventual correction.

Motor control and coordination

How the nervous system is organized to control and coordinate the neuromuscular function is much discussed and as yet unknown. It is an extraordinarily complex system, the capacity of which exceeds the most perfect of computers, and hypotheses on conscience, the thought process, motor planning and execution are impossible to prove. Such a complete organizational process involves structures such as: the cerebral cortex, which inhibits and excites the lower levels; the extrapyramidal system in charge of integrating the excitation and inhibition components, making them automatic by repetition; the corticospinal pyramidal path used to repeatedly excite the desired activity; and the basic spinal reflexes, which are the origin of all motor functions and sensitive feedback.

The human brain, unremarkable in appearance, and weighing approximately 1500 g, is evidently the most complex organization in the universe (Eccles 1969).

When referring to neuromuscular function, it is common to use the terms motor control, to define the excitation that voluntarily activates an isolated muscle, and motor coordination, a more complex neuromuscular activity that needs to integrate several elements to excite some muscles and inhibit others, to create patterns and sequences and thus to achieve functional body movements—something that is very important in sport.

The literature uses the terms motor control and coordination indistinctly, and includes many common models and theories concerning how it is organized and learned. In any circumstance, however, motor control is the result of a very important interaction between the individual, the activity and the surroundings (Fig. 13.1) (Acebes et al. 1996).

Measuring proprioceptive performance

Proprioceptive afferent signals take place and influence the motor response on several different

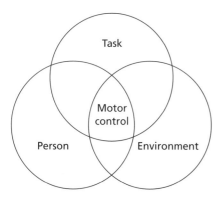

Fig. 13.1 Different elements that have an influence on motor control.

levels. Modulator influxes are added in the process of propagating and generating stimuli by means of the downward paths. Most of the interaction between motor and sensory responses takes place outside the voluntary perception level.

Psychophysical tests such as measuring the movement threshold or the capacity to reproduce an actively and passively preorientated angle are the test procedures used to assess proprioception. However, in sports our knowledge of proprioception is highly limited, for several reasons:

• It is not known how isolated proprioception mechanisms influence these tests. There are limited conclusions, for example, an improvement in a test result does not necessarily mean that there is a useful improvement in a person's proprioceptive function.

• The tests are performed while resting. It is not possible to measure the possible proprioceptive function that the individual is capable of under effort.

• To what extent are the tests understandable outside voluntary perception?

• Angular reproduction tests are not constant for individuals.

• Training has a partially paradoxical impact. It can worsen test results or influence different psychophysical test procedures in opposite ways. Training can also influence the results of psychophysical test procedures.

Electromyography can provide an orientated analysis of muscular function as the end-point of regulatory proprioceptive function. Conclusions concerning possible influences can be obtained by observing muscular movement within the framework of the sensory motor function, but it does not measure an immediate proprioceptive function. However, it does have some advantages, because:

• studies can be performed under conditions involving effort;

• the impact of training and the application of external stabilization aids, such as bandaging, can be studied by their effect on muscular action and regulation performance; and

• the pathological parameters of activation can be defined and identified.

Up to now, recognition procedure results have shown a decrease in the proprioception of major joints in relation to typical injuries and dysfunctions of the locomotive apparatus. It is difficult to evaluate the role of proprioception in the origin of injuries, since there are a lack of data concerning the proprioceptive situation before the injuries occured.

Studying the use of proprioception in sport, it is possible to obtain epidemiological data and results from prior examinations:

• From the findings of psychophysical and electromyographic examinations, it can be deduced that injuries produce alterations to the special somatosensory and proprioceptive characteristics of performance.

• Before a major injury occurs, there are frequently earlier injuries that have been damaging the proprioceptive structures.

• Directed proprioceptive training essentially reduces the frequency of injuries.

The effect of an injury on proprioception

The natural history of, for example, the rupture of the anterior cruciate ligament of an athlete's knee shows that, in spite of reconstructive surgical techniques and a good rehabilitation process

Table 13.2 Knee joint receptors.

Receptors	Location	Function

Ruffini corpuscles	Capsule
	Ligaments: LLI/LCA
	Cartilage
		Stable and dynamic mechanoreceptors
		Information on:
		    joint position
		    amplitude and speed of movement
		    intra-articular pressure
		Slow adaptation

Pacinian corpuscles	Intra and extra-articular fatty tissue
	Capsule
	Internal meniscus
	LLI
	Cartilage
		Stable and dynamic mechanoreceptors
		Information on:
		    end of the movement
		    sensitivity to acceleration and deceleration
		Rapid adaptation

Golgi–Mazzoni corpuscles	LCA/LCP/LLI/LLE Internal meniscus	Dynamic mechanoreceptors Information on external joint positions Slow adaptation
Free nerve endings	Capsule Ligaments Fatty tissue	Pain receptors Information on mechanical stimuli Slow adaptation

leading to a correct muscular situation, there is no guarantee that the treatment will be successful. This leads us to consider that there must be other factors, such as the enervation of the knee and the proprioceptive mechanisms, that are lost when the injury occurs (Table 13.2).

Capsular ligamentous elements, as primary passive structures, provide stability and normal kinematics to the knee joint. The presence of these receptor elements also means that, in addition to their mechanical function, they can act as dynamic organs by causing reflex synergic muscular activities.

The ligament injury, the resulting effusion, the immobilization required for treatment, and the following surgical trauma all produce alterations to proprioceptive sensitivity, creating confusing afferent messages that inhibit motor control and sensory motor programming, thus increasing the lack of stability by creating incorrect muscular responses. Knee stability cannot be restored without taking enervation into consideration (Jerosch & Prymka 1996; Lephart *et al.* 1997).

Proprioceptive re-education techniques

The treatments traditionally used for the recovery of injured athletes reprogramme the proprioceptive receptors and their afferent and efferent pathways. This is specifically the case for traditional kinesiotherapy, massage or modern isokinetic methods. They all stimulate the exteroceptive and proprioceptive systems.

In all these techniques, stretching, when correctly applied, has an important proprioceptive effect on the injured area, whether it be articular or muscular. Stretching not only gets the muscular receptors working, but also the articular level, improving integration of the body, which is fundamental in normal daily activities and sport (Commandre *et al.* 1996).

Proprioceptive techniques

Proprioceptive reprogramming can be achieved using the following techniques.

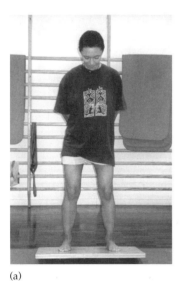

(a)

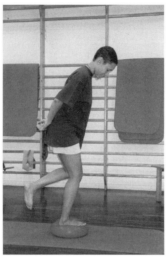

(b)

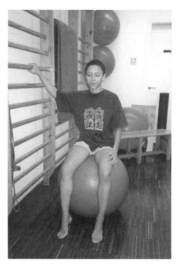

(c)

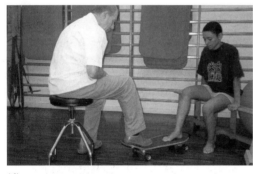

(d)

Fig. 13.2 Different proprioceptive training situations. (a) Balancing on unstable planes; (b) balancing on one foot; (c) balancing whilst sitting; (d) sliding the foot along an unstable plane.

• The use of unbalancing forces, using either unstable planes or applying destabilizers to an individual supported by a stable plane (Fig. 13.2). Both these kinds of imbalance are involved in sport, since the articular segment and the entire articular apparatus become involved in situations with components of either.

• Reprogramming can also be achieved with the proprioceptive neuromuscular facilitation techniques proposed by Kabat at the beginning of the 1950s, consisting of the use of superficial and deep information, such as the position of joints, tendons and muscles, contact with the therapist's hand, verbal orders and visual stimuli, all aimed at the work of the strongest muscle groups and leading to the functional improvement of other weaker, normally inhibited, groups.

Individuals make integrated movements that affect muscle groups that are used to working together. Complete kinetic chains work together following a series of rules: movement of the segments on the diagonal plane; a spiral component associated with each movement; and stretching stimuli which are used when applying maximum manual resistance.

For years, this method was essentially only used on patients with neurological disorders, but it is now frequently used in sports-relate pathologies.

THE UPPER LIMBS

The proprioceptive re-education of a limb is always global, integrating the joints and the entire limb in the locomotive apparatus, and taking into consideration the limb's function. Upper limbs are used for holding, picking up and throwing and lower limbs for walking, running, jumping and pushing oneself upwards. It is necessary to analyse what the segment has to achieve in each sport. Reprogramming a javelin thrower's arm is not the same as reprogramming a swimmer's arm (Fig. 13.3).

Exercises on unstable planes

Any of these exercises can be used, working in a closed kinetic chain. To increase the lack of stability, pressure is brought to bear on a Freeman board, and the exercise is performed in the quadruped position. Another variant is the use of a ball as a source of instability, while the individual is either standing or in a quadruped position. On occasion it is fundamental to throw the ball against a wall, forcing the individual to work to receive it.

Semiclosed and open kinetic chain exercises

Exercises using a stick held in both hands, while the physiotherapist unbalances it, are practical, very simple and can be graduated as required. This stimulates different positions, particularly in relation to the shoulder. This exercise can also be performed in a unilateral fashion.

The Kabat method

A basic exercise for the upper limbs is Kabat's diagonal movements, using the scapulohumeral joint as a pivot and starting with a flexion and cubital inclination of the wrist, a pronation of the forearm, an extension of the elbow and with the shoulder positioned with extension, abduction and internal rotation. Applying manual resistance, the movement is towards a radial extension and inclination of the wrist, supination of the forearm, with the elbow continuing to be

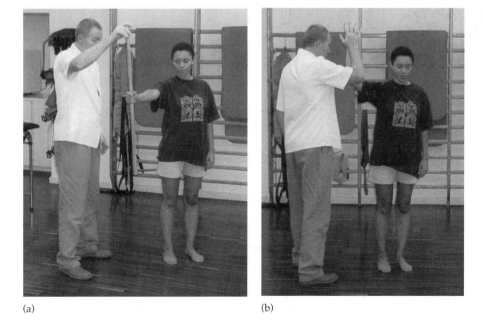

(a)   (b)

Fig. 13.3 (a) Proprioceptive training of the shoulder. (b) Proprioceptive training of the shoulder by pushing against the physiotherapist.

extended, and the shoulder moving towards flexion, adduction and internal rotation.

The second starting position can be a radial extension and inclination of the wrist, a pronation of the forearm, extension of the elbow, extension, adduction and internal rotation of the shoulder, moving towards a flexion and cubital inclination of the wrist, maintaining the elbow extended, and with the shoulder moving towards flexion, external rotation and adduction.

THE LOWER LIMBS

Using the Kabat technique with the upper limbs, two basic diagonal movements are used on which variations are then introduced. Something similar can be used after injuries to the lower limbs (Knoff & Voss 1968).

The first situation starts with a sole flexion and an eversion of the foot (with the knee bent or extended) with the hip extended with internal rotation, moving towards a dorsal flexion and inversion of the foot, and maintaining the knee in the original position, and the hip with flexion and external rotation (Blanc & Piur 1984; Bernier & Perrin 1998).

The second diagonal starts with a sole flexion and inversion of the foot, with the knee either bent or extended, and the hip extended with external rotation, moving towards an eversion and dorsal flexion of the foot, and flexion and internal rotation of the hip (Fig. 13.4).

Initially, the therapy starts with a perimaleolar massage, as there will probably be oedema, continuing with mobilization of the scar, if there is a scar, since scar tissue is occasionally adhered. Passive kinesiotherapy is then applied to all the ankle and foot joints, which helps to assess the state of the articular movements so that the athlete becomes aware of the state of his/her injured joint. These mobilizations should be smooth and never exceed the pain limit.

This is followed by active and selective unloaded work with the anterior tibial (flexion of the toes, varus of the foot and dorsal flexion of the ankle) and peroneals (plantar flexion of

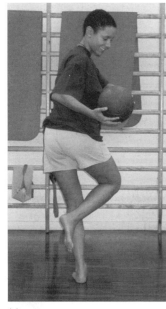

(a)

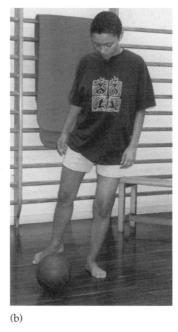

(b)

Fig. 13.4 (a) General proprioceptive training acting on a lower limb with upper limb work. (b) Standing proprioceptive work.

the ankle, flexion of the toes and varus of the foot). These exercises are performed both freely and with manual counter-resistance. The athlete should always perform the entire exercise in bare feet (Freeman 1965; Herveou & Messeau 1976; Herveou & Messeau 1981).

Stage 1

This exercise starts with learning crispation of the toes. The athlete should stand with the knees extended, trunk straight, feet parallel and in line with the coxofemoral joints and perpendicular to the frontal plane. The movement is towards a position in which the knees are extended and the trunk is straight and bent forwards, following a theoretical axis that passes through the malleoli. The purpose of this exercise is to work the musculature of the foot and adherence to the ground. It is the first level of proprioceptive information and the first state of alert.

Control of the anterior tibial is learned in the same way. The initial position is the same as for the previous exercise, but with a 30° flexion of the knees. The athlete bends forwards, imitating the initial stages of a fall, positioning the lower joints in an outwards turn. The physiotherapist should make sure that the contraction of the anterior tibial is intense and that the outer edge of the foot is supported (Fig. 13.5). The purpose of this exercise is the active maintenance of the internal longitudinal arch of the foot. It is the second level of proprioceptive information and the second state of alert.

Another exercise is with the two feet on the ground, knees extended, trunk straight, feet parallel and in line with the coxofemorals. The physiotherapist is positioned behind the athlete and on the side opposite the injury, pressing forwards and outwards.

Stage 2

What we have described above is the preparatory phase for the remaining exercises that work proprioceptively on the ankle, stimulating all the mechanoreceptors as much as possible. The exer-

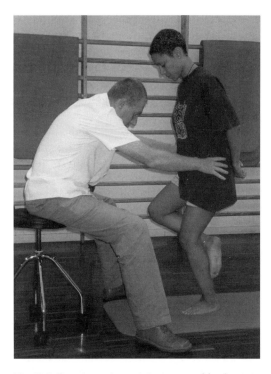

Fig. 13.5 Proprioceptive training on unstable planes with the physiotherapist's help.

cises reproduce all the situations of the foot when it is in contact with the ground when walking, running and jumping. Therefore, the position of the foot during the exercises is very important, with unipodal support during the first half step, which is when the load is greatest.

The toes are crispated, the anterior tibial is tensed to maintain the internal longitudinal arch, the big toe is firmly positioned on the ground and the foot is perpendicular to the frontal plane. Contact with the ground is thus at the heel, the outer edge of the foot, the metatarsal heads, the tips of the toes and the entire plantar face of the big toe. Cutaneous information is maximal and reproduces the foot's three support phases when walking. The knee is bent outwards at 30° to maximize the information captured by the proprioceptive mechanoreceptors, with the ligaments relaxed and maximum dynamic ankle stability.

Work with unipodal support starts at the second or third session of treatment. The athlete positions the injured limb in front of the healthy one, separated by a normal step length, reproducing the correction position of the foot (toes crispated, the anterior tibial tensed and the foot perpendicular to the frontal plane), with the knee bent to 30°, then returning to the initial position. The difficulty of the exercise can be increased by increasing the angle at which the knee is bent or extended.

Stage 3

At the third session, the athlete progressively starts the Freeman (BAPS) board exercises on the three axes of the rectangular plane. When the exercises on the rectangular plane are no longer difficult, work should start on the circular plane (Gagey 1993).

After the second week of therapy (after approximately 10 sessions of rehabilitation) the athlete should start jumping, first on the floor, then from the floor to the board and then from board to board, adding exercises involving catching a ball on the floor and on the Freeman board (Freeman 1965; Heurte *et al.* 1991).

At the last therapy sessions the athlete can run on a treadmill, beginning sports training combined with continuation of medical rehabilitation.

Adapting proprioception to training

Medicine's role in sport is the treatment and, above all, prevention of athletic injuries. We must attempt, therefore, to adapt proprioception to training systems (Raybaud *et al.* 1988; Caraffa *et al.* 1996). Individual attention is not always possible or desirable for athletes; a structure accessible to several athletes at the same time needs to be considered. It is possible to combine sports training and proprioceptive training by installing an 'athlete's programme area' next to the usual training area. These programme areas, which use proprioceptive re-education methods and techniques, can vary in infinite ways and be adapted to different sports.

Unbalanced surfaces can be grouped together, and when athletes have good stability on this equipment they can go on to other surfaces where the instability is greater. At the end of the progression, unipodal exercises can be performed with a ball, medicine ball and/or sandbag.

The material required is commonly found in rehabilitation centres:
• A rectangular board on two hemispheres, which will selectively work on the internal, external and anteroposterior muscular groups of the lower limb, depending on the position adopted.
• A circular board with a central spherical wedge, which works on proprioception in a broader sense. It regulates lack of balance, depending on the size of the hemisphere. It is even better if it is coated with a kind of synthetic lawn material, which adds cutaneous information to the proprioceptive reflex.
• A hanging balancing board, which provides maximum difficulty both for the lower limbs and for the trunk.

Within this framework, the athlete could work for 5 min on the balancing boards, going from the simplest to the most complex, ending with unipodal support and catching a ball. The training could continue with unipodal exercises on a soft carpet, where the athlete moves forward on the balancing bench to jump on a trampoline. From here he or she might move to the circumflex boards, after crossing a common area jumping from platform to platform.

Coordination training

Improving coordination depends on repeating the positions and movements associated with different sports and correct training. It has to begin with simple activities, performed slowly and perfectly executed, gradually increasing in speed and complexity. The technician should make sure that the athlete performs these movements unconsciously, until they finally become automatic.

In the first place, coordination training requires the athlete to be willing to undertake the activity

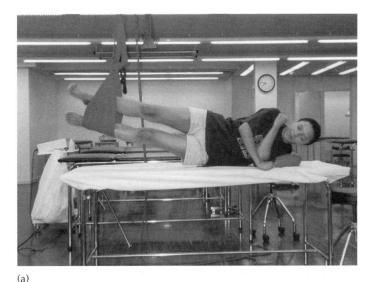

(a)

(b)

Fig. 13.6 (a) Spinal column proprioceptive training whilst lying on one side. (b) Spinal column proprioceptive exercise whilst crawling.

or to rest whenever he/she wishes; continuous perception information of the activity is needed, with perfect peripheral sensitive receptors from the subcortical centres. This creation of an automatic movement can only be achieved by voluntary repetition.

The basis of coordination training is the inhibition of the motor neurones that are not involved in the movement desired. Although direct training is not possible, this can be maintained by precisely executing certain activities. For this training, the individual has to be old enough to understand and follow instructions, be capable of learning and cooperating, and be capable of concentrating and avoiding fatigue. The receptors, paths and centres have to be intact and there must be a movement span of at least 30°, free of pain, at the joint affected by the muscle. Pain will lead to inhibition and, therefore, lack of coordination (Cerda *et al.* 1996).

Conclusions

For treatment to be effective it has to be applied early. The purpose of re-education, depending on the aetiology and severity of the injury, is to restore the athlete's functional possibilities. It has to lead to a rapid return to physical activity compatible with the competition level.

Proprioceptive re-education has to get the muscular receptors working, in order to provide a rapid motor response (Scott *et al.* 2000). The treatment has to be adapted to each individual, considering the type of injury and the stress to which the athlete will be exposed when practising his or her sport.

There is no test for proprioceptive training. Its success can only be measured under controlled conditions in which the training is assessed and a reduction of the injury is confirmed (Quante & Hille 1999; Coarasa Lirón de Robles 2001).

Proprioceptive re-education is not a synonym of exercises on unstable planes. It re-educates 'unstable' athletes who are going to practise sport on unstable planes (Lorza 1991, 1998; Lephart *et al.* 1997; Guegan & Nicolas 1999; Romano 1999).

It is important to use proprioception when treating athletic injuries (Fig. 13.6). Global work has to be carried out on the injured limb, using the body's own mechanisms, which are capable of being reprogrammed when practising sport again. It has to be carried out in an early stage and cannot guarantee that there will be no further relapses.

References

Acebes, O., Fernandez-Gubieda, M., Bascuñana, H., San Segundo, R. & Aguilar, J.J. (1996) El control motor y la coordinación. *Rehabilitación* **30**, 395–404.

Asirón Yribarren, P. (1991) *Propiocepción. Bases Fisiológicas*. Rehabilitación y Deporte, Pamplona: 37–56.

Bernier, J.N. & Perrin, D.H. (1998) Effects of coordination training on proprioception of the functionally unstable ankle. *Journal of Orthopaedics and Sports Physical Therapy* **27** (4), 264–275.

Blanc, Y. & Piur, M. (1984) Influence de la position du pied sur les contractions évoqueés des muscles moteurs de genou. *Annales de Kinesitherapie* **5**, 107–204.

Burgess, R.C. & Clark, F.J. (1969) Characteristics of knee joint receptors in the cat. *Journal of Physiological (London)* **203**, 317.

Burgess, R.C. & Wei, J.Y. (1982) Signaling of kinesthetic information by peripheral sensory receptors. *Annual Review of Neuroscience* **5**, 171–187.

Caraffa, A., Cerulli, G., Projetti, M., Aisa, G.Y., Rizzo, A. (1996) Prevention of anterior cruciate ligament injuries in soccer. A prospective controlled study of proprioceptive training. *Knee Surgergy, Sports Traumatology, Arthroscopy* **4** (1), 19–21.

Cerda, M., Abril, C., Puig, J.M., San Segundo, R. & Aguilar, J.J. (1996) Ejercicios terapéuticos para tratamiento del control y la coordinación motora. *Rehabilitación* **30**, 436–442.

Coarasa Lirón de Robles, A. (2001) Propiocepción en la rehabilitación del LCA. In: *Minutes of the 8th FEMEDE Congress, Zaragoza*. Spanish Federation of Sports Medicine, Pamplona: 137–142.

Commandre, F.A., Fourre, J.M., Davarend, J.P., Raybaud, A. & Formanirs, E. (1996) Re-education and rehabilitation of the lesions of the athletes locomotive system. *Cinesiologie* **35**, 9–23.

Dietz, V. (1987) Role des afferences péripheriques et des reflexes spinaux dans la fonction locomotrice humaine normale et pathologique. *Revue de Neurologie* **143** (4), 241–254.

Eccles, J.C. (1969) The dynamic loop hypothesis of movements control. In: *Information Processing in the Nervous System* (Leibovic, K.N., ed.). Springer-Verlag, New York: 245–269.

Freeman, M. (1965) Coordination exercises the treatment of functional instability of the foot. *Physiotherapy* **5**, 393–395.

Gagey, P.-M. (1993) La plate-forme de rééducation posturale. *Annales de Kinesitherapie* **6** (20), 331–334.

Gley, E. (1914) *Tratado de Fisiología*. Edition Salvat, Barcelona.

Grigg, P., Hoffman, A.H. & Fogarty, K.E. (1982) Properties of Golgi-Mazzoni afferents in cat knee joint capsule, as revealed by mechanical studies of isolated joint capsule. *Journal of Neurophysiology* **47**, 31–40.

Guegan, C. & Nicolas, K. (1999) Proprioception. *EPS* **275**, 81–83.

Herveou, C. & Messeau, L. (1976) *Technique de Rééducation et d'Education Proprioceptive du Genou et de la Cheville*. Edition Maloine, Paris.

Herveou, C. & Messeau, I. (1981) *Technique de Rééducation et d'Education Proprioceptive du Genou et de la Cheville, Reprogrammation Neuro-Motice*. Edition Maloine, Paris.

Heurte, A., Pennec, J.-P. & Bidault, J.-C. (1991) Le plateau proprioceptif informatise. *Kinesitherapie Scientifique* **307**, 19–21.

Jerosch, J. & Prymka, M. (1996) Proprioception and joint stability. *Knee Surgery, Sports Traumatology, Arthroscopy* **4** (3), 171–179.

Knoff, M. & Voss, D. (1968) *Facilitation Neuro-Musculaire Propioceptive*. Edition Prodem, Brussels.

Lephart, S.M., Pincevero, D.M., Giraldo, J.L. & Fu, F.H. (1997) The role of proprioception in the management and rehabilitation of athletics injuries. *American Journal of Sports Medicine* **25** (1), 130–137.

Lorza, G. (1991) *Propiocepción Técnica*. FEMEDE Collection of Monographs on Sport Medicine. Rehabilitación y Deporte, Pamplona: 57–67.

Lorza, G. (1998) La reeducación propioceptiva en la prevención y tratamiento de las lesiones en el baloncesto. *Archivos de Medicina del Deporte* **15** (68), 517–521.

Quante, M.Y. & Hille, E. (1999) Propiozeption: eire kritische analyse zum stellenwert in der sportmedizin. *Deutsche Zeitschrift für Sportmedizin* **50** (10), 306–310.

Raybaud, P., Gonzalez Iturri, J.J., Bertolino, M., Castillo, C. & Commandre, F.A. (1988) Propioceptividad y prevención en traumatología del deporte o 'el recorrido del deportista'. *Archivos de Medicina del Deporte* **5** (17), 49–51.

Romano, L. (1999) La reducazione propioceptiva. SDS. *Rivista di Cultura Sportiva* **17** (41–42), 120–123.

Scott, M., Lephart, F. & Fu, H.(2000) *Proprioception and Neuromuscular Control in Joint Stability*. Human Kinetics, Champaign, IL.

Sonjen, G.G. (1986) *Neurofisilogia*. Edition Panamericana.

Strumpell, A. (1924) *Tratado de Patología y Terapeútica Especiales de las Enfermedades Internas*, Vol. 2. Edition Seix Barral.

Thounnard, J.L., Paghki, P., Willens, P., Benoit, J.C. & De Nayra, J. (1986) La pathogenie de l'entorse de la cheville: test d'une hypothese. *Medica Physica* **9**, 141–146.

Chapter 14

Functional Rehabilitation and Return to Training and Competition

W. BEN KIBLER AND T. JEFF CHANDLER

Introduction

The goal of function-based rehabilitation pro-grammes is the return of the athlete to optimum athletic function. Optimal athletic function is the result of physiological motor activations creating specific biomechanical motions and positions using intact anatomical structures to generate forces and actions. Sport-specific function occurs when the activations, motions and resultant forces are specific and efficient for the needs of that sport. We use the 'critical point' framework (Fig. 14.1) to understand sport specificity. Every sport has metabolic, physiological and biomech-anical demands inherent in the way the sport is played, at whatever level of skill or intensity. Every athlete brings a specific musculoskeletal base to interact with the demands. Performance in the sport and injury risk are the results of the interaction. Sport-specific functional rehabilita-tion should focus on restoration of the injured athlete's ability to have sport-specific physiology and biomechanics to interact optimally with the sport-specific demands.

Rehabilitation protocols are structured around frameworks of progressions of exercises, loads and applied and generated forces as the athlete improves his or her ability to generate and control sport-specific forces. Our rehabilitation protocol includes three phases: acute, recovery and functional (Fig. 14.2) (Kibler *et al.* 1992). The patient progresses through each phase in a 'flow' dependent upon reaching certain criteria of injury healing and achievement of control of certain physiological and biomechanical functions. The acute phase is a broad, relatively non-specific phase with goals of:

1 Protection or healing of injured tissues.
2 Improvement of general flexibility and strength.
3 Improvement in the distant links in the kinetic chains involved in the sport or activity.

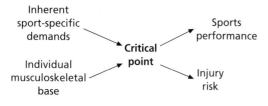

Fig. 14.1 The 'critical point' framework showing the relationship between sports demands and the musculoskeletal base in determining performance and injury risk.

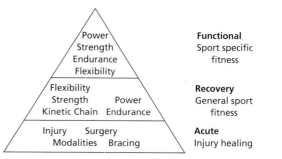

Fig. 14.2 Phases of the rehabilitation process. The start of rehabilitation includes all causes of injury, but the end focuses on return to function.

The recovery phase is a relatively long phase with goals of:

1 Preparation for maximum physical activity.

2 Improvement in kinetic chain linkage sequencing.

3 Normalization of any distant kinetic chain breakages such as inflexibility or strength imbalance.

4 Setting up the strength and power base for sport-specific progressions.

The functional phase is a focused phase, with the goals of sport-specific flexibility, strength, physiological activations, biomechanical motions and functional progressions.

The functional progressions should simulate the actual activities required in the sport. Return to play criteria are based on successful completion of the functional phase goals. The functional phase marks a transition between *re*habilitation and *pre*habilitation, which can be defined as conditioning strategies in the formerly injured athlete to prepare him or her for the stresses and demands inherent in the sport, and which must be faced in return to sport (Kibler & Chandler 1994). Prehabilitation focuses on sport-specific musculoskeletal areas that have been shown to be weak or susceptible to injury, or have actually been injured, in a specific sport (Chandler 1995). In some sports, the musculoskeletal system adapts to repetitive use by manifesting areas of muscle weakness or muscle tightness, or both. For example, long-distance runners frequently are found to have hamstring and gastrocnemius inflexibility, baseball and tennis players are found to have shoulder internal rotation deficits, and female soccer and basketball players have weakness of their glutei and hamstrings. These deficits are still present after injury, and may be even worse as a result of the injury or treatment. The purpose of the prospective programme is to condition those areas of high tensile load and high injury risk, or those that are the 'weak link' after injury, in a particular sport. Prehabilitation exercises consist of strength, power, range of motion and endurance exercises for the musculoskeletal areas and movements identified in a particular sport. This chapter will describe the activities that should take place in the functional phase.

The other two phases have been discussed in earlier chapters.

Upon entry into the functional phase, the athlete must have healing of the anatomical lesion, restoration of the distant links in the kinetic chain, general flexibility, endurance and strength, and be able to achieve the motions and positions necessary to play the sport or activity. The therapist and doctor must also know the demands of the sport or activity and the level of preparedness of the musculoskeletal base to work towards sport-specific progressions.

Sport-specific demands

There are many similarities in the demands sporting activities in general place on athletes. Most sports require some level of energy expenditure to generate the forces necessary to move the body, ball or other object toward a certain goal (Fig. 14.3). Most require some stability of one part of the body to achieve some movement of another part (Fig. 14.4). Most require some degree of flexibility of some body parts (Fig. 14.5). However, each sport has its own set of inherent demands, and these demands may change with the level of skill, intensity or frequency with which the sport is played. Therapists and doctors need to know these parameters in order to prehabilitate the athlete properly. Many different systems may be set up to profile sports and their demands. They may be based on anatomical requirements (range of motion required, strength required), metabolic requirements (aerobic or anaerobic activity) or amount of contact (collision, frequent contact or minimal contact).

We use an evaluation system that profiles the physiological requirements and the biomechanical kinetic chains necessary to play the sport (Kibler 1990). This method allows good discrimination between sports and generates enough information about the specific sport to plan an adequate prehabilitation programme that will be sufficiently specific for the sport.

The five physiological parameters we use include flexibility, strength, power (force × distance

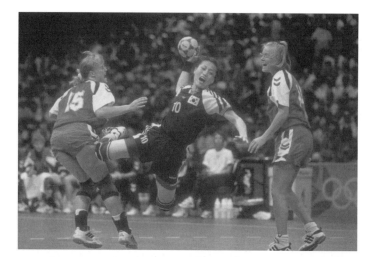

Fig. 14.3 Team handball: Atlanta 1996, Korea versus Denmark. (© Doug Pensinger, Allsport.)

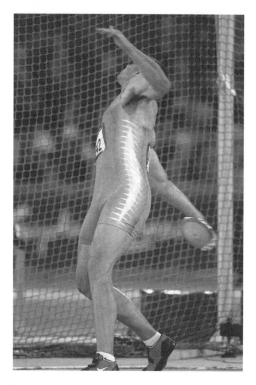

Fig. 14.4 Discus: Sydney 2000, Franz Kruger of South Africa in the men's discus final. (© Matthew Stockman, Allsport.)

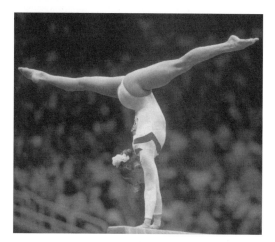

Fig. 14.5 Gymnastics: Atlanta 1996, Shannon Miller (USA). (© Allsport.)

(e.g. aerobic endurance in golf); 2, the parameter is important in performance or injury risk reduction (e.g. flexibility in tennis or basketball); and 3, the parameter is essential for maximum performance (e.g. aerobic endurance in running, strength in weightlifting). Each sport will then have a profile that can be used to meet the demands. Table 14.1 lists some sports and their resulting profiles.

Similarly, each sport can be characterized by the kinetic chains necessary to perform the sport. Kinetic chains are patterned, coordinated sequences of body segment activation and motion

per unit of time), anaerobic and aerobic endurance. We grade each sport from 1 to 3 based on the parameter's importance in the sport: 1, the parameter is important for general body fitness

Table 14.1 Individual sport profile.

	Flexibility	Strength	Power	Anaerobic	Aerobic
Basketball	2	2	3	3	3
Tennis	3	2	3	3	2
Golf	3	2	3	1	1
Soccer	2	2	3	3	3
Swimming	2	2	3	3	3
Running	2	1	2	1	3
Sprinting	3	2	3	3	1
Bicycling	2	2	3	3	3
Volleyball	2	2	3	3	1

Table 14.2 Sport kinetic chains.

Running	Ground → Leg → Hip/trunk → Opposite leg → Ground
Throwing	Ground → Leg → Hip/trunk/opposite leg → Shoulder → Arm
Serving	Ground → Legs → Trunk → Shoulder → Arm
Golf	Ground → Legs → Trunk → Shoulder/arm → Wrist
Kicking	Ground → Plant leg → Trunk/opposite hip → Kick leg → Ball
Swimming	Water → Hand/wrist → Arm/shoulder → Trunk/legs → Arm → Water
Shooting ball	Ground → Legs → Arm/wrist → Ball

that are used to accomplish athletic tasks. Running has a slightly different kinetic chain than sprinting. Tennis has a different kinetic chain than baseball pitching. Kicking a soccer ball has a different kinetic chain than jumping after a basketball. Table 14.2 lists some of the most common sports and their predominant kinetic chain patterns.

When the physiological and biomechanical requirements of the sport or activity are categorized, exercises and progressions of load and intensity can be employed to prepare the body for the sport. A runner will need back and leg flexibility exercises, progressive aerobic training with longer duration of training bouts, and eccentric strength training of the legs to absorb the closed chain loads in the stance phase. An ice hockey player will need anaerobic training for short bursts of activity and power training in both the arms and legs. A baseball pitcher will need arm and back flexibility, lower body strength, power training to develop force, and eccentric training for the arm to control deceleration loads.

Functional musculoskeletal prehabilitation exercises can be strenuous as they replicate the motions, positions, forces, intensities and muscle activations inherent in the sport. The athlete's body should have enough general athletic fitness to allow these vigorous activities without undue injury risk. The anatomical lesion should be healed. The physiological muscle activations, flexibility and endurance capabilities should be capable of withstanding the strength and power exercises.

The physician and therapist should monitor and test for these parameters as rehabilitation progresses and as the athlete goes into the prehabilitation protocols. For throwing athletes, the general criteria should include hip and trunk control over the planted leg, trunk rotational flexibility and strength, control of scapular elevation and protraction, functional glenohumeral internal rotation, and rotator cuff co-contraction strength (Kibler *et al.* 2000). For running athletes, general criteria should include gastrocnemius, quadriceps and hamstring flexibility, hip and trunk control over the planted leg, trunk extensor strength and aerobic capacity.

Athletes frequently have areas of inflexibility and weakness in other parts of the kinetic chain that may contribute to the injury or to decreased performance, and should be included in the prehabilitation exercises. The frequency of these distant alterations may be as high as 50–85% in association with injury (Ekstrand & Gilquist 1982; Kibler *et al.* 1991; Knapik *et al.* 1991; Warner *et al.* 1992; Burkhart *et al.* 2000).

Specific examples—prehabilitation protocols

The prehabilitation protocols should be based on progressions of flexibility, strength exercises, increasing loads and durations, and progress from closed chain to open chain configurations. This is illustrated by specific protocols for: (i) tennis/baseball, for overhead activities; (ii) running, for long distance and long duration; and (iii) soccer, for high-intensity power running and jumping.

Tennis/baseball

PREHABILITATION PLAN

The athlete should begin a shoulder flexibility and strengthening programme focusing on

increasing internal rotation range of motion and external rotation strength. Flexibility exercises are performed after the throwing activity is complete for the day. Due to the high tensile loads developed in the shoulder external rotators and due to the inflexibility of the athlete in this area, a flexibility programme is warranted. For strengthening, the goals of the training programme are to increase the strength of the scapular stabilizers and shoulder external rotators while maintaining explosiveness in those muscles. Plyometric/agility drills are incorporated into the prehabilitation programme as they may reduce the risk of injuries related to these ballistic movements. In addition to the prehabilitation programme, it is assumed the athlete participates in a general resistance training programme two or three times per week.

At this stage of healing and rehabilitation, physical therapy modalities (heat, ice, ultrasound, stimulation) are usually not indicated. Very little tissue alteration is expected at this stage of healing that would be modified by these modalities. Some heat may be used to help in increasing tissue pliability before the exercise bout, and cold may be occasionally used if there is some swelling postexercise.

WEEKS 1–2

Flexibility (daily, after activity):

Cross body stretch, scapula stabilized	3×30 s
Internal rotation, scapula stabilized	3×30 s
Triceps stretch	3×30 s
Racquet stretch (Fig. 14.6)	3×30 s

Strength ($3–5 \times$ week):

Shoulder external rotators/scapula retraction with tubing	3×25 reps (moderate speed)
Rows with dumbbells/tubing, elbows down	3×15 reps
Reverse flies with dumbbells/tubing	3×15 reps

Plyometric/agility ($3–5 \times$ week):

Five dot drill (Fig. 14.7)	2×20 foot contacts
Hexagon drill (Fig. 14.8)	3×15 s, double leg

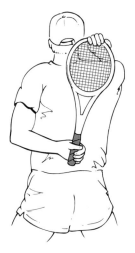

Racquet stretch
Use racquet as
rigid rod between
both hands to
rotate shoulder

Fig. 14.6 The racquet stretch. Use the racquet as a lever to rotate the shoulder into internal and external rotation (figure seen from behind).

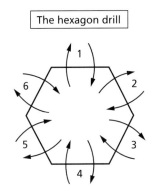

The hexagon drill

Fig. 14.8 The hexagon drill. Do in the sequence shown and repeat three times.

Line drill (Fig. 14.9)	2×20 double leg foot contacts
	2×20 single leg foot contacts
Footwork ladder, bounding (Fig. 14.10)	2×20 double leg foot contacts
	2×20 single leg foot contacts
Footwork ladder, quick feet	4×20 low-intensity foot contacts
Footwork sprints (carioca, shuffle, back pedal, cross-over step, skip, high knee, etc.)	$5-8 \times 9$ m

WEEKS 3–4

Flexibility (daily, after activity):

Cross body stretch, scapula stabilized	2×30 s
Internal rotation, scapula stabilized	2×30 s
Triceps stretch	2×30 s
Racquet stretch	2×30 s

5-dot drill

```
        1        2 Right leg  3 Left leg  4 Both feet
4    5       1–2      2          1          1
             ↓        ↓          ↓          ↓
    3        3        3          3          3
   •  1m     ↓        ↓          ↓          ↓
1    2       5        5          4          5
             ↓        ↓          ↓          ↓
  0.5m                4          5          4
                      ↓          ↓          ↓
                      3          3          3
                      ↓          ↓          ↓
                      1          2          2
```

Do each sequence with 5 repetitions

Fig. 14.7 The five dot drill. Each sequence should be done in the order listed and completed five times.

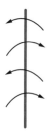

Line drill
Any 'line' will do; tennis court side line, baseball foul line, soccer touch line, basketball side line. May go forwards or backwards, landing on one foot or both feet, or jump over/jump back across the line

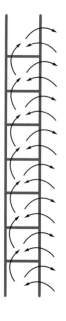

Ladder drill
Use a rope or other material, or draw on the surface to make the 'ladder'. Jump in and out of the squares, there are many variations possible for this drill

Fig. 14.9 The line drill. Jump back and forth across a line, which could be a tennis court side line, baseball foul line, soccer touch line, etc. Land on both feet (double leg) or one foot (single leg).

Fig. 14.10 (*right*) The footwork ladder drill. Use a rope, some other material or draw on the surface to make a 'ladder'. Jump in and out of the rectangular areas; many different drills can be done.

Strength (3–5 × week):

Shoulder external rotation/scapula retraction with tubing	4 × 25 reps (high speed)
Rows with dumbbells/tubing, elbows down	4 × 25 reps (high speed)
Shoulder internal rotators with tubing	4 × 25 reps (high speed)
Medicine ball forehand	2 × 25 reps
Medicine ball backhand	2 × 25 reps
Medicine ball serve	2 × 25 reps

Plyometric/agility:

Five dot drill	2 × 20 foot contacts
Hexagon drill	4 × 10 s, single and double leg
Line drill	2 × 20 double leg foot contacts
	2 × 20 single leg foot contacts
Footwork ladder, bounding	2 × 20 double leg foot contacts
	2 × 20 single leg foot contacts
Footwork ladder, quick feet	3 × 20 low-intensity foot contacts
Footwork sprints (carioca, shuffle, back pedal, cross-over step, skip, high knee, etc.)	10–15 × 4.5 m

WEEKS 5–6

Flexibility (daily, after activity):

Internal rotation, scapula stabilized	2 × 30 s
Racquet stretch	2 × 30 s

Strength (2–4 × week):

Shoulder external rotation/scapula retraction with tubing	2 × 25 reps (high speed)
Shoulder internal rotation with tubing	2 × 25 reps (high speed)

Plyometrics/agility:

Five dot drill	2 × 20 foot contacts
Hexagon drill	5 × 10 s, single and double leg
Line drill	2 × 20 double leg foot contacts
	2 × 20 single leg foot contacts
Footwork ladder, bounding	2 × 20 double leg foot contacts
	2 × 20 single leg foot contacts
Footwork ladder, quick feet	3 × 20 low-intensity foot contacts
Footwork sprints (carioca, shuffle, back pedal, cross-over step, skip, high knee, etc.)	10 × 4.5 m

Running

PREHABILITATION PLAN

It is suggested that the athlete should start prehabilitation on a more forgiving surface for training purposes whenever possible, such as grass or a rubber track. The main goal of the prehabilitation programme is to allow the athlete to progress at 10–25% increases in work load, which are usually safe progressions. Strengthening the ankle while trying to improve ankle range of motion is warranted. Flexibility of the hamstrings and gastrocnemius is stressed. Low-intensity plyometric and eccentric activities may help prepare the athlete to withstand the repetitive loads of running, as well as improve explosiveness for the kick at the end of the race.

WEEKS 1–4

The athlete is running 1.6–4.8 km, 3–4 days per week.

Flexibility (daily, after activity):

Lying hamstring stretch	3 × 30 s
Standing quadriceps stretch	3 × 30 s
Leg twists for iliotibial band	3 × 30 s
Wall calf stretch	3 × 30 s
Trunk sit and reach	3 × 30 s

Strength (4–5 × week):

Squats (light resistance)	3 × 20 reps
Lunges with light dumbbells	3 × 20 reps
Weighted heel raise	3 × 20 reps

Plyometrics/agility (3 × week, non-running days on grass):

Five dot drill	3 × 30 foot contacts
Line drill	3 × 30 double leg foot contacts

WEEKS 5–8

The athlete is running 4.8–8 km on Monday and Wednesday and 8 km on Friday and Saturday.

Flexibility (daily, after activity):

Lying hamstring stretch	3×30 s
Standing quadriceps stretch	3×30 s
Leg twists	3×30 s
Wall calf stretch	3×30 s
Trunk sit and reach	3×30 s

Strength (2–$3 \times$ week):

Squats (light resistance)	3×10 reps
Lunges with light dumbbells	3×10 reps
Weighted heel raise	3×10 reps

Plyometrics/agility (non-running days on grass):

Five dot drill	2×20 foot contacts
Line drill	2×20 single leg foot contacts
Bounding drill	2×10–15 foot contacts

WEEKS 9–10

The athlete is running 8–16 km on Monday and Wednesday and 16–24 on Saturday.

Flexibility (daily, after activity):

Lying hamstring stretch	2×30 s
Standing quadriceps stretch	2×30 s
Wall calf stretch	2×30 s

Strength ($2 \times$ week):

Squats (light resistance)	2×10 reps
Lunges with light dumbbells	2×10 reps
Weighted heel raise	2×10 reps

Plyometrics/agility (non-running days on grass):
Fartlek progressions—alternating low-intensity/high-intensity running bouts (20 m jog → 10 m run → 10 m sprint)

Soccer

PREHABILITATION PLAN

Soccer requires aerobic endurance, anaerobic capacity and power. It is common that injuries may recur if prehabilitation is not complete, because of the varied and large loads inherent in the demands.

WEEKS 1–3

Flexibility (daily, after activity):

Lying hamstring stretch	2×30 s
Standing quadriceps stretch	2×30 s
Leg twists	2×30 s
Wall calf stretch	2×30 s
Trunk sit and reach	2×30 s

Strength ($3 \times$ week, bodyweight as resistance):

Squats	2×20 reps
Forward lunges	2×20 reps
Side step/cross step lunges	2×20 reps
Heel raise	2×20 reps

Plyometrics/agility ($3 \times$ week):

Five dot drill	2×20 foot contacts
Line drill	2×20 double leg foot contacts
Footwork ladder, bounding	2×20 double leg foot contacts
Footwork ladder, quick feet	3×30 low-intensity foot contacts

WEEKS 4–6

Flexibility (daily, after activity):

Lying hamstring stretch	2×30 s
Standing quadriceps stretch	2×30 s
Wall calf stretch	2×30 s
Standing knee to chest	2×30 s

Strength (medicine ball or dumbbells as resistance):

Squats	3×15 reps
Forward lunges	3×15 reps
Side step/cross step lunges	3×15 reps
Heel raises	3×15 reps

Plyometrics/agility ($3 \times$ week):

Five dot drill	2×30 foot contacts
Line drill	2×20 double leg foot contacts
	2×20 single leg foot contacts
Footwork ladder, bounding	2×20 double leg foot contacts
	2×20 single leg foot contacts
Footwork ladder, quick feet	4×30 low-intensity foot contacts
Footwork springs (carioca, shuffle, back pedal, cross-over step, skip, high knee, etc.)	5–8×18 m

WEEKS 7–10

Flexibility (daily, after activity):

Lying hamstring stretch	2×30 s
Standing quadriceps stretch	2×30 s
Wall calf stretch	2×30 s
Standing knee to chest	2×30 s

Strength ($3 \times$ week, medicine ball or dumbbells as resistance):

Squats	2×10 reps
Forward lunges	2×10 reps
Side step/cross step lunges	2×10 reps
Heel raises	2×10 reps

Plyometrics/agility ($3 \times$ week):

Five dot drill	2×20 foot contacts
Line drill	2×20 double leg foot contacts
	2×20 single leg foot contacts

Criteria for return to sports

The injured athlete must be anatomically healed and must complete all of the rehabilitation stages to be considered for return to sport. Understanding the inherent demands allows an objective set of criteria for return. Throwers must have sport-specific functional range of motion of arm joints, stable scapula, trunk core stability and plyometric power development in the leg, no matter where their original injury occurred. Runners must have leg flexibility, trunk core stability and aerobic endurance, no matter where their original injury occurred (Kibler *et al.* 2000). All injured athletes must then complete sport-specific functional progressions of throwing, running, jumping, kicking or swimming. These exercises demonstrate that the athlete has the physiology and biomechanics necessary to withstand the inherent demands of the sport.

Some authors have advocated return to sport based on quantitative criteria such as quadriceps/hamstring ratios in runners or internal rotation/external rotation ratios in throwers. These ratios are usually based on isokinetic data, which have not been conclusively shown to be associated with true muscle capability. These ratios can be helpful in determining weaknesses,

but do not represent total capabilities, and should not be used as sole determinants of return to play. It is more important to know if the athlete can do all of the functions required in play, rather than if the athlete can generate torque at one joint.

It may appear that the criteria for return to sport are rigid or easily determined. Actually, the criteria should be employed with some leeway, based on the athlete and the situation. The athlete should not be allowed to 'play yourself into shape', with no guidelines or input. This allows deleterious kinetic chain substitutions and increases the chances of reinjury (Devlin 2000). However, the athlete should not be 'rushed' through the prehabilitation protocol, because the sport-specific exercises do impose significant demands, once again increasing the chances of reinjury.

Experience has taught us the value of gradual return to play, with emphasis on steady progression of exercises, strict attention to the preparedness of the musculoskeletal base for new exercises, involvement of the kinetic chain, and resolution of both the local and distant alterations that may exist in association with the injury (Kibler *et al.* 1991, 1992).

Return to play is completed by a sport-specific functional progression of doing the specific

Table 14.3 Interval throwing programme starting off the mound.

Stage 1: fastball only		Use interval throwing to 36 m phase as warm-up
Step 1:	Interval throwing	
	15 throws off mound 50%	
Step 2:	Interval throwing	
	30 throws off mound 50%	
Step 3:	Interval throwing	All throwing off the mound should be done in
	45 throws off mound 50%	the presence of your pitching coach to stress
Step 4:	Interval throwing	proper throwing mechanics
	60 throws off mound 50%	
Step 5:	Interval throwing	
	30 throws off mound 75%	
Step 6:	30 throws off mound 75%	Use speed gun to aid in effort control
	45 throws off mound 50%	
Step 7:	45 throws off mound 75%	
	15 throws off mound 50%	
Step 8:	60 throws off mound 75%	
Stage 2: fastball only		
Step 9:	45 throws off mound 75%	
	15 throws in batting practice	
Step 10:	45 throws off mound 75%	
	30 throws in batting practice	
Step 11:	45 throws off mound 75%	
	45 throws in batting practice	
Stage 3		
Step 12:	30 throws off mound 75% warm-up	
	15 throws off mound 50% breaking balls	
	45–60 throws in batting practice (fastball only)	
Step 13:	30 throws off mound 75%	
	30 breaking balls 75%	
	30 throws in batting practice	
Step 14:	30 throws off mound 75%	
	60–90 throws in batting practice 25% breaking balls	
Step 15:	Simulated game: progressing by 15 throws per work-out	

activity. Table 14.3 illustrates a sport-specific throwing progression (Andrews & Wilk 1996), while Fig. 14.11 illustrates a sport-specific soccer progression (Kibler & Naessens 1996).

Conclusions

Optimal return to sport requires not only rehabilitation of the general athletic fitness parameters for sport, but also the specific parameters for fitness in a particular sport or sporting activity. Devising a sport-specific rehabilitation pro-

gramme requires knowing the end-point—the set of anatomical, physiological and biomechanical parameters the athlete will need in order to meet the demands inherent in participation in that sport. Sport profiling is key to this knowledge. The functional phase of the rehabilitation protocol must emphasize acquisition of sport-specific parameters, and then shades into prehabilitation, a maintenance programme to continue to improve sport-specific fitness. Criteria for return to play must emphasize gradual return to sport-specific functional progressions.

Soccer field run

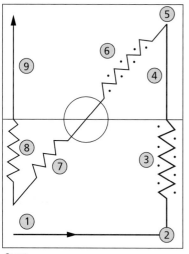

1 Sprint
2 Jump and head a ball
3 Run around cones
4 Run backwards
5 Pick up soccer ball
6 Dribble around cones
7 Three running jumps
8 Plyometric jumps over lines
9 Sprint

Fig. 14.11 Return to soccer functional programme. The drill encompasses all of the soccer-specific demands.

References

Andrews, J.R. & Wilk, K.E. (1996) *Throwing Progressions for Return to Baseball*. American Sports Medicine Institute, Birmingham, Alabama.

Burkhart, S.S., Morgan, C.D. & Kibler, W.B. (2000) Shoulder injuries in overhead athletes. The 'dead arm' revisited. *Clinical Sports Medicine* **19**, 125–159.

Chandler, T.J. (1995) Exercise training for tennis. *Clinical Sports Medicine* **14**, 33–46.

Devlin, L. (2000) Recurrent hamstring symptoms in rugby. *Sports Medicine* **29**, 279–287.

Ekstrand, J. & Gilquist, J. (1982) The frequency of muscle tightness and injuries in soccer players. *American Journal of Sports Medicine* **10**, 75–78.

Kibler, W.B. (1990) *The Sports Preparticipation Exam*. Human Kinetics, Champaign, IL.

Kibler, W.B. & Chandler, T.J. (1994) Sports specific conditioning. *American Journal of Sports Medicine* **22**, 424–432.

Kibler, W.B. & Naessens, G.C. (1996) Soccer pre-participation physical exam. In: *The US Soccer Sports Medicine Book* (Garrett, W.E., Kirkendall, D.T. & Contigulia, S.R., eds). US Soccer Federation, Chicago, Illinois: 147–167.

Kibler, W.B., Goldberg, C. & Chandler, T.J. (1991) Functional biomechanical deficits in running athletes with plantar fasciitis. *American Journal of Sports Medicine* **19**, 66–71.

Kibler, W.B., Chandler, T.J. & Pace, B.K. (1992) Principles of rehabilitation after chronic tendon injuries. *Clinical Sports Medicine* **11**, 661–673.

Kibler, W.B., McMullen, J. & Uhl, T.L. (2000) Shoulder rehabilitation strategies, guidelines, and practice. *Operative Techniques in Sports Medicine* **8**, 258–267.

Knapik, J.J., Bauman, C.L., Jones, B.H. *et al.* (1991) Preseason strength and flexibility imbalances associated with athletic injuries in female college athletes. *American Journal of Sports Medicine* **19**, 76–81.

Warner, J.J.P., Micheli, L., Arslenian, L.E. *et al.* (1992) Scapulothoracic motion in normal shoulders and shoulders with glenohumeral instability and impingement syndrome. *Clinical Orthopaedics and Related Research* **285**, 199–210.

Chapter 15

Orthoses in the Prevention and Rehabilitation of Injuries

WILLIAM MICHEO AND ALBERTO ESQUENAZI

Introduction

Advances in fabrication, increased availability and patient interest over the past few decades have contributed to the proliferation of orthotic use in sports and other areas of medicine. At the present time a more complete scientific understanding of the functional mechanism of orthoses and how the body responds to them is needed to further increase the efficacy of this intervention. The usefulness of bracing for the prevention or treatment of lower limb joint instability, particularly of the knee, has been controversial, with clinical and biomechanical data pointing in opposite directions (Cawley *et al.* 1991). In addition, a lot of the information available to the clinicians about orthotics and their use in sports medicine is provided by the manufacturers of the devices.

Advances in applied biomechanics, motion and gait analysis have helped considerably by allowing critical parameters to be accurately measured in the athlete, thus infusing objectivity in the process of orthotic prescription and the clinical management of injury (Esquenazi & Talaty 1996; Zheng & Barrentine 2000).

However, the question of exactly what is the best orthotic device for a given injury, and how a brace may provide improved function for an athlete participating in sport, is still not completely clear. Prescribed orthoses may impair some of the normal biomechanical functions that coexist in the injured limb or may force compensation in other anatomical sites. For example, a knee brace

prescribed to enhance mediolateral joint stability may produce a compensatory overactivation of the hamstrings that increases the likelihood of tendonitis (Esquenazi & Talaty 1996). In addition, they may increase energy expenditure or raise intramuscular pressure in the anterior leg compartments of the athletes that use them (Highgenboten *et al.* 1991; Styf *et al.* 1992).

The process of orthotic prescription is still subjective and evolving; it is dependent on the clinician's understanding of the injury, acquired skill and knowledge of the principles of physics and biomechanics. In addition, it requires a working knowledge of brace types, materials, functional design and the requirement of the sport, which in general are not part of routine clinical training.

Development of new materials and fabrication techniques in the last decade have greatly increased the range of applicability of orthoses to a wide variety of clinical situations in sports medicine. Due to this, braces are lighter, stronger, better fitting, more durable and perhaps more effective. These advances in brace construction allow clinicians to generate almost any combination of biomechanical features, that may be specific for a particular clinical problem and most beneficial for the athlete (Esquenazi & Talaty 1996).

Terminology and classification

The International Standards Organization of the International Society of Prosthetics and Orthotics has defined an orthosis as 'an externally applied device used to modify structural and functional characteristics of the neuromusculoskeletal system'. Orthoses are applied to the external surface of the body to achieve one or more of the following: to relieve pain, resist abnormal joint motion, reduce axial load, stabilize musculoskeletal segments, prevent or correct joint deformity and improve function while permitting joint(s) movement (Redford 2000).

Orthotics in the past have been classified into two major categories: static and dynamic. Static orthoses are rigid and give support without allowing movement. Dynamic orthoses allow a certain degree of movement and are fabricated with a combination of rigid materials and movable parts such as joint, cables, rubber bands or springs. Sometimes, dynamic orthoses are also termed functional orthoses (Redford 2000).

Depending on the clinical situation, the desired effect and the biomechanical characteristics, orthoses are considered *corrective* or *accommodative*. Corrective devices are used to improve the position of the joint by modifying the alignment of skeletal structures. Accommodative devices attempt to maintain a given position and prevent further joint deterioration.

Furthermore, orthoses for use in sports— particularly those for the knee and ankle—have been classified as either *prophylactic, functional* or *rehabilitative* depending on the clinical situation in which they are used (Wirth & DeLee 1990) (Table 15.1). Prophylactic bracing is intended to prevent or reduce the severity of injury to healthy joints. Ankle prophylactic bracing has been used in basketball, volleyball and soccer (Thacker *et al.* 1999).

Functional braces are designed to control normal joint motion as well as to attempt to resist abnormal joint rotation and translation (Wirth & DeLee 1990; Cawley *et al.* 1991). Most functional braces are intended to address knee or ankle joint instability caused by ligamentous injury. A common clinical situation in which a functional brace is used is in the patient with a non-operated anterior cruciate ligament (ACL) injury who desires to continue to participate in sports (Micheo *et al.* 1995).

Table 15.1 Classification of orthotics.

Design	Biomechanical characteristics	Clinical function
Static	Corrective	Preventive
Dynamic	Accommodative	Functional
		Rehabilitation

Rehabilitation braces are primarily intended to reduce pain and protect the joint immediately after an injury or during the initial postoperative period. These braces attempt to control the joint range of motion and provide protection in case of inadvertent loading that may result in injury (Wirth & DeLee 1990). These types of orthoses, along with early functional rehabilitation, have been used for the management of the injured medial collateral ligament of the knee (Reider *et al.* 1993).

In 1975 orthotic terminology was formally adopted to allow a simplified, standard, clear communication language among different clinicians. The terminology adopted encourages anatomical level description starting with the most proximal joint, followed by the orthotic adjective, rather than eponyms or proper names. If the orthosis is to involve the foot, ankle and knee it is termed knee–ankle–foot orthosis (KAFO). The particular material used and the desired functional effect of the orthoses should also be included as part of the design (Goldber & Hsu 1997).

Biomechanics

The major joints of the body can be seen as semi-constrained motion units with feedback control that respond to internal and external forces and allow a stable, complex, three-dimensional joint motion in both the loaded and unloaded conditions. During dynamic activity, powerful opposing muscle groups (flexors and extensors) exert moments of force working synergistically with soft tissue restraints (ligaments, capsule and tendons) as well as the surface geometry of the bones to position the joint for optimal loading

(Esquenazi *et al.* 1997; Zheng & Barrentine 2000). Orthotic systems usually function with a three-point force system in order to control joint movement (Buttler *et al.* 1983). Devices with a long lever arm and wide, close-fitting cuffs which distribute force over a large area have improved physical characteristics to control joint translation (Redford 2000). For example, a knee orthosis that extends up in the thigh and distally to the calf will restrain the flexion or extension motion based on its alignment. Rotational, translation and transverse forces are difficult to control with an orthotic system since orthoses achieve joint motion control through force transmission from the bone to the soft tissue and on to the brace structure, which allows brace migration and makes the system not rigid. These limitations in force control about a joint are particularly troublesome in patients with injury-related strength or proprioception loss (Janshen 2000).

Brace design should allow forces to be distributed over the largest area possible in order to reduce pressure concentration (force over area) and potential secondary soft tissue injuries (Buttler *et al.* 1983). Friction and shear stress should be controlled by appropriate construction and accommodating the soft tissue which interfaces between the brace and the joint it will act upon.

Fabrication

Materials for fabrication include metal, leather, elastic fabrics, low temperature thermoplastics, high temperature thermoplastics, composites and graphite. Plastics have the benefit of being lightweight, adjustable, cosmetic and having total contact in custom braces. Total contact construction is important to reduce an undesirable concentration of forces over soft tissues or pressure-intolerant areas such as bony prominences.

Composite materials and metal orthoses have the advantage of increased durability and, in the hands of a skilled orthotist, still maintain built-in adjustability. With the advent of new products such as carbon graphite and extruded plastic materials, we now have the additional advantage of maximum tension strength with lightweight

design. The latter, when used for sports orthotics, results in a lighter, stronger and more durable device. The choice of materials in the fabrication of orthotics is expanding rapidly and a detailed review of them is beyond the scope of this chapter.

Orthotics can be custom fabricated or bought off the shelf, with off-the-shelf orthotics being the most commonly prescribed braces today. In some cases, because of the patient's anatomy, difficulties with fit, size of the individual and joint incongruity, custom orthoses are required (Esquenazi & Talaty 1996).

When fabricating orthoses attention should be given to accommodating bony prominences, to alignment with the anatomical axis and to reducing ligamentous stress. The difficulty of application, maintaining adequate suspension and comfort are also of importance in achieving compliance with the use of these devices (Loke 2000).

A complete orthotic prescription should include the patient's diagnosis, consider the type of footwear to be used, include the joints it encompasses and specify the desired biomechanical alignment, as well as the materials for fabrication. Communication with the orthotist, who will fabricate or fit the brace, is of utmost importance in order to obtain a good clinical result.

Clinical application

The successful use of an orthotic device depends on matching brace function with the patient's functional needs. Appropriate orthotic application will result in restraint forces that oppose an undesired motion (Kilmartin & Wallace 1994). Often pathology of the muscle, tendon or ligament results in multiple deviations of the normal joint movement process. Primary causes are often masked by compensations and secondary deviations, which sometimes makes the clinical intervention difficult. Emphasis has been placed on initially identifying the primary causes of the particular disorder as the point from which to begin the clinical intervention (Esquenazi & Talaty 1996; Esquenazi *et al.* 1997).

Understanding clearly the pathology and the resultant compensations, the orthotic needs for a specific sport, how a brace may be used to meet these needs, and what effect the brace exerts on the overall performance of the mechanical system and the athlete are areas where research is in progress. The potential, protective and preventive use of orthoses in the athlete who has not been injured is controversial and further investigation is needed to clarify their role in this area.

Foot orthotics

Heel cord and/or plantar fascia tightness, calf weakness, increased pronation or a high arch are all conditions that alone or in combination can increase the likelihood of foot- and knee-related injuries in athletes (Fig. 15.1). At high risk for these injuries are athletes who participate in sports that require running or jumping (Frontera *et al.* 1994).

Optimizing the biomechanical posture of the foot structures, improving lower limb flexibility and strength, correcting or accommodating the presence of any abnormality in the architecture of the foot and improving shock absorption are all key interventions to prevent disabling injuries (Lee *et al.* 1987; Schwellnus *et al.* 1990; Redford 2000). Although statistics are not available, it is plausible that more prescriptions are written for foot orthotics than for all other orthoses combined. The use of orthoses has been advocated to improve foot posture and reduce the incidence of lower limb injuries during running or jumping (Fig. 15.2) (Orteza *et al.* 1992; Kilmartin & Wallace 1994). Limited information is available in the scientific literature to prove or refute the efficacy of foot orthotics for this type of activity.

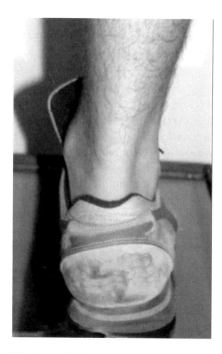

Fig. 15.1 A pronated foot.

Prefabricated orthoses (off the shelf) are less expensive devices that can be adjusted to provide adequate control or correction. In the hands of the experienced practitioner prefabricated orthotics are a very effective tool in the management of abnormal biomechanics of the foot. In some instances because of the wide variation in foot configuration, size and pathology, and when time and economic factors permit, custom orthotics should be considered as a better treatment option. As the name indicates custom orthotics are made specifically for an individual with their

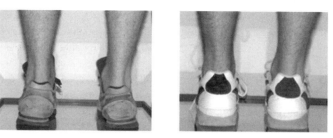

Fig. 15.2 Corrected foot pronation with moulded carbon graphite foot orthoses.

particular functional needs in mind. On-site fabrication by a skilled, certified orthotist or other trained clinician is preferable to referral to an outside site.

When prescribing foot orthotics for sports, knowledge of the patient's complaint, the pathology in question, functional anatomy, biomechanics, orthotic components, materials, sport requirements and, finally, recognition of the anticipated functional outcomes are essential for proper prescription (Orteza *et al.* 1992). Consideration should be given to the fact that external loads act as dynamic forces that may require different orthotic prescription and materials for different activities (Cornwall & McPoil 1999; Hertel *et al.* 2001; Subotnick 2001).

Foot orthoses are designed to be corrective or accommodative devices. Corrective devices that are meant to improve the position of the foot by correcting the alignment of skeletal structures can be manufactured from a variety of materials. Rigid materials such as thermoplastics, acrylic laminates and carbon graphite composites are used frequently for this (Fig. 15.3a). Cork and polyethylene are examples of materials used for semirigid orthotic devices (Hertel *et al.* 2001). The patient with a pronated flexible foot and metatarsal stress fracture may benefit from the use of a semirigid orthotic device as part of a complete rehabilitation programme (Chandler & Kibler 1993; Cornwall & McPoil 1999).

Accommodative devices made of soft, open or closed cell foams alone or in combination with semiflexible materials are meant to provide cushioning and support to an already deformed limb structure (Fig. 15.3b) (Subotnick 2001). They prevent further deformity while attemping to improve function and to control the direction and/or alignment of the joint movement. Individuals with rigid high arched feet and recurrent injury such as Achilles tendonitis or plantar fascitis are candidates for a soft orthotic device (Mascaro & Swanson 1994).

Appropriate posting, longitudinal or transverse arch build-ups, heel lifts, pressure relief areas or other special modifications, as well as application of different materials in the same orthotic

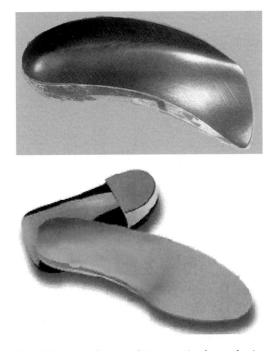

Fig. 15.3 (a) A carbon graphite corrective foot orthosis, and (b) a moulded accommodative foot orthosis.

device, can be integrated in the design and combined at the time of fabrication (Subotnick 2001). There are several factors to consider when selecting materials used in custom orthotic fabrication; these include the type of sport, the physical demands and the length of time the orthosis is to be used. For example, a triathlete or long-distance runner may need a device that is rustproof and designed to function with perspiration or wet skin. If the brace is intended for use for a few weeks a prefabricated device may suffice; however, if intended for longer term use (several months) then a more durable custom brace constructed out of carbon graphite may need to be considered.

The amount of corrective or controlling forces to be applied and the amount of axial loading, as well as the amount of cushioning that is desirable without introducing mediolateral ankle instability, should be considered (Schwellnus *et al.* 1990; Brown *et al.* 1996; Hertel *et al.* 2001). One example of this custom application is the use of TPE® (thermoplastic elastomer) for the longitudinal

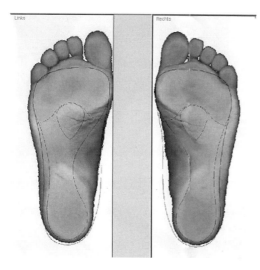

Fig. 15.4 Computer-aided foot orthotic design.

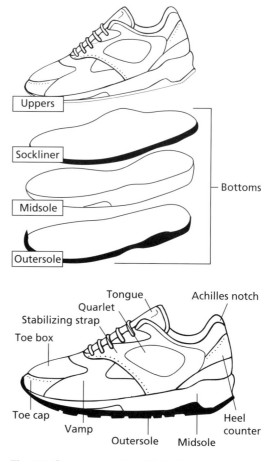

Fig. 15.5 Components of an athletic shoe.

arch, Pelite® as a moulded substrate and Poron® for shock absorption, all in the same foot orthotic.

In the very active athlete, accommodative orthoses may need to be replaced often to adjust for material deterioration, while in the child or teenager, replacement should be done to accommodate for growth. The cost of these custom-made devices, depending on regional variations and availability, has a wide spectrum. For the less complex accommodative devices price is not significantly different to that for prefabricated ones. In some areas, fabrication and delivery from the time of moulding can be accomplished in less than 48 h. This time may be further reduced with the use of computerized design and manufacturing systems (Fig. 15.4). These two factors—cost and fabrication time—need to be considered in the selection of custom orthotics.

The shoe is an integral part of any lower extremity orthotic that includes the foot, as it will serve as the foundation for the device and will directly impact on its function. The correct shoe size should be measured with the athlete standing after a period of exercise, since with weight-bearing and exercise the foot configuration will change. The shoe should be manufactured out of a breathable material, have a supportive counter and deep toe box with a wide heel and a flexible toe break (Fig. 15.5) (Janisse 1993; Johnson 2001). The users of fluid-filled heel chambers should keep in mind the possibility of increased ankle mediolateral instability. A removable insert with longitudinal arch support is a good option, and if a foot orthosis is to be used, the shoe insole should be removed.

When a custom orthosis is ready it should be evaluated on the patient to assure proper fit and function. When these characteristics are achieved, supervised wearing time should be gradually increased.

In prescribing orthotics for paediatric patients, such as in runners, tennis or soccer players, consideration should be given to the fact that throughout childhood growth and development act as dynamic forces that require frequent orthotic re-evaluation and modification. Not infrequently, as the patient approaches adolescence, cosmetic considerations and peer pressure supersede functional considerations, which impacts on orthotic use, compliance and function.

Ankle orthotics

The ankle sprain is one of the most common injuries in athletes, particularly in sports where participants frequently jump and land on one foot or are expected to make sharp cutting manoeuvres, for example basketball, soccer, football and volleyball (Lee *et al.* 1987; Frontera *et al.* 1994). Because ankle sprains are common and may result in days or weeks lost from practice and competition, efforts have been made to prevent such injuries through directly protecting the athlete with better shoes, ankle wrapping, taping or bracing (Tropp *et al.* 1985; Thacker *et al.* 1999).

Ankle braces range from simple off-the-shelf models that provide light support to custom hinged models that help control significant ankle instability. The important function is to limit plantar flexion and inversion, which is the position of instability for the ankle. For example, an articulated ankle foot orthosis with plastic moulded side pieces allows dorsiflexion and plantar flexion but very little inversion or eversion (Wilkerson 1992).

Several interventions that could lower the rate of occurrence of ankle sprains in a variety of sports have undergone scientific review (Tropp *et al.* 1985). Clinical trials in soccer and volleyball players suggest that training agility, flexibility, specialized ankle disc training and education reduce the risk of ankle sprain (Thacker *et al.* 1999).

In the past, taping the ankle has been the preventive method of choice for coaches and trainers in many sports. Data from controlled trials indicate that taping can prevent ankle sprains, despite the fact that tape loosens in approximately 10 min and provides little or no measurable support to the inverting ankle within 30 min (Liu & Jason 1994; Manfroy *et al.* 1997). This residual protection may be associated with increased proprioception that allows the peroneal muscles to react more rapidly to inhibit extreme ankle inversion.

Clinical studies have not shown that the height of the shoe affects the incidence of ankle injury (Barrett *et al.* 1993). This, in addition to the high cost of taping to prevent ankle injury, has led to the widespread use of ankle orthoses in the treatment and prevention of ankle injury. Semirigid orthoses provide external support, may enhance proprioception and may be adjusted more easily than tape (Thonnard *et al.* 1996; Baier & Hopf 1998). Data from randomized controlled trials demonstrate the effectiveness of some of these devices, especially for the prevention of reinjuries, although clinical research indicates that some devices will be more effective or more acceptable to athletes than others (Thacker *et al.* 1999). For example, lace-up (Fig. 15.6a) or elastic ankle supports are inexpensive and reusable but may be uncomfortable and do not provide uniform compression. Stirrup-type orthoses have been effective in reducing the recurrence of ankle injury and are acceptable to wearers (Fig. 15.6b) (Surve *et al.* 1994). However, they may be expensive and because of difficulty with fit may decrease performance levels.

Based on the available medical literature as well as the clinical experience of the authors, athletes who suffer an ankle sprain should complete supervised rehabilitation before returning to practice or competition, and those athletes suffering a moderate or severe sprain should wear an appropriate orthosis for at least 6 months. Research suggests that the benefit of the orthosis may persist for up to 1 year after injury (Thacker *et al.* 1999). It is not clear that there is a benefit of using an orthosis if the athlete has not been injured.

Knee orthoses

In the autumn of 1984, the Sports Medicine Committee of the American Academy of Orthopaedic Surgeons conducted a symposium on knee bracing to classify the types of knee braces available and to review the existing research. The Sports

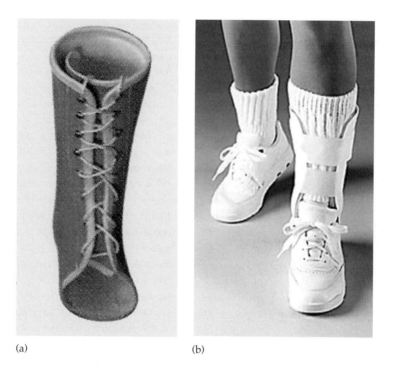

(a)   (b)

Fig. 15.6 (a) An ankle–foot leather lace-up orthosis, and (b) a stirrup ankle orthosis.

Medicine Committee developed three categories to describe the various types of knee braces available: prophylactic, rehabilitative and functional (Wirth & DeLee 1990; Cawley *et al.* 1991).

Prophylactic knee braces are those that are designed specifically to prevent or reduce the severity of injury to the knee resulting from an externally applied force. They are not designed to provide increased knee stability in the knee with a disrupted ligament. These braces are used almost exclusively in American football in an attempt to prevent ligament injuries. They are designed either with lateral or bilateral uprights, hinges and thigh as well as calf bands (Osternig & Robertson 1993; Munns 2000). Though prophylactic braces are used to protect the medial collateral ligament they may preferentially protect the ACL (Paulos *et al.* 1991). Prophylactic braces continue to be manufactured and used; however, their efficacy for use in Olympic sports has yet to be resolved in the minds of many clinicians. In addition, they may increase the risk of injury at other joints of the extremity such as the ankle.

Rehabilitation braces or postoperative knee braces are those braces designed to be applied immediately following injury or ligament reconstruction (Wirth & DeLee 1990; Munns 2000). These braces are characterized by greater length and usually incorporate a means for providing selective range of motion control by the use of hinges that can limit motion or be locked in one position (Reider *et al.* 1993). Typically, they consist of circumferential wraps and straps attached to medial and lateral side bars with a hinge attachment at the level of the knee joint line. If rotational control is desired they may require attachment to a footplate. These devices are commonly used and are widely accepted within the sports medicine community. A note of caution for the prescriber of the brace is that motion at the knee joint may exceed the limits set by the hinges by 10–20° and this needs to be considered in managing the patient.

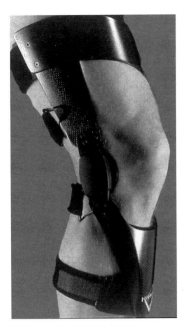

Fig. 15.7 A functional knee orthosis.

Functional knee braces are those orthoses that are designed specifically to provide mechanical stability in knees with disrupted ligaments (Fig. 15.7). These braces have straps or cuffs and knee hinges, and function by limiting anterior tibial translation, knee hyperextension and, to a lesser degree, rotation. These functional knee braces are routinely used in the chronically unstable knee and most physicians recommend their use in this application (Bonamo *et al.* 1990; Gotlin & Huie 2000). While functional knee braces continue to be applied on ligament-deficient knees, they are also commonly used in knees with reconstructed ligaments. Thus, functional knee braces are applied as prophylactic devices to provide strain or overload protection to reconstructed, healing ligaments or grafts.

The preponderance of existing brace research addresses functional knee braces. It has attempted to measure tibial translation using a variety of methods including both manual displacements and knee arthrometer systems. Many published studies demonstrate that knee bracing does reduce anterior tibial translation in varying degrees under low, non-physiological loading conditions. Many

authors have commented in the literature that functional knee braces do not provide increased mechanical stability under higher loads such as the physiological loads associated with sport (Cherf & Paulos 1990; Cawley *et al.* 1991).

It is interesting that in clinical and biomechanical studies that also conducted a subjective evaluation of the orthoses, over 90% of the patients reported significant functional improvement when using a functional knee brace (Cook *et al.* 1989; Cawley *et al.* 1991; Anderson *et al.* 1992). This is despite the fact that laboratory research clearly shows that the use of a functional knee brace may not protect the ligament at the physiological loads associated with sports, will have a significant cost in terms of energy expenditure and may lead to reduced performance (Highgenboten *et al.* 1991).

Cook *et al.* (1989) found that the application of a functional knee brace to an ACL-deficient knee enabled patients to generate torque and shear forces during a cutting manoeuvre that were near those generated by normal, non-ACL-deficient subjects and significantly better than cutting manoeuveres performed by unbraced ACL-deficient limbs (Cherf & Paulos 1990; Hertel *et al.* 2001).

The stabilizing effect of functional knee braces has been correlated with knee stability and muscle firing patterns (Anderson *et al.* 1992; Wojtys 1993). When anterior tibial translation loads were applied to the partially loaded limb, reductions in tibial translation of 15–30% with muscles relaxed and 60–80% with the muscles contracted were documented. In addition, a slowing of muscle reaction time or a latent period between the onset of the load and the firing of the muscles was reported (Cawley *et al.* 1991; Wojtys 1993). It is interesting that the braces, which best controlled tibial translation, also exhibited the longest latent period for muscle firing.

Many clinicians are in agreement that functional knee bracing serves an important role in the treatment of non-reconstructed knee ligament injuries (Bonamo *et al.* 1990; Micheo *et al.* 1995). In general, studies that performed subjective evaluation of functional knee braces found a positive response in those patients wearing orthoses.

Proprioception and proprioceptive deficits resulting from disruption of the knee ligaments has been a hotly debated topic within the orthopaedic and sports medicine community since the discovery of mechanoreceptors within the substance of both the ACL and the medial collateral ligament of the knee as well as the joint capsule (McNair *et al.* 1996; Birmingham *et al.* 2000). While there may be an interrelationship between neurosensory and neuromuscular control systems, and proprioception may provide positional joint awareness, it is not clear what is the mechanism for this phenomenon in the injured athlete. In theory, functional knee bracing may enhance position sense until the intrinsic neurosensory mechanisms are re-established and provide overload protection to the healing tissues.

For conditions that involve the patellofemoral joint, such as runner's knee, a pullover knee sleeve with various types of cut-outs that are designed to support or stabilize the patella can be helpful (Paluska & McKeag 1999). For patellar dislocation or subluxation, a patellar-stabilizing brace that has a cut-out sleeve and heavier buttressing is indicated (Cherf & Paulos 1990). In patients with patellar tendonitis or jumper's knee, an infrapatellar counterforce orthosis may be used (Fig. 15.8). The theory behind the use of this type of counterforce bracing is that it inhibits full muscular contraction and decreases the force on the partially injured musculotendinous unit (Crossley *et al.* 2001).

A treatment modality for patellofemoral pain that has gained recent acceptance is patellar taping. This technique tries to correct patellar malalignment, including subluxation, tilt and rotation, permitting progression in a rehabilitation programme of quadriceps muscle strengthening. Some clinical studies have shown good results in pain reduction and quadriceps muscle recruitment; however, radiological studies show that although the technique appears to position the patella medially this position is not maintained after exercise (Larsen *et al.* 1995; Kowall *et al.* 1996).

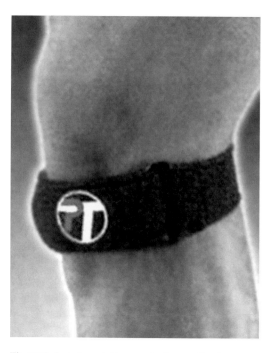

Fig. 15.8 An intrapatellar counterforce orthosis.

Low back orthoses

Low back pain is very common with a high incidence reported in men and women. The incidence of spinal injuries related to sporting activities has been estimated at 10–15%. Sports in which back injuries are among the most frequent reported injuries include golf, gymnastics, football, rowing, wrestling, weightlifting and tennis (Tall & DeVault 1993). The prevalence, however, varies with the patient's age, the sport played and with the position played. In gymnastics, the incidence of back injuries is estimated to be 11% (D'Hemecourt *et al.* 2000).

The most common injury site has been reported to be the soft tissues. However, depending on the biomechanical demands of the sport, discogenic or posterior element injuries have also been described. Sports that place repeated flexion and rotation demands on the spine may lead to disc-related symptoms, while those that place repeated hyperextension demands on the spine may lead to posterior element injury such as spondylolysis (Kaul & Herring 1994; Standaert *et al.* 2000).

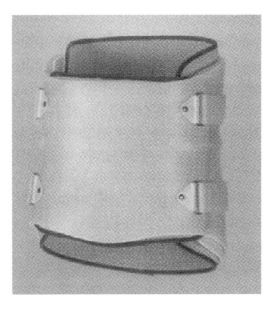

Fig. 15.9 A lumbosacral overlap orthosis.

Young patients usually present with injury to the posterior elements while older athletes present with injury to the disc (Blanda *et al.* 1993; Gerbino & Micheli 1996; Young *et al.* 1997).

Bracing has been routinely used for management of spondylolysis (Blanda *et al.* 1993; Stinson 1993; Kaul & Herring 1994). Micheli has recommended the use of a rigid polypropylene brace (modified Boston overlap brace) constructed in 0° of lumbar flexion, prescribed for 23 h per day for up to 6 months (Fig. 15.9) (Gerbino & Micheli 1996). In the case of an acute spondylolysis, or even in chronic cases, where immobilization was attempted in order to achieve healing, his protocol has recently been modified to weaning from the brace as early as 4 months if there is evidence of healing by computed tomography scanning (D'Hemecourt *et al.* 2000). The use of less rigid materials, in combination with the avoidance of repeated hyperextension until the patient is asymptomatic, has been advocated by others, including our own clinical group with good results (Standaert *et al.* 2000).

The use of bracing for the treatment of discogenic symptoms is more controversial (Stillo *et al.* 1992; Young *et al.* 1997). A soft brace or corset may be used in the initial stages for patient comfort with correction of posture and reduction of gross motion as the mechanism of action of the orthosis. If the patient's symptoms are severe and worsen with a flexed posture, the use of a brace in 5° of extension has been advocated by some clinicians (Gerbino & Micheli 1996).

Treatment of stable compression vertebral fractures routinely includes the use of extension bracing. Depending on the location of the fracture, a thoracolumbar–sacral (TLSO) or lumbar–sacral orthosis (LSO) in extension is used. A custom-made TLSO or a Jewett-type extension brace may be used from 4 to 12 weeks depending on bony healing (Nachemson 1987).

Upper extremity orthoses

Hand and upper extremity injuries are among the most common injuries sustained by athletes. Unfortunately, there is a tendency to minimize their severity as the hand does not bear weight and the injuries rarely render the athlete unable to compete (Alexy & De Carlo 1998). Wrist and hand injuries are fairly common and described to occur in 3–9% of all athletic injuries (Rettig & Patel 1995).

Injuries can be traumatic or related to overuse. The most common problems of the elbow include tendonitis (lateral, medial and posterior), nerve dysfunction and ligamentous injuries. Lateral epicondylitis or tennis elbow is the most common overuse problem about the elbow in athletes (Plancher *et al.* 1996a; Sánchez 2001). Tenosynovitis of the wrist is quite common in sports; de Quervain's syndrome (tenosynovitis of the first dorsal compartment) and extensor carpi ulnaris tendonitis are commonly seen in racquet sports and weightlifting (Rettig & Patel 1995).

The scaphoid is the most commonly injured carpal bone, accounting for 70% of all carpal fractures (Alexy & De Carlo 1998). The injury results from a fall on the hand with the wrist dorsiflexed greater than 90° and may be seen in a variety of sports. Dislocation of the proximal interphalangeal joint is also a common traumatic injury of the hand.

Nerve injuries can also occur associated with overhead sports, for example volleyball. Ulnar neuropathy at the level of the elbow can be seen in baseball pitchers, and median neuropathy at the level of the carpal tunnel can occur in racquet sports such as tennis and racquetball (Plancher *et al.* 1996b).

Orthoses can be used to manage acute and overuse injuries of the wrist and hand. Stable scaphoid fractures can be managed with a short forearm to thumb spica cast followed by the use of a thumb spica splint. Some athletes can return to sports participation with the use of a playing cast or a padded thermoplastic splint if there is evidence of healing (Alexy & De Carlo 1998). Dislocations of the proximal interphalangeal joint can be treated with closed reduction and the use of a digital extension block splint in approximately 30° of flexion (Sailer & Lewis 1995). After 3 weeks the patient may progress to the use of buddy taping until the patient has pain-free full range of motion.

Tendonitis of the first dorsal compartment can be treated with the use of a thumb spica splint in combination with steroid injection and physical therapy. A short course of immobilization with a wrist–hand orthosis in 15–20° of wrist extension can be considered for other types of acute tendonitis of the wrist.

Counterforce bracing with the use of a forearm support band may be used for the treatment of lateral epicondylitis. The orthosis should be used just distal to the elbow to alter the tension forces on the wrist extensor muscles (Fig. 15.10) (Tropp *et al.* 1985; Plancher *et al.* 1996a). As previously stated, the counterforce brace inhibits full muscle contraction thus decreasing the forces applied to the partially injured musculotendinous unit. It has also been shown to decrease elbow angular acceleration and decrease electromyographic muscle activity of the forearm muscles (Sailer & Lewis 1995; Plancher *et al.* 1996a).

Ulnar neuropathy at the level of the elbow cubital tunnel can be treated with protection using an elbow pad to avoid direct pressure over the nerve, or in severe cases with an elbow orthosis

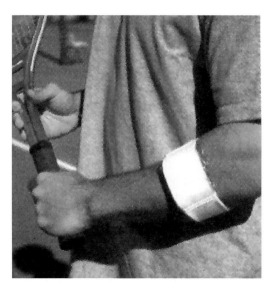

Fig. 15.10 An elbow counterforce orthosis.

made of rigid thermoplastic material in 45° of flexion. In the early stages of recovery the orthosis should be worn during most of the day and as the patient's symptoms improve it should be used only at night (Plancher *et al.* 1996a). Median entrapment at the level of the wrist should be treated with a splint that immobilizes the wrist in 0–5° of wrist extension. The orthosis should be worn at night and during the day when performing provocative activities that increase symptoms.

Future research

Research is underway with a different focus, which considers the effect of the orthotic intervention on each segment of the whole body, as well as on the total body response. This will help to clarify the brace–body interaction. Questions are being addressed such as what is the best orthotic alignment (arc of motion allowed), what is the global effect of the brace on the body, how does the body response to a brace change over time, and how do subject perceptions correlate to more quantitative outcome measures? Research can play an important role in advancing the use of orthoses by: (i) isolating key facets of orthotic function; (ii) the introduction and refinement of analytical methods that provide a more explicit and quantitative measure of the action of the brace and body response; and (iii) the application of these methods to a detailed analysis of the entire system response rather than just the local effect at the site of the intervention.

An area where research is currently being conducted is intersegmental dynamic analysis. Knowledge of the highly coupled nature of human body dynamics is important in understanding the total body movement pattern, how adaptations are made to this pattern, and the origins of its dysfunction (Esquenazi & Talaty 2000; Talaty *et al.* 2001). Gage (1991) states 'It is time to start thinking of the balance between joints. Many muscles span more than one joint and if a surgeon performs a procedure at the knee, it will also have an effect on the ankle and the hip'. His experience, like that of many clinicians, has indicated an awareness of the coupled nature of body interactions. While it may be easier to make the physical connection in the case of a biarticulate muscle, this principle applies to *all* muscles. The same principles apply to orthotic intervention. Research in our laboratory attempts to understand orthotic function and effects on this level (Talaty *et al.* 2001). To this end, tools have been developed which allow decomposition of the net effects of muscle groups on each segment in the body and an understanding of how these component effects sum to produce the overall effect. The role of our work is to take a rigorous technique and apply it to produce results, which can be generalized to better understand the specific dysfunction and what 'type' of optimized orthotic device should be used.

In addition to this biomechanical and gait laboratory research, clinical trials to appropriately assess the role of orthotics in sports medicine need to be performed. In the future, combining laboratory and biomechanical data with the results of well-structured clinical studies will allow sports medicine practitioners to have better information in order to address the orthotic needs of their patients.

References

Alexy, C. & De Carlo, M. (1998) Rehabilitation and use of protective devices in hand and wrist injuries. *Clinics in Sports Medicine* **17**, 635–655.

Anderson, K., Wojtys, E.M., Loubert, P.V. & Miller, R.E. (1992) A biomechanical evaluation of taping and bracing in reducing knee joint translation and rotation. *American Journal of Sports Medicine* **20**, 416–421.

Baier, M. & Hopf, T. (1998) Ankle orthoses effect on single-limb standing balance in athletes with functional ankle instability. *Archives of Physical Medicine and Rehabilitation* **79**, 939–944.

Barrett, J.R., Tanji, J.L., Drake, C. *et al.* (1993) High-versus low-top shoes for the prevention of ankle sprains in basketball players. *American Journal of Sports Medicine* **21**, 582–585.

Birmingham, T.B., Kramer, J.F., Krirkley, A. *et al.* (2000) Knee bracing after ACL reconstruction: effects on postural control and proprioception. *Medicine and Science in Sports and Exercise* **33**, 1253–1258.

Blanda, J., Bethem, D., Moats, W. *et al.* (1993) Defects of pars interarticularis in athletes: a protocol for nonoperative treatment. *Journal of Spinal Disorders* **6**, 406–411.

Bonamo, J.J., Fay, C. & Firestone, T. (1990) The conservative treatment of the anterior cruciate deficient knee. *American Journal of Sports Medicine* **18**, 618–623.

Brown, M., Rudicel, S. & Esquenazi, A. (1996) Measurement of dynamic pressures at the shoe–foot interface during normal walking with various foot orthosis using a new version of the FSCAN system. *Foot and Ankle International* **17**, 152–156.

Buttler, P.B., Evans, G.A., Rose, G.K. *et al.* (1983) A review of selected knee orthoses. *British Journal of Rheumatology* **22**, 109–120.

Cawley, P.W., France, E.P. & Paulos, L.E. (1991) The current state of functional knee bracing research. *American Journal of Sports Medicine* **19**, 226–233.

Chandler, T.J. & Kibler, W.B. (1993) A biomechanical approach to the prevention, treatment and rehabilitation of plantar fasciitis. *Clinics in Sports Medicine* **15**, 344–352.

Cherf, J. & Paulos, L.E. (1990) Bracing for patellar instability. *Clinics in Sports Medicine* **9**, 813–821.

Cook, F.F., Tibone, J.E. & Redfern, F.C. (1989) A dynamic analysis of a functional brace for anterior cruciate ligament insufficiency. *American Journal of Sports Medicine* **17**, 519–524.

Cornwall, M.W. & McPoil, T.G. (1999) Plantar fasciitis: etiology and treatment. *Journal of Orthopaedic and Sports Physical Therapy* **29**, 756–760.

Crossley, K., Bennell, K., Green, S. *et al.* (2001) A systematic review of physical interventions for patellofemoral pain syndrome. *Clinical Journal of Sport Medicine* **11**, 103–110.

D'Hemecourt, P.A., Gerbino II, P.G. & Micheli, L.J. (2000) Back injuries in the young athlete. *Clinics in Sports Medicine* **19**, 663–679.

Esquenazi, A. & Talaty, M. (1996) Alignment of custom orthoses: FO to HKAFO. *Biomechanics* **111** (9), 29–34.

Esquenazi, A. & Talaty, M. (2000) Gait analysis: technology and clinical application. In: *Physical Medicine and Rehabilitation*, 2nd edn (Braddom, R.L., ed.). W.B. Saunders, Philadelphia: 93–108.

Esquenazi, A., Talaty, M., Seliktar, R. *et al.* (1997) Dynamic electromyography during walking as an objective measurement of lower limb orthotic alignment. *Journal of Basic and Applied Myology* **7** (2), 103–110.

Frontera, W.R., Micheo, W.F., Amy, E. *et al.* (1994) Patterns of injuries in athletes evaluated in an interdisciplinary clinic. *Puerto Rico Health Sciences Journal* **13**, 165–170.

Gage, J.R. (1991) *Gait Analysis in Cerebral Palsy.* MacKeith Press, London.

Gerbino, P.G. & Micheli, L.J. (1996) Low back injuries in the young athlete. *Sports Medicine and Arthroscopy Review* **4**, 122–131.

Goldber, B. & Hsu, J.D. (eds) (1997) *Atlas of Orthoses and Assistive Devices*, 3rd edn. Mosby, St Louis.

Gotlin, R.S. & Huie, G. (2000) Anterior cruciate ligament injuries. *Physical Medicine and Rehabilitation Clinics of North America* **11**, 895–915.

Hertel, J., Denegar, C.R., Buckley, W.E. *et al.* (2001) Effect of rearfoot orthotics on postural sway after lateral ankle sprain. *Archives of Physical Medicine and Rehabilitation* **82**, 1000–1003.

Highgenboten, C.L., Jackson, A., Meske, N. *et al.* (1991) The effects of knee brace wear on perceptual and metabolic variables during horizontal treadmill running. *American Journal of Sports Medicine* **19**, 639–643.

Janisse, D. (1993) The art and science of fitting shoes. *Foot and Ankle* **13**, 257–262.

Janshen, L. (2000) Neuromuscular control during gymnastic landings. In: *Proceedings of XVIII International Symposium on Biomechanics in Sports* (Hong, Y. & Johns, D.P., ed.). Hong Kong: 154–157.

Johnson, J.A. (2001) The running shoe. In: *Textbook of Running Medicine*, 1st edn (O'Connor, F.G. & Wilder, R.P., eds). McGraw-Hill, New York: 589–594.

Kaul, M.P. & Herring, S.A. (1994) Rehabilitation of lumbar spine injuries in sports. *Physical Medicine and Rehabilitation Clinics of North America* **5**, 113–156.

Kilmartin, T.E. & Wallace, W.A. (1994) The scientific basis for the use of biomechanical foot orthoses in the treatment of lower limb sports injuries—a review of the literature. *British Journal of Sports Medicine* **28**, 180–184.

Kowall, M.G., Kolk, G., Nuber, G.W. *et al.* (1996) Patellar taping in the treatment of patellofemoral pain. *American Journal of Sports Medicine* **24**, 61–66.

Larsen, B., Andreasen, E., Urfer, A. *et al.* (1995) Patellar taping: a radiographic examination of the medial glide technique. *American Journal of Sports Medicine* **23**, 465–471.

Lee, K.H., Matteliano, A., Medige, J. *et al.* (1987) Electromyographic changes of leg muscles with heel lift: therapeutic implications. *Archives of Physical Medicine and Rehabilitation* **68**, 298–301.

Liu, S.H. & Jason, W.J. (1994) Lateral ankle sprains and instability problems. *Clinics in Sports Medicine* **13**, 793–809.

Loke, M. (2000) New concepts in lower limb orthotics. *Physical Medicine and Rehabilitation Clinics of North America* **11**, 477–496.

Manfroy, P.P., Ashton, J.A. & Wojtys, E.M. (1997) The effect of exercise, prewrap, and athletic tape on the maximal active and passive ankle resistance to ankle inversion. *American Journal of Sports Medicine* **25**, 156–163.

Mascaro, T.B. & Swanson, L.E. (1994) Rehabilitation of the foot and ankle. *Orthopedic Clinics of North America* **25**, 147–160.

McNair, P.J., Stanley, S.N. & Strauss, G.R. (1996) Knee bracing: effects on proprioception. *Archives of Physical Medicine and Rehabilitation* **77**, 287–289.

Micheo, W.F., Frontera, W.R., Amy, E. *et al.* (1995) Rehabilitation of the patient with an anterior cruciate ligament injury: a brief review. *Boletín Asociación Medica de Puerto Rico* **87**, 29–36.

Munns, S.W. (2000) Knee orthoses. *Physical Medicine and Rehabilitation State of the Arts Reviews* **14**, 423–433.

Nachemson, A.L. (1987) Orthotic treatment for injuries and diseases of the spinal column. *Physical Medicine and Rehabilitation State of the Art Reviews* **1**, 11–24.

Orteza, L.C., Vogelbach, W.D. & Denegar, C.R. (1992) The effect of molded orthotics on balance and pain while jogging following inversion ankle sprains. *Journal of Athletic Training* **27**, 80–84.

Osternig, L.R. & Robertson, R.N. (1993) Effects of prophylactic knee bracing on lower extremity joint position and muscle activation during running. *American Journal of Sports Medicine* **21**, 733–737.

Paluska, S.A. & McKeag, D.B. (1999) Using patellofemoral braces for anterior knee pain. *The Physician and Sports Medicine* **27**, 81–82.

Paulos, L.E., Cawley, P.W. & France, E.P. (1991) Impact biomechanics of lateral knee bracing. *American Journal of Sports Medicine* **19**, 337–342.

Plancher, K.D., Halbrecht, J. & Lourie, G.M. (1996a) Medial and lateral epicondylitis in the athlete. *Clinical Sports Medicine* **15**, 283–305.

Plancher, K.D., Peterson, R.K. & Steichen, J.B. (1996b) Compressive neuropathies and tendinopathies in the athletic elbow and wrist. *Clinics in Sports Medicine* **15**, 331–371.

Redford, J.B. (2000) Orthotics and orthotic devices: general principles. *Physical Medicine and Rehabilitation State of the Art Reviews* **14**, 381–394.

Reider, B., Sathy, M.R., Talkington, J. *et al.* (1993) Treatment of isolated medial collateral ligament injuries in athletes with early functional rehabilitation. *American Journal of Sports Medicine* **22**, 470–477.

Rettig, A.C. & Patel, D.V. (1995) Epidemiology of elbow, forearm, and wrist injuries in the athlete. *Clinics in Sports Medicine* **14**, 289–297.

Sailer, S.M. & Lewis, S.B. (1995) Rehabilitation and splinting of common upper extremity injuries in athletes. *Clinics in Sports Medicine* **14**, 411–446.

Sánchez, C. (2001) Epicondylalgias, differential diagnosis. *Archivos de Medicina del Deporte* **18**, 43–51.

Schwellnus, M.P., Jordan, G. & Noakes, T.D. (1990) Prevention of common overuse injuries by the use of shock absorbing insoles. *American Journal of Sports Medicine* **18**, 636–641.

Standaert, C.J., Herring, S.T. & Halpern, B. (2000) Spondylolysis. *Physical Medicine and Rehabilitation Clinics of North America* **11**, 785–803.

Stillo, J.V., Stein, A.B. & Ragnarsson, K.T. (1992) Low-back orthoses. *Physical Medicine and Rehabilitation Clinics of North America* **3**, 57–94.

Stinson, J.T. (1993) Spondylolysis and spondylolisthesis in the athlete. *Clinics in Sports Medicine* **12**, 517–528.

Styf, J.R., Nakhostine, M. & Gershuni, D.H. (1992) Functional knee braces increase intramuscular pressures in the anterior compartment of the leg. *American Journal of Sports Medicine* **20**, 46–49.

Subotnick, S.I. (2001) Foot orthotics. In: *Textbook of Running Medicine*, 1st edn (O'Connor, F.G. & Wilder, R.P., eds). McGraw-Hill, New York: 595–603.

Surve, I., Schwellnus, M.P., Noakes, T. *et al.* (1994) A fivefold reduction in the incidence of recurrent ankle sprains in soccer players using the sport-stirrup orthoses. *American Journal of Sports Medicine* **22**, 601–606.

Talaty, M., Seliktar, R. & Esquenazi, A. (2001) Inter-segmental effects of an ankle foot orthoses on joint rotation. In: *Proceedings of the XVIIIth Congress of the International Society of Biomechanics, ETH Zurich, Switzerland*. Interrepro AG.

Tall, R.L. & DeVault, W. (1993) Spinal injury in sport: epidemiologic considerations. *Clinics in Sports Medicine* **12**, 441–448.

Thacker, S.B., Stroup, D.F., Branche, C.M. *et al.* (1999) The prevention of ankle sprains in sports. *American Journal of Sports Medicine* **27**, 753–760.

Thonnard, J.L., Bragard, D., Willems, P.A. *et al.* (1996) Stability of the braced ankle: a biomechanical investigation. *American Journal of Sports Medicine* **24**, 356–361.

Tropp, H., Askling, C. & Gillquist, J. (1985) Prevention of ankle sprains. *American Journal of Sports Medicine* **13**, 259–262.

Wilkerson, L.A. (1992) Ankle injuries in athletes. *Primary Care* **19**, 377–392.

Wirth, M.A. & DeLee, J.C. (1990) The history and classification of knee braces. *Clinics in Sports Medicine* **9**, 731–741.

Wojtys, E.M. (1993) Should ACL braces be used in sports? In: *19th Annual Meeting, AOSSM, Sun Valley, Idaho*.

Young, J.L., Press, J.M. & Herring, S.A. (1997) The disc at risk in athletes: perspectives on operative and non-operative care. *Medicine and Science in Sports and Exercise* **29** (S) 222–232.

Zheng, N. & Barrentine, S.W. (2000) Biomechanics and motion analysis applied to sports. *Physical Medicine and Rehabilitation Clinics of North America* **11**, 309–322.

THE LIBRARY
SWINDON COLLEGE
NORTH STAR

Index